Immunogenetics and Immunodeficiency

Immunogenetics and Immunodeficiency

Edited by B. Benacerraf

*Fabyan Professor of Comparative Pathology
Harvard Medical School*

University Park Press
Baltimore

Published by
University Park Press,
Chamber of Commerce Building,
Baltimore, Maryland, USA

Published in Great Britain by
MTP
St. Leonard's House,
Lancaster,
England

Library of Congress Cataloging in Publication Data
Main entry under title:

Immunogenetics and immunodeficiency.

1. Immunogenetics. I. Benacerraf, Baruj, 1920–
[DNLM: 1. Immunologic deficiency syndromes.
2. Immunogenetics. QW541 I57]
QR184.I45 1975   616.07'9   75-25774
ISBN 0-8391-0835-4

Made and printed in Great Britain

Contents

List of Contributors

BARUJ BENACERRAF
Department of Pathology,
Harvard Medical School,
Boston, Mass. 02115, U.S.A.

G. BIOZZI
Section de Biologie,
Fondation Curie—Institut du Radium,
26, rue d'Ulm 75231,
Paris, Cedex 05, France

Y. BOUTHILLIER,
Section de Biologie,
Fondation Curie—Institut du Radium,
26, rue d'Ulm 75231,
Paris, Cedex 05, France

BLAS FRANGIONE,
Irvington House Institute,
Department of Medicine,
New York University Medical Centre,
550 First Avenue,
New York, N.Y. 10016, U.S.A.

J. A. FRELINGER,
Department of Human Genetics,
Ann Arbor, Michigan, U.S.A.

DAVID H. KATZ,
Department of Pathology,
Harvard Medical School,
Boston, Mass. 02115, U.S.A.

THOMAS KINDT
The Rockefeller University,
New York, N.Y. 10021, U.S.A.

HENRY G. KUNKEL
The Rockefeller University,
New York, N.Y. 10021, U.S.A.

D. MORTON,
Section de Biologie,
Fondation Curie—Institut du Radium,
26, rue d'Ulm 75231,
Paris, Cedex 05, France

FRED S. ROSEN,
Department of Pediatrics,
Harvard Medical School,
Boston, Mass. 02115, U.S.A.

D. C. SHREFFLER,
Department of Human Genetics,
Ann Arbor, Michigan, U.S.A

C. STIFFEL,
Section de Biologie,
Fondation Curie—Institut du Radium,
26 rue d'Ulm 75231,
Paris, Cedex 05, France.

Preface

The identification of the genes which determine biological phenomena, and the study of the control they exert on these phenomena, has proven to be the most successful approach to a detailed understanding of their mechanism. The greatest advances in molecular biology have relied upon the application of the methodology of genetics to the elucidation of the fundamental processes of life at the cellular level.

The same statement may be made concerning our understanding of immunological phenomena. The genetic approach has again proven extremely productive and has permitted us to identify many fundamental questions in immunobiology and to resolve some of them successfully. Among the problems with which the young discipline of immunogenetics has been concerned are the structural genes of the immunoglobulin chains. These genes have been identified by their control of allotypic antigenic determinants on the constant segment of H chains of different classes, on the constant segments of L chains and on both the constant and variable regions of rabbit H chains. These studies have provided the first evidence for the control of a single polypeptide chain by two distinct structural genes. Much has been learned concerning the genes coding the C and V regions of immunoglobulin chains (a) from the study of the inheritance of allotypic and idiotypic determinants on these chains discussed by Kunkel and Kindt and (b) from the analysis of the amino acid sequence in immunoglobulin chains from individual myeloma proteins and abnormal paraproteins, discussed by Frangione.

The study of transplantation antigens and of the genes which control their expression on cell surfaces has been one of the most important and successful contributions of immunogenetics. A considerable debt is owed to Gorer and to Snell for their pioneer work in this field, which permitted the identification of the major histocompatibility complex (MHC) and of minor histocompatibility loci in the mouse and for the development of congenic resistant strains of mice selected to differ only at the MHC, the H-2 complex. These studies proved to be invaluable when it became known that the MHC of mammals controlled many essential immunological functions, in addition to histocompatibility antigens, such as the ability to make specific immune responses to distinct thymus-dependent antigens, the capacity to develop mixed leukocyte reactions in culture, and the ability to regulate immune responses through the control of essential antigen-dependent cellular interactions between macrophages and T cells and T cells and B cells. More recently, the MHC was demonstrated also to control such important defence mechanisms as the levels of many complement components and in certain cases the structural genes for component proteins of the complement systems. The MHC of mammals appears therefore to constitute possibly the most important control centre for immunological defence mechanisms. Frelinger and Shreffler have described the properties of the MHC and of their products in the mouse and other laboratory animals and in man. Benacerraf and Katz have focused their attention upon the functions of genes in the I region of the MHC responsible for the control of specific immune responses to thymus-dependent antigens and also for the critical cell interactions through which this control is effected.

The discovery that the products of the SD loci of the MHC in man, the histocompatibility antigens, are very intimately associated in a molecular complex with a small polypeptide chain, B_2 microglobulin, which shows a sequence analogy with the basic immunoglobulin unit suggests a relationship between these two systems. The recent demonstration that T cell products coded for by the I region of the H-2 complex of the mouse bind specifically to the antigen which stimulated their synthesis and therefore possess antibody activity, although they are not immunoglobulins, indicate that the relationship between immunoglobulins and their genes and the products of the MHC should be profitably explored further.

The development of both humoral and cellular immune responses involves very complex phenomena which require the activities of many regulatory genes concerned with the differentiation of the T cells, B cells, and macrophages, and also with the synthesis and secretion of specific immunoglobulin antibodies of different classes and of T cell products, in addition to the structural genes for immunoglobulins and the MHC. The essential role which these regulatory genes play in the development of immune responses is clearly demonstrated by the immunological deficiency diseases discussed by Rosen. These immunodeficiency diseases result in the majority of cases from defects in regulatory genes controlling the differentiation of B cell functions, T cell functions, or both, and not in structural genes of either immunoglobulin chains or the MHC.

An animal model to investigate the number of these regulatory genes and their operation would be very useful. Such a model has indeed been provided by the studies of Biozzi and associates discussed in this volume.

In conclusion, Immunogenetics is a very young science but a thriving one. We have attempted to discuss some of the major advances in this field, but did not try nor could be expected to describe all the accumulated knowledge in Immunogenetics. Also we must accept the inescapable fact, which is common to books in all active fields such as ours that numerous advances and important discoveries are presently being made in many laboratories which will make this volume rapidly inadequate and eventually obsolete. We may nevertheless console ourselves that we have attempted for the first time to bring together various aspects of immunogenetics which should be found to interrelate increasingly as the fascinating story unfolds.

May 1975   Baruj Benacerraf

1

Structure of Human Immunoglobulins and their Variants

BLAS FRANGIONE

1.1 INTRODUCTION

The heterogeneity of immunoglobulins is the result of three types of amino acid sequence variability: isotypic, allotypic and idiotypic variants (Figure 1.1).

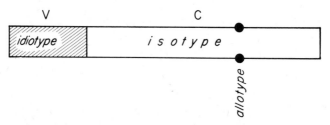

Figure 1.1 Localization of the three different types of heterogeneity of human immunoglobulin heavy chains. V: variable region, C: constant region.

Isotypes: Defines different classes, subclasses and types of immunoglobulin polypeptide chains. They are present in all individuals of the same species and they are the product of different structural genes.

Allotypes: Allotypes are defined as intraspecies inherited antigenic determinants. They are present in some, but not all members of a species and in molecules of the same isotype. They result from the existence of multiple forms (alleles) of immunoglobulin genes at individual gene loci.

Idiotypes: Are markers for certain antibodies and myeloma proteins. They represent antigenic determinants present in the variable region and have been shown to include the binding site. The significance of this third source of diversity is at present controversial.

This review will deal mainly with the three levels of heterogeneity present in human immunoglobulin heavy chains since those of the light chain have been extensively reviewed[1-3]. Furthermore it will describe in some detail studies on the primary structure of variants of human myeloma proteins and will suggest mechanisms for their generation which are similar to mutants which have been observed in microorganisms.

1.2 HUMAN IMMUNOGLOBULINS: NOMENCLATURE AND CLASSIFICATION

The nomenclature used in this review incorporates all recommendations and revisions suggested by the series of committees organized by the World Health Organization (through June, 1972)[4].

1.2.1 Classes and chains

In 1972 it was recommended that the symbol Ig be used to designate immunoglobulins. There are five major classes of Ig molecules in man (IgG, IgA, IgM, IgD and IgE), which can be distinguished by the primary structure of their heavy (H) chains (Table 1.1). The class of H chain in each class of Ig is

Table 1.1   Major classes of immunoglobulins

Characteristic	IgG	IgA	IgM	IgD	IgE
Mol. weight	150 000	160 000–350 000	900 000	160 000	190 000
Sed. coeff. (S)	7	7(9–15)	19	7	8
Serum level (mg/ml)	12	2	1	0.03	0.0003
Carbohydrate (%)	2.5	10	10	10	12
Valence	2	2	10		
Special functions	Complement and heterologous skin fixation. Placental transfer	External secretions. Local protection	Complement fixation		Reagin activity

designated by the corresponding Greek letter as shown in Table 1.2. More recently, it has been found that IgG, IgA and possibly IgM can be further divided into subclasses based on specific antigenic markers present on the H chains. Subclasses are indicated by arabic numerals following the letter denoting the class. The corresponding H chains are named $\gamma1$, $\gamma2$, $\gamma3$, $\gamma4$, $\alpha1$, $\alpha2$, $\mu1$ and $\mu2$ respectively (Table 1.2).

Light (L) chains exist in two different types: κ (kappa) and λ (lambda), which can be readily distinguished immunologically. They are not class-specific and both types occur in all classes. In human IgG, the amount of κ chains is approximately twice that of λ chains. Subclasses have been found only for the λ type, and at the present time they are referred to in terms of those specific antigenic markers which distinguish them, e.g. Oz+, Oz−, Kern+, Kern− (Table 1.2).

3

Table 1.2 Human immunoglobulin chains (Isotypes)

	Common L chains		Unique H chains					Other chains	
	κ	λ	γ IgG	α IgA	μ IgM	δ IgD	ϵ IgE	J — IgA polymers s IgA and IgM	SC* — s IgA
Present		All Igs							
Molecular formula			$(\gamma_2\kappa_2)$ or $(\gamma_2\lambda_2)$	$(\alpha_2\kappa_2)$ or $(\alpha_2\lambda_2)$	$(\mu_2\kappa_2)$ or $(\mu_2\lambda_2)$	$(\delta_2\kappa_2)$ or $(\delta_2\lambda_2)$	$(\epsilon_2\kappa_2)$ or $(\epsilon_2\lambda_2)$	IgA polymers $(\alpha_2\kappa_2)_{2-3}$-J / $(\alpha_2\lambda_2)_{2-3}$-J ; $(\mu_2\kappa_2)_5$-J / $(\mu_2\lambda_2)_5$-J	$(\alpha_2\kappa_2)_2$SC-J or $(\alpha_2\lambda_2)_2$SC-J
Molecular weight†	22.5	22.5	53	55	70	65	70	15	70
Isotypic variants	None	Oz+, Oz−, Kern+, Kern−	$\gamma1$ $\gamma2$ $\gamma3$ $\gamma4$	$\alpha1$ $\alpha2$	$\mu1$ $\mu2$	—	—	—	—
Variable subgroups	$V_\kappa I$ $V_\kappa II$ $V_\kappa III$	$V_\lambda I$ $V_\lambda II$ $V_\lambda III$ $V_\lambda IV$ $V_\lambda V$	$V_H I$ $V_H II$ $V_H III$	$V_H I$ $V_H II$ $V_H III$	$V_H I$ $V_H II$ $V_H III$	$V_H I$ $V_H II$ $V_H III$	$V_H I$ $V_H II$ $V_H III$		
Number of constant domains	1	1	3	3	4	4	4	—	—

* Secretory component
† × 10^{-3}

4

In addition to L and H chains, certain classes of Ig molecules contain other, non-homologous chains. Thus, IgA in external secretions of man and several other species contains a chain not present in serum IgA. The designation 'secretory component' for the additional polypeptide chain is used, and the entire molecule is termed secretory IgA (sIgA). IgM, polymeric serum IgA and sIgA molecules contain an antigenically and physicochemically distinctive polypeptide, termed the J chain.

1.2.2   Regions, domains and fragments

Each Ig chain consists of two regions designated the variable, 'V' and constant, 'C' region. The V region is the amino terminal (N-terminal) portion of the L and H chain (approximately 110–120 residues), which can be made up of many different amino acid sequences, even within one subclass. On the other hand, the C region is the carboxyl terminal (C-terminal) portion of the chain and has the same primary structure as all other chains of the same class, subclass and type, although its length differs in different classes of H chains. The particular Ig chain in which these regions are studied are designated by subscripts, e.g. V_κ, C_κ, V_H, $C_{\gamma1}$, etc.

Sequence analyses have demonstrated that C_κ and C_λ contain about 110 residues, C_γ is three times larger and C_μ and C_ϵ four times larger. The homology regions of the H chains (each about 110 residues in length) are designated by arabic numerals counting from the N-terminal direction e.g. $C_{\gamma1}$, $C_{\gamma2}$, $C_{\gamma3}$ (Figure 1.2). The various C regions are evolutionarily related with each other. Due to the amino acid sequence and the presence of one intrachain disulphide bond, each homology region folds in a somewhat similar conformation, a compact globular domain.

Ig domains

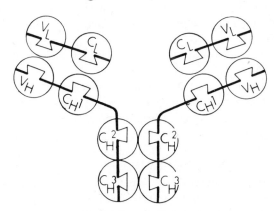

Figure 1.2   The domains of an IgG molecule. L: light chain, H: heavy chain.

1.3 PRIMARY STRUCTURE OF HUMAN IMMUNOGLOBULINS

1.3.1 Variable region

Variable regions associated with L and H chains sharing certain similarities in their amino acid sequence can be classified as belonging to a single group. Within a group a number of subdivisions can be made such that V regions of any one subgroup resemble one another more closely than members of other subgroups. A particular scheme of subgroups is somewhat arbitrary and some authors consider the term 'subgroup' confusing. Three subgroups of κ chain and five subgroups of λ chain are identified: $V_\kappa I$, $V_\kappa II$ and $V_\kappa III$; $V_\lambda I$, $V_\lambda II$, $V_\lambda III$, $V_\lambda IV$ and $V_\lambda V$ (for amino acid sequences see references 1, 2). The V regions of H chains can be also classified into at least three subgroups, $V_H I$, $V_H II$ and $V_H III$, which appear to be non-class-specific (Table 1.2).

More than ten complete V regions from human myeloma H chains have been sequenced as shown in Figure 1.3. Certain positions are highly conserved. In fact, about 65% of the variable region of human H chains shows limited sequence variation, and 20% is invariant, regardless of subgroup assignment[3]. Within a subgroup most variations involve amino acid interchanges due to single base replacements in the corresponding codon.

Other V region positions vary to a greater extent, and have been designated 'hypervariable' regions. Three broad regions of sequence hypervariability are apparent in the H chains: residues 31–37, 51–68 and 101–110 (Figure 1.3). In L chains the hypervariable regions are residues 25–34, 50–56 and 89–97. The hypervariable regions of both the H and L chains are believed to be related to the antigen binding site.

The problem of antibody diversity is as controversial as it was ten years ago in spite of our knowledge of Ig structure and genetics. Two quite distinct models of how this diversity might arise have been proposed[1,2,5-7].

(1) *The germ-line theory*: According to this model the primary structure of every V region an animal can produce is encoded in its DNA. Every vertebrate genome contains many thousands of different V genes with divergence due to natural selection of favourable random point mutations, duplications and recombinations.

(2) *Somatic mutation theories*: in contrast only a small number of germ-line genes are hypothesized in this model. These genes mutate during mitotic cell division and they increase rapidly during ontogeny, either by antigenic-driven selection or by random drift of selectively neutral mutations. These theories do agree on an exceptional feature of the Ig genes: the existence of separated gene coding for V and C regions. The model assumes that, in order to be transcribed, a V gene must be brought adjacent to a C gene to form a single functioning cistron (VC gene). The joining mechanism is not known although it has been assumed to be equivalent to a genetic translocation[2].

V_H I

Eu (γ1): PCA-Val-Gln-Leu-Val-Glu-Ser-Gly-Ala-Glu-Val-Lys-Lys-Pro-Gly-Ser-Ser-Val-Lys-Val-Ser-Cys-Lys-Ala-Ser
Ca (γ1): ——————Arg——————————Ala——————————————Ile——————————Thr
Ste (γ1): ————His————Ser——————————Ala————Met————Arg
Zuc (γ3): ————Val——————————Asp-Leu-Val——————Gly————Ser

V_H II

Daw (γ1): PCA-Val-Thr-Leu-Arg-Glu-Ser-Gly-Pro-Ala-Leu-Val-Arg-Pro-Thr-Gln-Thr-Leu-Thr-Leu-Thr-Cys-Thr-Phe-Ser
Ou (μ): ——————Thr——————Lys————Pro
He (γ1): ————Lys————Asn————Thr————Lys————Leu
Cor (γ1): ————Lys————Lys

V_H III

Tei (γ1): Glu-Val-Gln-Leu-Val-Glu-Ser-Gly-Gly-Gly-Leu-Val-Gln-Pro-Gly-Gly-Ser-Leu-Arg-Leu-Ser-Cys-Ala-Ala-Ser
Was (γ1): ——————Leu
Nie (γ1): PCA————Gln——————————Val————Arg
Jon (γ3): Asp——————————Lys
Zap (α1): ————Ala——————————Gly
Tur (α1): ————Leu
Gal (μ): ————Asp————Arg
Wei (γ1): Asp————Met————Ala————Lys————Glu————Val
Caa (γ1): ————Ala————(- -)————Val
Wat (γ2):
Til (γ2, μ): ————Leu————Ile
Vin (γ4):
Eva (μ): ————(- -)————Glu-(- -)————Val
Lay (μ): Ala————Leu
Pom (μ): ————Leu
Ben (μ): ————Ala
Ski (α1): ————Asx————Thr————Lys————Ala
Low (α2): ————Lys————Gly
Jor (α2): ————Glx
Sha (ε): ————Met————Lys————Val————Val
Avi (α2): ————Glu————Lys————( )

7

50

$V_H I$

Eu (γ1) Gly-Gly-Thr-Phe-Ser-Arg-Ser-Ala-Ile-( )-Ile-Trp-Val-Arg-Gln-Ala-Pro-Gly-Gln-Gly-Leu-Glu-Trp-Met-
Ca (γ1) ———Thr——————His-Tyr————Met—————
Ste (γ1)
Zuc (γ3)

$V_H II$

Daw (γ1) Gly-Phe-Ser-Leu-Ser-Gly-Glu-Thr-Met-Cys-Ala-Ala-Trp-Ile-Arg-Gln-Pro-Pro-Gly-Glu-Ala-Leu-Glu-Trp-Leu-
Ou (μ) ————Thr-Ser-Arg————Arg——————Ser————Lys—————
He (γ1) ——Leu————Thr-Thr-Asp-Gly-Val-Ala————Gly————Gly————Arg—————
Cor (γ1) ————Ser-Thr-Gly——————Gly——————Lys-Gly—————

$V_H III$

Tei (γ1) Gly-Phe-Thr-Phe-Ser-Thr-Ser-Ala-Val-Tyr-( )Trp-Val-Arg-Gln-Ala-Pro-Gly-Lys-Gly-Leu-Glu-Trp-Val-
Was (γ1) ——————Ser————Asp————Met————( )—————
Nie (γ1) ——————————Arg-Tyr-Thr-Ile-His-( )—————
Jon (γ3) ——————————Ala-Trp-Met-Lys-( )—————
Zap (α1) ——————————Thr-Ser-Arg-Phe-( )—————
Tur (α1) ——————————Arg-Val-Leu-Ser-Ser-( )—————
Gal (μ) ——————(Asx, Val, Leu, Asx-Asx, Phe)Met-Thr-( )—————
Wei (γ1) ——————Leu————Tyr-Gly-Met-Asx—————
Caa (γ1) ——————————Asx-Asx-Tyr—————
Wat (γ2) ——————Asx————Tyr-Thr-Met-Val—————
Til (γ2, μ) ——————————Tyr-Val-Met—————
Vin (γ4) ————Val——————Asn-Trp-Met—————
Eva (μ)
Lay (μ) ——————————Ala————Met-Ser—————
Pom (μ) ——————————Ser————Met—————
Ben (μ) ——————————Thr-Phe-Met——( )
Ski (α1) ——————————Leu-Gly-Asx-Tyr-Glx-Met-Asx
Low (α2) Val————————Phe————Tyr-Val-Met-Asx
Jor (α2) ——————————Asx-Tyr-Ser-Met-Asx
Sha (ε)
Avi (α2)

75

$V_H I$

Eu (γ1) Gly-Gly-Ile-Val-Pro-Met-Phe-Gly-Pro-Pro-Asn-Tyr-Ala-Gln-Lys-Phe-Gln-Gly-Arg-Val-Thr-Ile-Thr-Ala-Asp-
Ca (γ1)
Ste (γ1)
Zuc (γ3)

$V_H II$

Daw (γ1) Ala-Trp-Asp-Ile-Leu-Asn-Asp-Asp-Lys-Tyr-Tyr( )Gly-Ala-Ser-Leu-Glu-Thr-Arg-Leu-Ala-Val-Ser-Lys-Asp-
Ou (μ) ——Arg( )——Asx-Asx-Asx-Asn ——Trp-Ser-Thr ——Arg Ser- Ile ——Asn-
He (γ1) ——Leu-Leu-Tyr-Trp ——Asp-Lys-Arg-Phe-Ser-Pro ——Lys-Ser ——Thr ——Thr-Arg
Cor (γ1) ——Arg( )——Asx-Trp ——Asp-Lys ——Tyr-Asx-Thr ——Thr

$V_H III$

Tei (γ1) Gly-Trp-Arg-Tyr-Glu-Gly-Ser-Ser-Leu-Thr-His-Tyr-Ala-Val-Ser-Val-Gln-Gly-Arg-Phe-Thr-Ile-Ser-Arg-Asn-
Was (γ1) Ala ——Lys ——Gln-Glu-Ala ——Asn-Ser ——Phe ——Asp-Thr ——Asn
Nie (γ1) Ala-Val-Met-Ser-Tyr-Asx-Gly-Asx-Asn-Lys ——Asp ——Asn
Jon (γ3) Val ——Val ——Gln-Val-Val-Glu-Lys-Ala-Phe ——Asn ——Asn
Zap (α1) Glu-Phe ——Val-Gln ——Ala-Ile- Ser ——Asp ——Ala
Tur (α1) Ser-Gly ——Leu-Asn-Ala ——Asn-Leu ——Phe ——Ala
Gal (μ) Ala-Asn-Ile-Lys-Glx-Asx-Gly ——Glx-Glx-Asx ——Val-Asp ——Lys ——Asp-
Wei (γ1)
Caa (γ1)
Wat (γ2)
Til (γ2, μ)
Vin (γ4)
Eva (μ)
Lay (μ)
Pom (μ)
Ben (μ)
Ski (α1)
Low (α2)
Jor (α2)
Sha (ε)
Avi (α2)

9

$V_H I$ 100

Eu (γ1) Glu- Ser- Thr- Asn- Thr- Ala- Tyr- Met- Glu- Leu- Ser- Ser- Leu- Arg- Ser- Glu- Asp- Thr- Ala- Phe- Tyr- Phe- Cys- Ala- Gly-
Ca (γ1)
Ste (γ1)
Zuc (γ3)

$V_H II$

Daw (γ1) Thr- Ser- Lys- Asn- Gln- Val- Val- Leu- Ser- Met- Asn- Thr- Val- Gly- Pro- Gly- Asp- Thr- Ala- Thr- Tyr- Tyr- Cys- Ala- Arg-
Ou (μ) Asp————————————————Ile————————Ile- Asn——————————Val-
He (γ1) ————————————————————Ile- Thr————Thr- Asp- Met- Asp——————Val——————Val- His-
Cor (γ1) ————————Arg————————————Thr————( )Asp——————Val-

$V_H III$

Tei (γ1) Asp- Ser- Lys- Asn- Thr- Leu- Tyr- Leu- Gln- Met- Leu- Ser- Leu- Glu- Pro- Glx- Asx- Thr- Ala- Val- Tyr- Tyr- Cys- Ala- Arg-
Was (γ1) ——————————————————Asn- Arg——————————Ala-
Nie (γ1) ——————————Asn——————Arg-
Jon (γ3) ——————————Asn——————Ile——Val- Thr-
Zap (α1) ——————————————Asn- Thr- Gly————————Ala-
Tur (α1)
Gal (μ) ——————————————————————Gln- Ala——————————————————Leu-
Wei (γ1) Asn- Ala————————Ser————————Asn——————Arg- Val——————————Leu-
Caa (γ1)
Wat (γ2)
Til (γ2, μ)
Vin (γ4)
Eva (μ)
Lay (μ)
Pom (μ)
Ben (μ)
Ski (α1)
Low (α2)
Jor (α2)
Sha (ε)
Avi (α2)

10

Eu (γ1)   Gly- Tyr- Gly- Ile (   )Tyr- Ser- Pro- Glu- Glu- Tyr- Asn- Gly- Gly- Leu- Val
Ca (γ1)
Ste (γ1)
Zuc (γ3)

*V*_H *II*
Daw (γ1)   Ser- Cys- Gly- Ser- Gln (   )Tyr- Phe- Asp- Tyr- Trp- Gly- Gln- Gly- Ile- Leu- Val
Ou (μ)   Val- Val- Asn——Val-(   )Met- Ala- Gly——*Met——Val————Thr- Thr——
He (γ1)   Arg- His- Pro- Arg- Thr- Leu (   ) Ala———Val————Thr- Lys——
Cor (γ1)   Ile- Thr- Val- Ile- Pro- Ala- Pro- Ala- Gly—— Met——Val——Arg——Thr- Pro——

*V*_H *III*
Tei (γ1)   Val- Thr- Pro- Ala- Ala- Ala- Ser- Leu- Thr- Phe- Ser- Ala- Val- Trp- Gly- Gln- Gly- Thr- Leu- Val
Was (γ1)   Phe- Arg- Gln- Pro- Phe- Val- Gln ——Phe- Asp- Phe——
Nie (γ1)   Ile- Arg- Asp- Thr——Met(   )—Phe——His——
Jon (γ3)   ——Val- Val- Ser- Thr (   )Ser- Met- Asp——Pro——
Zap (α1)   Thr- Arg——Gly- Gly- Tyr (   )——Asp——
Tur (α1)   Leu- Ser- Val- Thr——Val (   )Ala- Phe- Asp——Lys——
Gal (μ)   Gly- Trp- Gly (   )Gly- Gly- Asp- Tyr——
Wei (γ1)
Caa (γ1)
Wat (γ2)
Til (γ2, μ)
Vin (γ4)
Eva (μ)
Lay (μ)
Pom (μ)
Ben (μ)
Ski (α1)
Low (α2)
Jor (α2)
Sha (ε)
Avi (α2)

Figure 1.3   Amino acid sequences of human V_H region subgroups. A straight line indicates that a residue is identical to that in the first sequence listed for that subgroup. ( ) Empty parentheses are gaps inserted to maximize homologies. (–) Undetermined amino acid residues. PCA, pyrrolidone carboxylic acid.* Protein Oμ has an insertion of four Tyr in a row at position 110. Patient Til had a biclonal gammopathy (IgG2, IgM). Both proteins appear to have the same V_H sequence (refs. 8–22).

1.3.2   Immunoglobulin G

In 1959, a proteolytic enzyme (papain) was used to split rabbit IgG into fragments which retained biological activity[23], and shortly thereafter it was shown that IgG molecules could be separated into H and L chains after reduction with mercaptoethanol[24]. In 1962 the now well-established four-chain model for IgG was proposed[25]. The molecule consists of identical pairs of H and L chains (MW = 50 000 and 25 000 respectively) connected by S—S bonds. Papain digestion produces two Fab (for antigen binding) fragments and one Fc (for crystallizable fragment) in the case of rabbit IgG. Each Fab fragment contains one L chain and approximately half of a H chain (Fd fragment), and is capable of binding one antigenic determinant. The Fc fragment is a dimer containing the C-terminal halves of the two H chains.

The region near the middle of the H chains were the inter-H chain disulphide bridges are located (hinge region) is very sensitive to enzymatic digestion, not only by papain, but by pepsin, trypsin and probably other enzymes as well. Each enzyme splits at a different site near the hinge region (the sites of splitting have been well established in human IgG1 and IgM, Figure 1.10). In addition, cyanogen bromide (CNBr), a reagent which splits peptide chains at methionine residues, attacks preferentially a methionine residue just to the C-terminal side of the inter-H chain bridges giving an $(Fab')_2$-like disulphide bridged dimer. With the exception of molecules carrying Gma allotypic markers[26], all IgG molecules contain at least three methionine residues in the Fc fragment; therefore, after CNBr cleavage one should expect four fragments: hinge, C_H2, C_H3 and an octadecapeptide from the carboxyl end. Gma molecules contain two methionine residues resulting from a mutation in position 358 (Leu for Met, see below); thus, C_H2 cannot be separated from C_H3 using this procedure.

Since it has now been established that antibodies of different specificities differ in primary structure, normal IgG consists of a population of many chemically distinct molecules. In certain instances, however, prolonged and intensive immunization has resulted in the formation of antibodies composed of one or a very few molecules with different amino acid sequence[27-31].

Myeloma proteins are Ig molecules that appear in the plasma of patients with multiple myeloma. The Ig derived from a neoplastic clone of plasma cells can compose 95% of the serum Ig, and this homogeneous protein can be readily purified for chemical studies. It is accepted that myeloma proteins are not abnormally structured proteins; rather they occur as a result of the clonal expansion of antibody-producing cells present in the normal population[32]. Myeloma proteins can be found in all known classes and subclasses of antibody molecules although each individual protein belongs to one class and subclass.

In 1969, the first complete amino acid sequence of a human IgG1 myeloma protein was reported[8] (Figure 1.4). One of the most striking features of the immunoglobulin molecule is the demarcation of its chains into connected regions that are associated with different functions: variations in the sequences of V_H and V_L regions for antigen binding, and at the same time conservation of sequence of C_H and C_L regions for other immunological functions.

1.3.2.1 Subclasses

Normal human IgG contains a mixture of four different subclasses of H chains, $\gamma1$, $\gamma2$, $\gamma3$ and $\gamma4$. The biological significance of the four types is still poorly understood, although it is known that IgG2 does not fix to the skin of guinea pigs[33] and IgG4 does not fix complement[34] (Table 1.3). Comparison of the amino acid sequences of 233 residues from the C-terminus of $\gamma1$ and $\gamma4$ chains (Figure 1.5) shows 14 residue differences, 11 of which are localized in the C_H2 domain. Nevertheless, the relationship between biological activity and difference in primary structure is still unclear, although C_H2 has been implicated in complement fixation[35,36]. IgG4 proteins are the most anionic among the IgG subclasses, and the Fc fragment is responsible for its unique electrophoretic mobility. The types of amino acid replacements observed in the Fc fragment of IgG4 (Figure 1.5) clearly explain such behaviour.

Partial amino acid sequences of the different subclasses of γ chains and isolation of their intrachain cystine bridges[6,37] (Figures 1.6 and 1.7), provided convincing evidence that the immunoglobulin molecule evolved by successive duplication of precursor genes[38,39] and that a loop of about 60 residues is a fundamental pseudo-subunit which is repeated 12 times in an IgG molecule[37]. Four pairs of such loops, one in the L and three in the H chains, are essentially invariant within each type and subclass (Figure 1.2). These findings fit very well with the domain hypothesis[8] which postulates that a homology region is folded in a compact domain stabilized by a single intrachain disulphide bond and linked to neighbouring regions by less tightly-folded stretches of polypeptide chains. X-ray crystallographic studies of Fab fragment of a human myeloma immunoglobulin[40] showed, as expected, that C_L, C_H1, V_L and V_H subunits are strikingly similar in their three-dimensional folding and that a centrally-located cleft divided the Fab into two structural domains, V and C. The structural subunits C_H1 and C_L in the C domain interact over a wider area and are more tightly packed than the V_H and V_L subunits in the V domain. In the V domain, the overall structural design was described as one in which the exposed hypervariable positions occur at adjacent bends of tightly packed, linear polypeptide chains.

1.3.2.2 Interchain bridges

It is noteworthy that the stretch in the H chain which contains the interchain disulphide bonds (hinge region) has no homologous counterpart in other positions of H or L chains. In fact the inter-H chain bridges present

Cγ1

PCA- Val- Gln- Leu- Val- Gln- Ser- Gly- Ala- Glu- Val- Lys- Lys- Pro- Gly- Ser- Ser- Val- Lys- Val- Ser- (Cys)- Lys- Ala- Ser- 25

Gly- Gly- Thr- Phe- Ser- Arg- Ser- Ala- Ile- Ile- Trp- Val- Arg- Gln- Ala- Pro- Gly- Gln- Gly- Leu- Glu- Trp- Met- Gly- Gly- 50

Ile- Val- Pro- Met- Phe- Gly- Pro- Pro- Asn- Tyr- Ala- Gln- Lys- Phe- Gln- Gly- Arg- Val- Thr- Ile- Thr- Ala- Asp- Glu- Ser- 75

Thr- Asn- Thr- Ala- Tyr- Met- Glu- Leu- Ser- Ser- Leu- Arg- Ser- Glu- Asp- Thr- Ala- Phe- Tyr- Phe- (Cys)- Ala- Gly- Gly- Tyr- 100

Gly- Ile- Tyr- Ser- Pro- Glu- Glu- Tyr- Asn- Gly- Gly- Leu- Val- Thr- Val- Ser- Ser- Ala- Ser- Thr- Lys- Gly- Pro- Ser- Val- 125

Phe- Pro- Leu- Ala- Pro- Ser- Ser- Lys- Ser- Thr- Ser- Gly- Gly- Thr- Ala- Ala- Leu- Gly- (Cys)- Leu- Val- Lys- Asp- Tyr- Phe- 150

Pro- Glu- Pro- Val- Thr- Val- Ser- Trp- Asn- Ser- Gly- Ala- Leu- Thr- Ser- Gly- Val- His- Thr- Phe- Pro- Ala- Val- Leu- Gln- 175

Ser- Ser- Gly- Leu- Tyr- Ser- Leu- Ser- Ser- Val- Val- Thr- Val- Pro- Ser- Ser- Leu- Gly- Thr- Gln- Thr- Tyr- Ile- (Cys)- 200

Asn- Val- Asn- His- Lys- Pro- Ser- Asn- Thr- Lys- Val- Asp- Lys- Arg- Val- Glu- Pro- Lys- Ser- (Cys)- Asp- Lys- Thr- His- Thr- 225

14

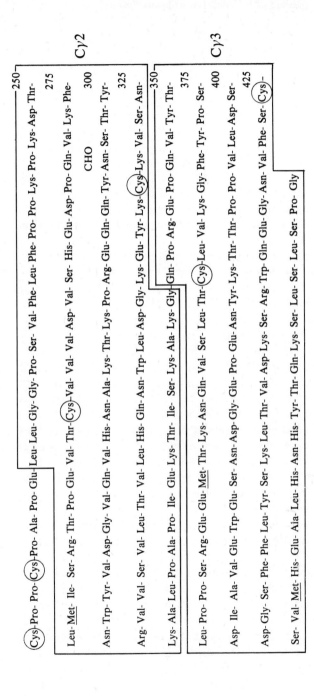

Figure 1.4 Complete amino acid sequence of the γ heavy chain of human IgG1 myeloma protein Eu[8]. Constant (C) domains are in boxes: $C_{\gamma 1}$ (residues 119–220), $C_{\gamma 2}$ (residues 234–341), $C_{\gamma 3}$ (residues 342–446). Half-cystinyl residues are circled. The section between $C_{\gamma 1}$ and $C_{\gamma 2}$ called the interdomain or hinge region (residues 220–233) contains the interchain disulphide bonds. Constant methionine residues are underlined.

Table 1.3 Biological properties of the subclasses of human IgG

	IgG1	IgG2	IgG3	IgG4
Complement fixation	+	±	+	0
Passive cutaneous anaphylaxis*	+	0	+	+
Placental transfer	+	+	+	+
Percentage distribution in normal sera	65–70	20	7–8	3–4

* In the guinea pig

remarkable variations in different subclasses of IgG[37] (Figures 1.8a and 1.8b). IgG1 and IgG4 molecules contain four interchain bridges. Two such bonds join the H chains to each other, and two bonds join H to L chains although the inter-H—L bridges occur in non-homologous sequences and in different positions.

IgG2 molecules are cross-linked by six interchain bonds, two joining H to L chains and the other four, binding both H chains. The half-cystine which binds H to L chains in IgG2 is found in similar sequences in γ3 and γ4 chains (Figure 1.8a). The sequence around the inter-H bonds of IgG2 that includes the four half-cystines are present in a section, eight residues long. This arrangement may explain in part the known resistance of IgG2 protein to papain digestion.

Previous studies of IgG3 myeloma proteins[41,42] showed them to contain seven interchain bonds: two binding H to L chains and five joining the H chains. A partial sequence of the hinge region of γ3 chain indicated an insertion of an extra fragment at the N-terminal end, although the length was not known. This fact, coupled with the observation that the molecular weight of γ3 H chain is 58–60 000 in contrast to about 50 000 for the γ1, γ2 and γ4 H chains[43,44], led to the suggestion[45] that the difference is due to a larger hinge region consisting of about 100 amino acid residues. Recently this extra fragment was isolated from the whole molecule[46] and from an unusual γ3 H chain disease (HCD) protein[47]. Based on its molecular weight (10–11 000), isolation of all the radioactively-labelled cysteine-containing tryptic peptides, amino acid composition and partial sequence, it appears that the extra fragment in the case of γ3 HCD proteins (OMM) represents a series of similar or identical duplications. Whether this is also true for the intact γ3 H chain remains to be investigated. In all classes of immunoglobulins, the half-cysteine residues that participate in the normal interchain disulphide bridge between L and H chains are always at the C-terminal end of the L chain. In human γ1 chains, the cysteine residue which joins H to L is at position 220[8]. However, in human γ2, γ3, γ4[37] and μ[13,21] chains, and in other species[48–50], the corresponding cysteinyl residue occurs at about position 130 (Figure 1.6). In the three-dimensional model of Fab[40], these three positions (C-terminus of L chain, positions 130 and 220 of H chain) are sufficiently close; about 6 Å, to allow for the alter-

Residue position	232	234	268	272	274	283	294	296	327	330–331	355	409	455
γ1–Eu	··· Pro	··· Leu	··· His	··· Gln	··· Lys	··· Gln	··· Gln	··· Tyr	··· Ala	··· Ala-Pro	··· Arg	··· Lys	··· Pro ···
γ4–Vi	··· Ser	··· Phe	··· Gln	··· Glu	··· Gln	··· Glu	··· Glu	··· Phe	··· Gly	··· Ser-Ser	··· Gln	··· Arg	··· Leu ···

Figure 1.5 Differences in amino acid sequence in C_H2 and C_H3 domains between γ1 and γ4 heavy chains[6,8].

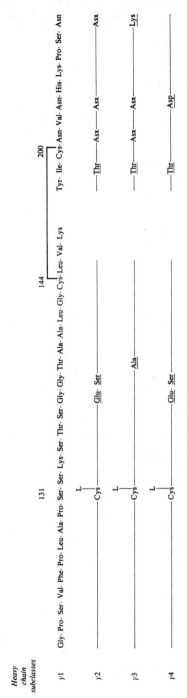

Figure 1.6 Sequences around the disulphide bridges in the C_H1 region of human immunoglobulins of different subclasses. Note that γ1 is the only H chain subclass that does not have the H—L disulphide bond at position 131[6]. Established points of differences between γ1, 2, 3, and 4 are underlined.

17

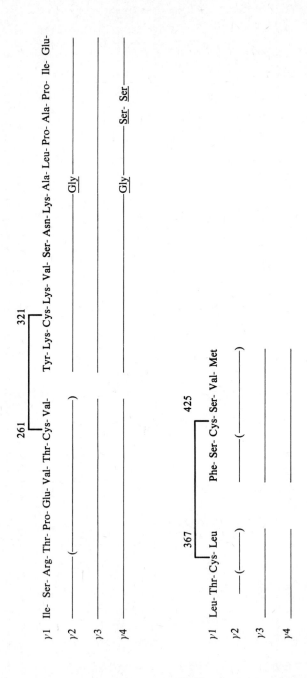

Figure 1.7 Sequences around disulphide bridges in the C_H2 and C_H3 domains of different γ chains[6].

native disulphide bonds without altering the folding of the polypeptide chains. These findings were previously suggested when an additional intrachain disulphide bond joining position 131–221, was described in rabbit IgG[48].

1.3.2.3 Chemical typing

Based on differences in sequence around interchain bridges, and their number, a simple method was developed for distinguishing chains[51]. High voltage electrophoresis of pepsin–trypsin digests of myeloma proteins, which has been partially reduced and alkylated with ^{14}C-iodoacetate, gave autoradiographic patterns which were characteristic for each type of H and L chain, and permitted the classification of both L and H chains by simple inspection (Figure 1.9). This method has the advantage of obviating the use of specific antisera

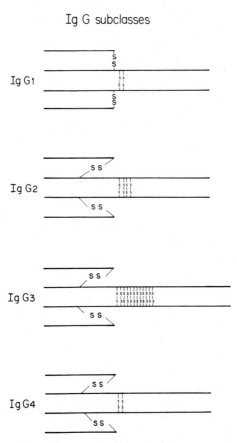

Ig G subclasses

Figure 1.8a Suggested arrangement of S—S interchain bridges in human IgG1, IgG2, IgG3, and IgG4. The exact number of interchain bonds in IgG3 is uncertain[37].

19

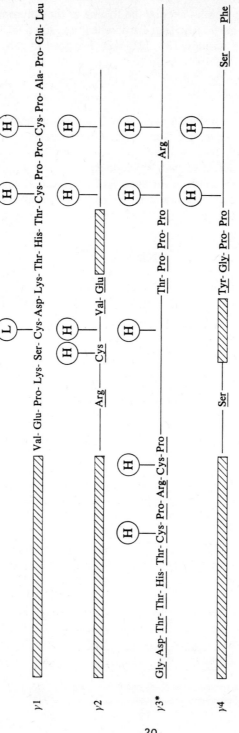

Figure 1.8b Amino acid sequence of the hinge region of different subclasses of human IgG. Solid lines indicate identity to γ1 chain. Shaded blocks indicate gaps to maximize homology. *The sequence of γ3 is taken from γ3 HCD protein OMM, where it was postulated that the hinge region contains a series of similar or identical duplications[47] (not shown). H and L indicate the position of interchain disulphide bonds. Established points of different between γ1, 2, 3, and 4 are underlined.

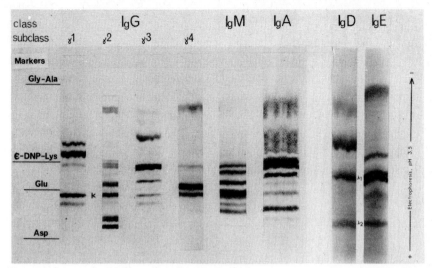

Figure 1.9 Autoradiographs obtained after electrophoresis at pH 3.5 of peptic–tryptic digests of partially reduced and carboxymethylated G myeloma proteins of different subclasses, IgM macroglobulins, and A, D and E myeloma proteins. κ: peptide derived from the C-terminal of L chains (κ type). λ1 and λ2 are two related peptides derived from the C-terminal of L chains (λ type). Each H chain gives a specific autoradiographic pattern due to differences in the peptides derived from the inter H—H or inter H—L disulphide bonds[51, 52, 124].

(which are not widely and readily available) and, in addition, it seems possible that differences in mobility of some of these peptides might provide easily detectable clues to unusual mutations.

1.3.2.4 Genetic markers

Allotypes or genetic markers are antigenic determinants on Ig molecules which are inherited in Mendelian fashion and are detected by immunological methods. They have been identified in most mammalian species.

Three sets of allotypic markers are recognized in human Ig, the closely linked Gm and Am factors and the independently inherited Inv system. In Table 1.4 are listed the current known factors. The alphabetical and numerical nomenclatures have been used in different laboratories in spite of the fact that the numerical nomenclature was recommended by WHO in 1965. It was suggested in the last WHO meeting (Rouen, 1974) to keep both for the time being and when possible to identify the chain on which a given allotype is found. The signatories agreed to employ numbers for the allotypes on the κ chains and α2 chains and to use Km instead of Inv.

A series of antigenic determinants which act as allotypes within a chain subclass can behave as an isotype on one or more of the remaining subclasses. These have been referred to as 'non-markers', but it was suggested that they be

Table 1.4 Human immunoglobulins (Allotypes)

Location H chain	Recommended designations		Previous designation	
	Alphameric	Numeric		
$\gamma 1$	Glm(a)	Glm(1)	Gm(a)	Gm(1)
	(x)	(2)	(x)	(2)
	(f)	(3)	(bw), (b2), (f)	(3) (4)
	(z)	(17)	(z)	(17)
$\gamma 2$	G2m(n)	G2m(23)	(n)	(23)
$\gamma 3$	G3m(b0)	G3m(11)	(b^β), (b^0)	(11)
	(b1)	(5)	(b), (b1),	(5) (12)
	(b3)	(13)	(b3), (Bet)	(13) (25)
	(b4)	(14)		
	(b5)	(10)	$(b\alpha)$, (b5)	(10)
	(C3)	(6)	(Gm-like), (c), (c3)	(6)
	(c5)	(24)	(Gm·like), (c), (c5)	(24)
	(g)	(21)	(g)	(21)
	μ	(26)	Pa	
	ν	(27)	Ray	
	(s)	(15)	(s)	(15)
	(t)	(16)	(t)	(16)
$\gamma 2$	A2m(a)	A2m(1)	Am(1), Am+	Am(2), Am−
	A2m(2)	A2m(2)		
L chain κ	Km(1)	Km(1)	Inv(l) Inv(1)	
	(2)	(2)	Inv(a), Inv(2)	
	(3)	(3)	Inv(b), Inv(3)	

referred to as 'isoallotypes'. The notation suggested for isoallotypes is shown in Table 1.5.

The Km factors are associated with κ type BJ proteins and κ type L chains, and since L chains are common to all classes of Ig, Km antigens can be found in IgG, A, M, D and E molecules, Km markers are inherited through a series of three alleles $Km^{1,2}$, Km^1 and Km^3. About 98% of Caucasoid individuals who have Km^1 antigen also have Km^2. Amino acid sequence studies have shown that $Km^{1,2}$ is associated with a leucine residue in the C region of κ chain (position 191) and that Km^3 is associated with a valine at the same position[6]. When the rare antigen Km^1 is present, valine is in position 153 instead of alanine[53] (Table 1.6).

Gm factors are associated with IgG molecules only, and are located on the C region. Although the serological specificities reside in the H chains, some of them require combinations with L chains to provide the quaternary structure necessary for their expression[26]. Amino acid interchanges, probably responsible for allotypic differences in human Ig H chains, are shown in Table 1.6. Arginine is found at position 214 and Glu, Met at positions 356 and 358 respectively, when the molecule is G1m(f,Na). Lysine is found at position 214 and Asp, Leu at position 356, 358 when the molecule is G1m(a, z). A Phe residue is found at position 436 when $\gamma 3$ chain is G3m(b1) and a Tyr residue is

Table 1.5   Suggested nomenclature for the isoallotypic markers of IgG

Location H chain	Recommended		Previous
	Alphameric	Numeric	
γ1, γ2, γ3	Na	N1	non-a
γ3	Nb0	N11	non-b0
γ3	Nb1	N5	non-b1
γ3	Ng	N21	non-g
γ1, γ3, γ4 (N4a)	N4a	N4a	4a
γ2, γ4 (N4b)	N4b	N4b	4b

Table 1.6   Location and amino acid differences between IgG molecules of different allotypes

Chain	Marker	Location	Residue(s)
κ	Km(1)	153 ... 191	Val ... Leu
κ	Km(1, 2)	153 ... 191	Ala ...Leu
κ	Km(3)	153 ... 191	Ala ...Val
γ1	Glm(z or 17)	214	Lys
γ1	Glm(a or 1)	356–358	Asp-Glu-Leu
γ1	Glm(f or 3)	214	Arg
γ1	Na or Nl	356–358	Glu-Glu-Met
γ4	N4b	309	Leu
γ4	N4b	309	deletion

found at the same position when the molecule is G3m(g). In γ4 chain, Leu is found in position 309 when the activity is N4a and that residue is deleted in N4b molecules[54]. For more details, see Chapter 2 of this volume.

1.3.3   Immunoglobulin M

IgM of man and other mammals has a molecular weight of about 900 000 (Table 1.1). Each molecule can be dissociated into five similar subunits (IgMs) each having a MW of about 180 000[55]. The subunits are joined through an intersubunit S—S bond on each μ chain to form a pentamer. A third chain has been described in polymeric Ig molecules[56,57] and called J chain because of its supposed function of joining monomers (see IgA).

There are ten L–H chain pairs and one J chain per molecule. Electron micrographs of IgM molecules clearly showed that five four-chain units are linked in a circle, and that the links are flexible so that the units may bend above and below the plane of the circle[58]. Human IgM antibody to *Salmonella typhi*[59] and a Waldenstrom macroglobulin with binding affinity for nitrophenyl groups[60] were shown to have ten binding sites with similar affinity. On the other hand rabbit IgM anti-hapten antibody[61] appeared to have a bimodal distribution of binding constants: five sites and single affinity and the other five had weaker affinity. This behaviour remains unresolved. $(Fc)_5\mu$ fragment can fix complement up to 19 times more effectively than intact IgM on a molar basis[62] and $C_{\mu4}$ domain appears to be responsible for this biological activity[63].

Structural studies are mainly done with proteins obtained from patients suffering from Waldenstrom's macroglobulinaemia. They serve as a model for structural analysis of IgM antibodies just as myeloma proteins and Bence-Jones proteins are models for IgG antibodies and light chains respectively. Trypsin at 60 °C splits human IgM at a single site on the μ chain (Figure 1.10) and gives an apparently homogeneous pentameric $(Fc)_5\mu$ fragment (MW 340 000). These fragments are linked by disulphide bonds and they dissociate into five identical Fc-like fragments after reduction[64]. Disulphide linked Fab dimers $(Fab')_2$ can be isolated by degrading the molecule with trypsin at 37°C[65] (Figure 1.10).

All the cysteine-containing peptides from a μ chain had been characterized (14 cysteine residues for each μ chain), and a disulphide-bonding model for human IgM has been proposed[13,66,67]; four bonds are interchain and ten intrachain. The interchain disulphide bridges are arranged as follows (Figure 1.11): one joins H to L; one joins H to H in the monomer subunit; one is intersubunit (located at the C-terminus of the $C_{\mu3}$ domain); and the fourth cysteine apparently joins either the J chain or the homologous cystine of the next monomer subunit (that is, it behaves either as a μ–J bond or as a second intersubunit bond, see J chain). The higher molecular weight of μ chain (70 000 daltons instead of 50 000) and the isolation of five intrachain cystine bonds indicated that each μ chain contains five domains instead of the four present in γ chains. Almost complete amino acid sequence studies of two human IgM proteins have shown[13,21] that two domains (V_H and $C_{\mu1}$) are in Fd, one ($C_{\mu2}$) is in the adjacent region which is degraded very easily with different enzymes, and two ($C_{\mu3}$ and $C_{\mu4}$) are in Fc. The amino acid sequence of μ chain from protein Oμ is shown in Figure 1.12 (protein Oμ belongs to the V_HII subgroup). The V_H region comprises about 120 residues. In fact protein Oμ has 124 residues in the V region since it has an insertion of four tyrosines at position 110 (see Figure 1.3).

In the switch region, that is, the juncture of V and C regions, μ and γ chains share very few residues and whether this section is a recognition site for the union of V and C genes remains open. The $C_{\mu1}$ region includes the disulphide bridge to the L chain, an intrachain bridge and the first carbohydrate group: C1. The sequence between Fd and Fc does not reveal any fragment that is rich in proline and cysteine residues like the hinge region of human γ and α chains. The most proline-rich sequence (although it lacks disulphide bridges) is the beginning of the $C_{\mu2}$ region. Most of $C_{\mu2}$ is degraded to peptides after trypsin digestion at 60 °C suggesting that there is an exposed and flexible region in IgM molecules resembling, therefore, the behaviour of the hinge region in other molecules.

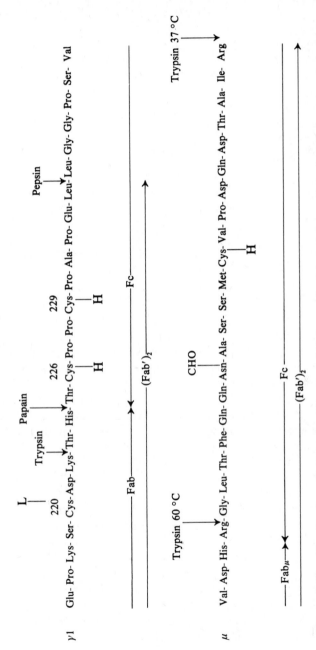

Figure 1.10. The site of specific cleavage of human μ chain by trypsin. Fab$_\mu$ and Fc$_\mu$ are defined as the fragments obtained by tryptic digestion of IgM at 60 °C, whereas (Fab')$_2\mu$ is the analogous dimeric fragment obtained with trypsin at 37 °C at which temperature Fc$_\mu$ is degraded to peptides[62,63]. Fc$_\mu$ is a pentamer because of the presence of intersubunit (IS) disulphide bonds (see text). Also shown is the site of specific cleavage of human $\gamma1$ chain by papain, trypsin and pepsin; the Fc fragment may be a monomer or dimer depending on the state of the H—H interchain bridges.

Ig M

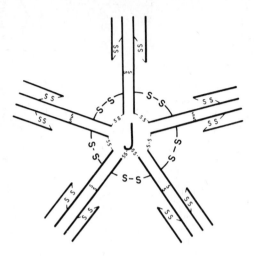

Figure 1.11   Suggested arrangement of S—S interchain bridges of human IgM.

Two basic types of oligosaccharide units are present in IgM proteins. One type (simple) contains mannose and N-acetylglucosamine, and the other (complex) contains mannose, N-acetylglucosamine, fucose, galactose and sialic acid. The locations of these groups were determined[13,68] and are shown in Figure 1.12. The $C_{\mu 3}$ region has two complex oligosaccharides (C2 and C3) and a simple one (C4). C3 and C4 are within an intrachain loop in the $C_{\mu 3}$ domain close to the intersubunit bond. Sequence studies showed these groups to have a common core structure which is identical to a glycopeptide isolated from IgG myeloma proteins[69].

The degree of homology between C_μ and C_γ is around 30%. The best fit seems to be between $C_{\gamma 1}$ and $C_{\mu 1}$ (33%), and between $C_{\gamma 3}$ and $C_{\mu 4}$ (43%). $C_{\mu 2}$ and $C_{\mu 3}$ have approximately 25% homology with $C_{\gamma 2}$. Again, as in the case of subclasses of γ chains, the greatest degree of homology centres around intrachain half-cystine residues. In contrast, the greatest disparity in primary structure exists between domains. Furthermore, 19 additional residues are present at the C-terminal end of μ chain. Partial amino acid sequence of chains[70,71] indicates that human μ and α chains have 55% identity in the last 40 residues, including the C-terminal end nonadecapeptide that is missing in γ chains (Figure 1.16). Our data on the sequence of α chain[72] do not support such a high degree of homology throughout the entire C regions of μ and α chains.

Pathological IgM macroglobulins can be classified into two groups depending upon the presence or absence of a particular antigenic determinant[73] present in the Fab$_\mu$ fragment. It correlates with the presence of two distinctive spots upon fingerprint analysis. Since the determinants were found in all 26 normal sera tests, it was suggested that they are expressions of isotypic variants ($\mu 1$ and $\mu 2$).

1.3.4 Immunoglobulin A

1.3.4.1 Subclasses

In recent years IgA has assumed great significance because although it is a minor constituent of serum it is the predominant Ig present in external secretions, and thus appears to play an important role in local defence mechanisms[75]. The basic structure of IgA is similar to that of other Igs in that it consists of two L chains and two H (α) chains which determine the properties characteristic of this class. However, higher molecular weight polymers are frequently found. Two antigenically distinguishable subclasses known as IgA1, and IgA2 have been recognized[76-78]. The antigenic differences are located on the α chains and are independent of L chain type and monomer–polymer-related structures. IgA1 constitutes about 93% of normal IgA globulins and about 7% of IgA2[79]. It was reported that IgA2 lacks the disulphide bonds linking H to L chains and instead consists of a pair of disulphide-bonded L chains which are bound to a pair of disulphide-bonded α chains by non-covalent bonds[80]. Moreover, a genetic marker was found to be associated with IgA2 globulins[81,82], (Table 1.4). It was shown that IgA2 belonging to the A2m(1) genetic variant lacks the disulphide bonds linking H to L but the other variant, A2m(2), has the usual H–L disulphide bonds characteristic of other Igs. The fact that 20 out of 22 IgA2 myeloma proteins, mostly from Caucasians, were A2m(1) explains the initial report that the H–L disulphide bond is absent in IgA2 molecules, which therefore dissociate in acid[83]. Chemical studies supported those findings and also showed that the H–L peptide of A2m(2) IgA proteins was the same as that in IgA1 proteins (Figure 1.13a) indicating an evolutionary relationship similar to that found in different subclasses of IgG[84].

The present status of human $\alpha 1$ and $\alpha 2$ chains is as follows. We now know the sequences around nearly all the half-cystine peptides involved in disulphide bridges[22,72,85,86], the complete sequence of the V region of two α chains[20] (Figure 1.3), the N-terminal sequence of the first 25–30 residues of the V regions of a number of unblocked α chains[18 20,22], and the C-terminal 40 residues[70,71] (Figure 1.16). These data account for almost half of $\alpha 1$ and $\alpha 2$ chains. Studies of cysteine-containing peptides have revealed an unusually high content of cysteine residues (between 17 to 18). One of the cysteine residues forms the H–L disulphide bridge. There are at least two interchain H–H bridges. Two additional cysteine residues in the hinge form intrachain bonds with cysteine residues in

PCA-Val-Thr-Leu-Thr-Glu-Ser-Gly-Pro-Ala-Leu-Val-Lys-Pro-Lys-Gln-Pro-Leu-Thr-Leu-Thr-Cys-Thr-Phe-Ser-
22

Gly-Phe-Ser-Leu-Ser-Thr-Ser-Arg-Met-Arg-Val-Ser-Trp-Ile-Arg-Arg-Pro-Pro-Gly-Lys-Ala-Leu-Glu-Trp-Leu-

Ala-Arg-Ile-Asx-Asx-Asx-Lys-Phe-Tyr-Trp-Ser-Thr-Ser-Leu-Arg-Thr-Arg-Leu-Ser-Ile-Ser-Lys-Asn-Asp-
97

Ser-Lys-Asn-Gln-Val-Val-Leu-Ile-Met-Ile-Asn-Val-Asn-Pro-Val-Asp-Thr-Ala-Thr-Tyr-Tyr-Cys-Ala-Arg-Val-

V | C   L

Val-Asn-Ser-Val-Met-Ala-Gly-Tyr-Tyr-Tyr-Tyr-Met-Asp-Val-Trp-Gly-Lys-Gly-Thr-Thr-Val-Thr-Val-Ser-
140

Ser-Gly-Ser-Ala-Ser-Ala-Pro-Thr-Leu-Phe-Pro-Leu-Val-Ser-Glu-Asn-Ser-(Asx,Pro,Ser,Ser,Thr)Val-Ala-
153
C1

Val-Gly-Cys-Leu-Ala-Glx-Asp-Phe-Leu-Pro-Asp-Ser-Ile-Thr-Phe-Ser-Trp-Lys-Tyr-(Asn,Asx,Ser,Asx,Lys)Ile-

Ser-Ser-Thr-Arg-Gly-Phe-Pro-Ser-Val-Leu-Arg-Gly-Gly-Lys-Tyr-Ala-Ala-Thr-(Ser,Glx)Val-Leu-Leu-Pro-Ser-
213

Lys-Asp-Val-Met-Gln-Gly-Thr-Asp-Glu-His-Val-Cys-Lys-Trp-Val-Gln-His-Pro-Asn-Gly-Asx-Lys-Gln-Lys-Asx-

Val-Pro-Leu-Pro-Val-Ile-Ala-Glu-Leu-Pro-Pro-Lys-Val-Ser-Val-Phe-Val-Pro-Pro-Arg-Gly-Phe-Phe-Gly-
259

Asx-Pro-Arg-Lys-Ser-Lys-Ile-Cys-Gln-Ala-Thr-Gly-Phe-Ser-Pro-Arg-Gln/Val-Trp-Ser-Leu-Arg-Glu-Gly-Lys-

Gln-Val-Gly-Ser-Gly-Val-Thr-Asx-Thr-Asx-Val-Glx-Ala-Glx-Ala-Lys-Glx-Ser-Gly-Pro-Thr-Thr-Tyr-Lys-
320

Val-Thr-Ser-Thr-Leu-Thr-Ile-Lys-Glx-Ser-Asp-Trp-Leu-Gly-Glu-Ser-Met-Phe-Thr-Cys-Arg-Val-Asp-His-Arg-

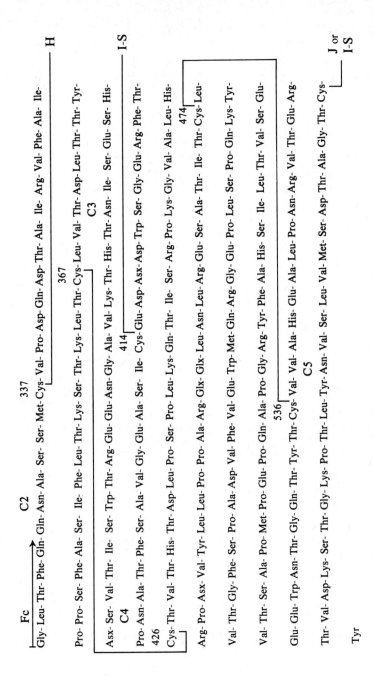

Figure 1.12 Amino acid sequence of the μ heavy chain of human IgM macroglobulin Ou[13]. The positions of interchain and intrachain bonds and carbohydrate units are identified. V: variable, C: constant, IS: intersubunit, J: J chain, C1, C2, C3, C4 and C5: Carbohydrate groups in the constant region.

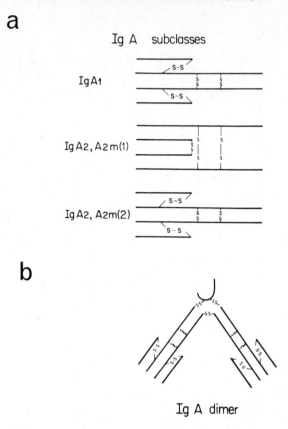

Ig A dimer

Figure 1.13a   Suggested arrangement of interchain disulphide bonds in human IgA of different subclasses and genetic markers. The C-terminal half-cystine residue of the α chain in the monomer is probably part of an intrachain bond.

Figure 1.13b   Dimeric IgA: J chain is linked to the C-terminus of two α chains (one from each monomer). The presence of an intersubunit bond in polymeric forms has not been detected yet.

the Fc and Fd fragment, respectively. While most of the remaining cysteine residues appear to be involved in intrachain bridges, it seems likely that some are bridged to the J chain or the secretory component, or join subunits.

In the last 40 residues the $\alpha 1$ and μ chains have 55–60% homology including the C-terminal nonadecapeptide tail that is missing in the γ and ϵ chains (Figure 1.16). (The C regions of μ and $\gamma 1$ chains have only 30–35% homology). An analysis of the distribution of V_H subgroups among IgA indicates that, unlike the situation in the IgG and IgM classes, the V_H III subgroup predominates (65% to 75% in IgA and approximately 20% in IgG and IgM)[89].

1.3.4.2 Hinge region

Sequence studies of the hinge region of IgA1 molecules show that like other hinge regions, they are rich in cysteine and proline residues; however, the hinge region of IgA1 differs in having at least 16 residues with an unusual sequence that consists of two identical stretches of eight residues and contains several identical CHO groups. It is possible that a triplication has occurred or alternatively that a smaller fragment (four residues) was duplicated six times (Figure 1.14). Comparison with the sequence of the hinge peptide derived from an IgA2 protein shows that they are identical in the first eight residues and in the last five, but that the hinge region of IgA2 lacks CHO and has a gap of about 13 residues just in the place where the duplication of a small fragment was shown in IgA1[85].

Only the amino composition of the hinge region of the IgA2, A2m(2) molecule is known and it appears similar to the one present in IgA2, A2m(1) since it lacks CHO, serine and threonine[90].

The arrangement of disulphide bridges in the hinge regions of IgA1 and IgA2 myeloma proteins was studied using diagonal electrophoresis, and a tentative model was proposed[91]. It seems likely that the arrangement of the disulphide bridges of the two hinges is similar in spite of their remarkable structural differences. When the hinge regions of IgA1, IgA2 and IgGs are aligned, striking homologies can be seen particularly with IgG3 [47].

1.3.4.3 Carbohydrate

Of all the Ig classes present in man, only IgA [92,93] and IgD [94] have both N-acetylgalactosamine- and N-acetylglucosamine-containing oligosaccharide units. The structures of the two asparagine-linked oligosaccharide units of an IgA1 myeloma protein were defined[95], and the peptide structure and linkage points of five O-glycosidically-linked oligosaccharide units present in the hinge were also described. The peptide structure appears to be identical to the one determined for the hinge region glycopeptide isolated previously[84]. The locations of the oligosaccharide units of this glycopeptide clearly show (Figure 1.14) that IgA2 could not have any of these units because all the serines involved in O-glycosidic linkages were absent. With the exception of a terminal N-acetylgalactosamine at the N-terminus, the location and structure of the five O-glycosidically-linked oligosaccharide units of the glycopeptide preserve the symmetry present in the sequence of the hinge region. These studies established that the oligosaccharide groups found in human Igs differ as regards the type of structure, the number of each type per H chain, and the actual sequence, suggesting that the carbohydrate moieties may play an as yet unidentified role in the biologic functioning of each Ig class.

1.3.4.4 IgA protease

Enzymatic proteolysis of human IgA yields Fab fragments while the Fc is

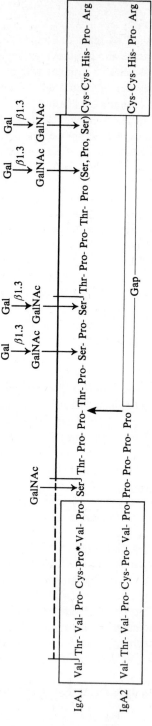

Figure 1.14 Amino acid sequences of the 'hinge' region of IgA1 and IgA2 myeloma proteins[85]. Homologous regions are in boxes: thick line indicates a duplication, or a triplication if mutants are allowed (dotted lines). The heavy arrow indicates the site of cleavage of α1 chains by IgA protease[98]. The hinge region of IgA2 is resistant, probably due to the lack of a Pro—Thr bond and the presence of five Pro residues. The α2 hinge lacks CHO groups and has a deletion of 13 residues. Also shown are the structure and location of the O-glycosidically linked units[95]. *Position where normal synthesis resumes after an internal deletion in protein DEF (see Heavy Chain Variants).

degraded into small peptides. Recently, it was reported[96,97] that normal faeces contain an IgA fragment corresponding to Fc$_\alpha$ and that faeces contain a proteolytic enzyme which cleaves serum and secretory IgA to yield both fragments. The enzyme was termed IgA protease because enzymatic activity has thus far been found only against IgA. IgA protease can be obtained from centrifuged suspensions of faeces or from culture fluids of *Streptococcus sanguis*. The specificity of the enzyme is quite restricted. It does not appear to cleave IgG or M. It cleaves the Pro—Thr bond[98] in the hinge region of IgA1 (Figure 1.14). This bond is absent in IgA2 because of a deletion and apparently the enzyme does not split IgA2. The presence of Fc$_\alpha$ fragments in normal faeces suggests a role for this enzyme in the secretory immune system. Of considerable interest from the evolutionary point of view is that the enzyme is produced by bacteria in those regions of the alimentary tract heavily populated by bacteria, mainly the mouth and the colon. This may account for the increased ratio of IgA2/IgA1 in secretions as compared to serum.

1.3.4.5 J Chain

Recent studies on polymeric Igs have shown the presence of a polypeptide chain, the J chain, in addition to the H and L chains that comprise the monomer unit[56,57]. The J chain is a covalent disulphide bridge within the polymers and its absence from all forms of monomeric Igs suggests that J chain plays an important role in initiating and maintaining the polymeric state. Initial studies using SDS–polyacrylamide gels and gel-filtration showed that J chain had the same mobility as L chain (25 000 daltons). However, a MW of 15 000 was obtained for rabbit J chain by equilibrium centrifugation[99] and subsequently, using non-dissociating buffer[100], a similar value was obtained for human J chain. Two models have been proposed[101]: (a) J chain links each monomer unit (bracelet model), and (b) J chain serves as a clasp between two monomers (clasp model).

To distinguish between these possibilities, several methods have been used: (1) stepwise reduction and differential radioalkylation which permitted cleavage of J chain S—S bonds to be correlated with the extent of depolymerization[102,103]; (2) CNBr cleavage of polymeric Igs[104,105]. These studies indicated that the J chain is disulphide-bonded to only two of the subunits of the polymeric Ig and that the remaining subunits in the higher polymers are directly disulphide-bonded one to the other. Furthermore, it was shown that J chain is linked to the penultimate cysteine residues of the C-terminal octadecapeptide of α[104,105] (Figure 1.13b) and probably μ chains[106]. Several cysteine-containing peptides were isolated from the J chain[107] and two of them appeared to be implicated in the linkage (unpublished observation) to the α chains. Although they are different from those present in H and L chains[22,57], fingerprinting analyses and studies of the cysteine-containing peptides of the J chain from different proteins are consistent with the conclusion that the J chain associated with different classes of Igs are identical.

1.3.4.6   Secretory IgA

Secretory IgA (sIgA) is present in mucous membrane secretions. It contains four different types of polypeptide chains: H (α), L, J and a distinct chain called secretory component (SC) which is not synthesized in plasma cells as the others are, but in the lining epithelial cells of mucous membranes[107]. SC is not normally found associated with any other protein; however, not all the SC in secretions occur as a part of sIgA—some exist in a free state. Bound secretory component (BSC) and free secretory component (FSC) have been isolated and compared in human[109] and rabbit[110], and within each species were reported to be similar in MW (71 000 for human) and antigenic determinants. Furthermore, identity of BSC and FSC was suggested by peptide maps and amino acid sequences of the first 14 residues[111] (Figure 1.15). At present it is not possible to speculate on the evolutionary origin of SC since it does not have homology to any known protein. Recent studies[112] suggested that a single intrachain disulphide bridge in FSC forms two interchain disulphide bridges when FSC is eventually joined to dimeric IgA (the exact at-

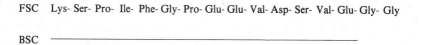

FSC   Lys- Ser- Pro- Ile- Phe- Gly- Pro- Glu- Glu- Val- Asp- Ser- Val- Glu- Gly- Gly

BSC   ——

Figure 1.15   N-terminal sequence of human free secretory component (FSC) and bound secretory component (BSC)[111].

tachment site in the IgA portion of sIgA is not yet known). It was postulated[113] that final assembly takes place within the epithelial lining cells of mucous membranes from SC synthesized in the epithelial cell and IgA entering the epithelial cell after secretion by a local immunocyte.

1.3.5   Immunoglobulin E

IgE represent a distinct class of Ig which plays a major role in atopic diseases[114]. The discovery of IgE myeloma proteins[115,116], which are the same as reaginic antibodies with respect to antigenic characteristics and skin fixing properties, has provided a good tool for studying IgE at the molecular level. IgE is a four-chain glycoprotein with a sedimentation coefficient of 8S and a MW of nearly 190 000. The carbohydrate content is about 12% and it is associated with the H chain (ε) only. The MW of the ε chain is about 70 000 daltons[117,118]. The role of IgE antibodies in immediate hypersensitivity reactions is due to their attachment to membrane receptors on mast cells and basophilic granulocytes[119]. This cytotropic activity has been shown to be located in the Fc fragment[120]. Studies have been performed in order to delineate some of the conformational properties of the intact molecule and its proteolytic fragments using circular dichroism (CD) as the probe, and to study conformational changes accompanying heating and reduction[121]. It was shown that heating of IgE at 56 °C for 30 min. results in an irreversible conformational transition. These changes have been localized to the C-terminal portion of the ε chain. The conformational changes seen upon reduction are likely to implicate more extensive regions of the molecule than those affected by heating although they are not well defined yet[122]. Each ε chain contains 15 half-cystine residues, four to five of which form interchain bonds[118,122]. It appears now that one of these interchain bridges joins H to L, two join H to H and the other two are a labile extra intrachain bond probably located in the Fd fragment[123]. The sequences of labile cysteine-containing peptides have been published[124].

A comparison of the molecular size of the polypeptide portion of ε chain and γ chain indicates that the former is larger by an amount corresponding to one domain, which fits very well with the presence of five intrachain bridges. The sequences around interchain bonds, as was the case in IgM molecules, are not homologous to those reported for γ and α chains, and in a chemical sense they do not resemble a hinge region. Thus both IgE and IgM appear to possess an extra domain instead of a hinge region.

Fragments consisting of the C-terminal domains have been isolated after CNBr cleavage, and the sequence has shown 34% homology with the analogous domain of γ1 chains[125]. A higher degree of homology (around 43%) is found when γ1 is compared with the corresponding stretch of the μ chain. This contrasts with the 23% homology between the analogous region of the ε chain and μ chain. These comparisons are shown in Figure 1.16.

1.3.6   Immunoglobulin D

Compared with other Igs, IgD is a relatively minor component, its average concentration in the serum being only about 30 μg/ml, 1/400 of the serum IgG concentration. The antigenic distinctiveness of IgD as in other Igs, lies in its heavy (δ) polypeptide chain[126,127]. Patients suffering from multiple myeloma only rarely produce IgD myeloma proteins, the frequency being about 2%, and they are predominantly of λ chain type[128,129]. IgD has a high carbohydrate content, approximately 11–14%, and has a sedimentation coefficient around 6–7S. The molecular weight estimated on different myeloma proteins and by different techniques has varied from 166 000 to 200 000 for the whole molecule and 60–70 000 daltons for the δ chain[130,131], which could correspond to three or four constant domains respectively. The carbohydrate of the δ chain is distributed among at least three glycopeptides[131], two containing glucosamine localized in the Fc fragment and one containing galactosamine localized in the Fd–Fc region. IgD has a remarkable susceptibility to degrada-

440 450 460

μ Lys-Gln-Thr-Ile-Ser-Arg-Pro-Lys-Gly-Val-Ala-Leu-His-Arg-Pro-Asx-Val-Tyr-Leu-Pro-Pro-Ala-Arg-Glx-

350

γ Glu-Lys————Lys-Ala————Gln-Pro-Arg-Glu-▨————Gln————Thr————Ser————Glu-

ε Met-Arg-Ser-Thr-Thr-Lys-Thr-Ser————Pro-Arg-Ala-Ala-Ala————Glu————Ala-Phe-Ala-Thr-Pro-▨▨-Glu-

470 480

μ Glx-Leu-Asn-Leu-Arg-Glu-Ser-Ala-Thr-Ile-Thr-Cys-Leu-Val-Thr-Gly-Phe-Ser-Pro-Ala-Asp-Val-Phe-Val-Glu-

γ Glu-Met-▨▨-Thr-Lys-Asn-Gln-Val-Ser-Leu————Lys————Tyr————Ser————Ile-Ala————

ε (Trp, Pro, Ser, Gly)————Asp-Lys-Arg————Leu-Ala————Ile-Gln-Asn————Met————Glu————Ile-Ser————Gln-

490 500 510

μ Trp-▨▨-Met-Gln-Arg-Gly-Glu-Pro-Leu-Ser-Pro-Gln-Lys-Tyr-Val-Thr-Ser-Ala-Pro-Met-Pro-Glu-Pro-Gln-Ala-

400

γ ————Glu-Ser-Asn-Asp————Glu-Asn————Lys————Thr-Pro————▨▨-Val-Leu-Asp-Ser-Asp-

ε ————Leu-His-Asn-Glu-Val-Gln-Leu-Pro-Asp-Ala-▨▨-Arg-His-Ser————Thr-Gln————▨▨-Arg-Lys-Thr-Lys-

520 530

μ Pro-Gly-Arg-Tyr-Phe-Ala-His-Ser-Ile-Leu-Thr-Val-Ser-Glu-Glu-Glu-Trp-Asn-Thr-Gly-Gln-Thr-Tyr-Thr-Cys-

α ————Ala-Ala————Asp————Lys————Asx————Phe-Ser————

γ Gly-Ser-▨▨-Phe————Leu-Tyr————Lys————Asp-Lys-Ser-Arg————Gln-Glu————Asn-Val-Phe-Ser————

ε Gly-Ser-Gly-Phe————Val-Phe————Arg————Glu————Thr-Arg-Ala————Glx-Glx-Lys-Asp-Glu-Phe-Ile————

36

540 550 560

μ Val- Val- Ala- His- Glu- Ala- Leu- Pro- Asn- Arg- Val- Thr- [box] Glu- Arg- Thr- Val- Asp- Lys- Ser- Thr- Gly- Lys- Pro- Thr-

α Met——Gly———— Leu- Ala- Phe———— [box] Gln- Lys———— Ile———— Arg- Leu- Ala—
440

γ Ser——Met———— His———— His- Tyr———— [box] Gln- Lys- Ser- Leu- Ser- Leu——Pro—

ε Arg- Ala- Val——Glx—— Ala- Ser- Pro- Ser- Gln—— Val- Gln———— Ala———— Ser- Val- Asn- Pro—

CHO
570

μ Leu- Tyr- Asn- Val- Ser- Leu- Val- Met- Ser- Asp- Thr- Ala- Gly- Thr- Cys- Tyr-

CHO

α His- Val————Val- Glu——Ala- Glu- Val- Asp—

Figure 1.16 Comparison of the amino acd sequence of the C-terminal domain of the μ chain with the analogous regions of $\gamma 1$ and ϵ chains. Forty residues from the C-terminal region of α chain are also shown[8,13,70,71,125]. Boxes indicate where gaps have been inserted to maximize homologies. The almost complete amino acid sequence of ϵ chain is now available[123].

37

tion which appears to be unique among Igs. This may account for its very short half-life in the body, 2.8 days[132]. In the serum the protein may be degraded to fragments similar to Fc and Fab almost completely in several days, even at 4 °C. Fc obtained after 'spontaneous' degradation and after proteolysis were immunologically identical and this was also true of the slow fragments, Fab. The sedimentation coefficients and Stokes radii of the intact protein and fragments were determined and the frictional coefficient ratios and molecular weight calculated. Both the intact molecule and the Fc fragment appear to be less compact than other intact Igs or Fc fragments. It was proposed that this difference in conformation may account in part for the increased susceptibility to proteolysis[133]. Cleavage by trypsin, plasmin and the spontaneously occurring fragmentation were localized at the C-terminal side of the glycopeptide containing galactosamine, and cleavage with papain, in the absence of reducing agent, at the N-terminal side of the same glycopeptide. Peptide maps suggested that the sites of cleavage are at least 15 amino acid residues apart[131]. IgD is cross-linked by three interchain bridges[124,134], two H–L and one H–H (Figure 1.17). The presence of only a single inter-H chain disulphide bond is unique among human Igs although it has been shown in rabbit IgG[48,136]. The sequence available for IgD is around the interchain bonds and the N terminus of the Fc fragment[135] (Figure 1.17).

Antigenic differences among IgD myeloma proteins have been interpreted as suggesting IgD subclasses[137]. Although no genetic markers are available for IgD, the correlation of serum level with allotype markers of $\gamma1$ and $\gamma3$ subclasses indicates close linkage between IgD and G heavy chain constant region genes[138].

In spite of similarities to other Igs, antibody activity in IgD has been difficult to demonstrate. Sera from some patients allergic to penicillin G contain IgD specific for the benzylpenicilloyl antigenic determinant[139]. Antibody activity to diphtheria toxoid, bovine γ-globulin and cell nuclei were also shown to be associated with IgD[140,141]. However, absorption of activity with

L
|
Pro- Ile- Ile- Ser- Gly- Cys- Arg-   1
Thr- Pro- Glu- Cys- Pro- Ser- His- Thr- Gln- Pro- Leu- Gly- Val   10

H

20
Tyr- Leu- Leu- Thr- Pro- Ala- Val- Gln- Asp- Leu- Trp- Leu- Arg- Asx- Lys- Ala- Thr- Phe- Thr- (Cys)-Phe-Val-   30

40
Val- Gly- Thr- Asx- Leu- Lys- Gly- Ala- Leu- Pro- Thr- (. . .)-Val- Glx- Leu- Gly- (Trp)-Tyr   50

Figure 1.17 Amino acid sequence around interchain bridges of human IgD and the N terminus of the Fc fragment[124,134,135]. Residue No. 1 indicates the beginning of Fc. ( ): tentative; (...): undetermined.

antiserum to IgD was not demonstrated. Although antibody activity has been ascribed to IgD, the biologic function is still unknown. It may be that IgD has a special function as a membrane receptor on B lymphocytes (see below). IgD in its native and aggregated forms lacks the structural features necessary for skin binding and complement fixation[142,143]. Analysis of human cord sera showed that it contained IgD, and comparison of the concentrations of maternal vs. cord serum IgA, M and D suggested that the fetus is capable of synthesizing IgD[144].

IgD has been found to be present on the membrane of a variable proportion of peripheral blood lymphocytes in human adults and recently on a much higher percentage of newborn (cord) blood lymphocytes[145,146]. In both cases the representation on cells was much greater than would be expected from only a consideration of the concentration of IgD in normal serum. Recently an IgD-like protein has been shown to be a major membrane Ig on mouse lymphocytes[147]. The result in humans also showed that most of the cells that carry IgD also bear IgM and *vice versa* although the amount of each Ig differed among the cells[146]. The finding that both IgD and M are simultaneously present on a high proportion of lymphocytes was unexpected since it does not follow the pattern of previous reports where restriction to one class was the general rule. The possibility that IgD was acquired by a cytophilic process was excluded by the finding that IgD-bearing cells were of one L chain type only, and by the demonstration of reappearance after proteolytic stripping of IgD on the membrane of lymphocytes in an IgD free culture medium. On the basis of these findings it was proposed that IgD functions as a lymphocyte antigen receptor[146].

1.4 VARIANTS OF HUMAN IMMUNOGLOBULIN

Biosynthetic studies have indicated that under normal conditions, the synthesis of H and L chains is approximately balanced and that plasma cells secrete primarily complete Ig molecules. However, in certain diseased states, unbalanced synthesis can occur. The most commonly encountered is the production of free L chains, although in general, they do not have structural abnormalities. The first examples of a structurally altered immunoglobulin occurred in 1963[148] with the recognition of the first patient with Heavy Chain Disease (HCD). While HCD still remains the most striking abnormality, a series of more subtly altered molecules have been described.

1.4.1 Heavy chain variants—Heavy chain disease proteins

Of the five recognizable classes of HCD in man, those corresponding to γ, α, and μ have already been found. To date, there are about 35 cases of γHCD, 50 of αHCD and 7 of μHCD. The clinical features of these disorders have been

Table 1.7 Some properties of γ, α, and μ heavy chain disease proteins

Property	γ	α	μ
Electroph. mob.	Fast γ–β	β	$\alpha 1$
S rate	2.8–4.0	4–11	10–11
MW (monomer)	25–58 000	35–42 000	35–55 000
Carbohydrate	High: 5–20%	More than 10%	More than 10%
L chain	Not present	Not present	Present 5 out of 7
J chain	Not present	Often present	In some
Subclasses	$\gamma 1$, $\gamma 2$, $\gamma 3$, $\gamma 4$	$\alpha 1$	—

reviewed recently[149–151]. The results of physicochemical studies of these molecules are summarized in Table 1.7. Thus far, antibody activity has not been detected. In patients with μHCD, the protein is found only in low concentration in the serum; in contrast, in γ and αHCD, the proteins occur in large amounts in serum and urine. L chains have not been detected in patients with γ and αHCD.

1.4.1.1 γ Heavy chain disease proteins

Most γHCD proteins are now recognized to have internal deletions of variable sizes. Based on the location of the deletion, a classification was proposed[150], (Table 1.8 and Figure 1.18).

(i) Deletion of part of the V region and $C_H 1$ domain with resumption of normal sequence in the middle of the H chain. Three proteins fall into this category: CRA ($\gamma 1$), GIF ($\gamma 2$) and ZUC ($\gamma 3$). Proteins ZUC and GIF have a normal N-terminal which in the case of ZUC consisted of 18 residues, and in the case of GIF about 100. CRA differs in having heterogeneity at the N-terminal, and furthermore the first ten residues do not fit with any known sequence. Preliminary observations indicate that the heterogeneity is due to the presence of at least two different sequences in approximately the first ten residues; from there on a single amino acid sequence can be detected. In each of these three proteins normal structure resumes at a glutamic acid residue which corresponds to residue 216[8] at the beginning of the interdomain region or hinge region (between $C_H 1$ and $C_H 2$ domains).

(ii) Deletion of the Hinge Region. Two crystallizable myeloma proteins have been described having a small deletion involving only the hinge[152–154]. Both belong to the $\gamma 1$ subclass and in non-dissociating solvents they have a MW of 145 000 daltons. However, when subjected to acid or urea, they yield L chain dimers and two free H chains. In the case of protein MCG, the deletion has been clearly mapped and shown to involve residues 216–230[153] (Table 1.8 and Figure 1.18). Dissociation without reduction is due to the absence of all the H chain half-cysteine residues involved in interchain binding, which in this subclass are clustered in the deleted fragment.

(iii) Deletion of part of the V region, the $C_H 1$ domain and the hinge region. Detailed chemical studies of one protein in this group, protein Hal, a $\gamma 4$ HCD

Table 1.8 Amino acid sequence of variants of human IgG with internal deletions

I—Proteins where normal sequence commences at residue 216

CRA (γ1)   [10↓216] Gly·(Leu₀.₇, Ile₀.₅, Phe, Asp₂.₉)·Arg·Thr·Thr·Glu·Pro·Lys·Ser·Cys·Asp·Lys·Thr·His·Thr·Cys·Pro·Pro·Cys·Pro·Ala-   [↓231]

GIF (γ2)   PCA·Val/Leu·Thr·Cys / Tyr·Cys·Ala (Glu, Ser, Leu) Lys/Val·Thr·Asn·Val·Ser·Glu·Arg —— Cys —— Val·Glu- . .   [CHO ±110↓216]

ZUC (γ3)   PCA·Val·Gln·Val·Val·Glu·Ser·Gly·Ala·Asp·Leu·Lys·Val·Lys·Pro·Gly·Gly·Ser·Ser·Glu ——————— Thr·Pro·Pro·Pro ——————— Arg-   [CHO 18↓216]

II—Protein where the deletion starts at residue 216

McG (γ1)   ( )Lys·Val·Asp·Lys·Arg·Val-   [215↓]

III—Protein where normal sequence commences at Met residue 252

HAL (γ4)

I—Proteins where normal sequence commences at residue 216

CRA (γ1)   Pro·Glu·Leu·Leu·Gly·Gly·Pro·Ser·Val·Phe·Leu·Phe·Pro·Pro·Lys·Pro·Lys·Asp·Thr·Leu·Met·Ile·Ser·Arg·Thr·Pro·Glu·Val·Thr·Cys·Val-   [252]

GIF (γ2)   ( )Met-

ZUC (γ3)   ———————————————————Met—

II—Protein where the deletion starts at residue 216

McG (γ1)   ———————————————————Met—   [252]

III—Protein where normal sequence commences at Met residue 252

HAL (γ4)   PCA(Glu,Thr)(Glu₂, Asp, Gly) Val·Leu·Ser·Met-   [10↓252]   [CHO]

An arrow indicates the residue where normal sequence starts after internal deletions.
Two arrows in protein McG indicate the size of the deletion.
The numbers, 216, 231 and 252, over the residues indicate the position corresponding to the sequence of γ¹ H chain[8].
PCA = pyrrolidone carboxylic acid.
CHO = carbohydrate. Note extra carbohydrate group in variants CRA, GIF, ZUC and HAL.
/ = no overlap; ± = approximate position.
( ) = no sequence available.
— = homology. Dots have been introduced to maximize homology.

41

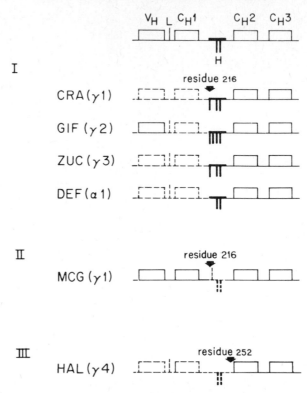

Figure 1.18 Comparison of the deletions detected in variants of human H chains and tentative classification. On top are represented the domains and disulphide bridges of normal γ and α chains. Thick lines indicate the position of the hinge region. Dotted lines localize the deletions. Normal sequences after internal deletions start at the indicated residues. For the sequence of γ1, γ2, γ3, and γ4 variants, see Table 1.8b, and for protein DEF, see Figure 1.14.

protein showed that normal sequence resumes at a methionine residue at position 252[155]. Since the deletion extends beyond the inter-H chain disulphide bonds, proteins of this type dissociate into monomeric forms in non-reducing, denaturing media. Three other proteins with internal deletions have not been as carefully studied in terms of reinitiation of synthesis but probably resemble variant Hal in having a deletion which includes the hinge[19,156—158].

(iv) Deletion of the Fc fragment or one of its domains: observed in α and μ chains (see below).

(v) Degraded heavy chains. These are HCD proteins which begin at the hinge region, a site which in native IgG is particularly susceptible to enzymatic cleavage. They appear to represent examples of proteolytic digestion of a larger precursor molecule althouth the putative precursor molecules have not been identified so far[159]. In this respect studies underway of proteins from the serum of a patient (OMM) with γ3 HCD in whom two related proteins of different size have been detected can be of great value. One is a polypeptide with a

MW of about 60 000 daltons after reduction, and the other with a MW of 39 000 daltons after reduction. The former appears to consist of virtually the entire H chain, and the latter consists of the hinge region and the Fc fragment[47,160]. While it is tempting to postulate that the smaller molecule is derived from the larger one by proteolysis, it is also possible that they represent a two-step mutation.

1.4.1.2 α Heavy chain disease proteins

αHCD appears as a condition primarily affecting the secretory IgA system. It is usually characterized by a lymphoplasmacytic proliferation involving the small intestine, and its geographic distribution suggests that environmental factors play a role in the aetiology and pathogenesis. (Most patients with αHCD originated from areas with high rates of infestation by intestinal micro-organisms, e.g. North Africa, Middle East and Far East[161,162].) All of the 50 αHCD proteins studied belong to the α1 subclass. Their MWs range between 35–42 000 daltons for the monomer, and their CHO content is very high. Antigenic and some chemical analysis provided evidence for the existence of an intact Fc fragment[163]. Since the N-terminus in most of them was shown to be heterogeneous, the question arose whether αHCD proteins are normal α chains which undergo postsynthetic intracellular or extracellular degradation or whether they contain a primary defect followed by secondary proteolysis. Careful structural studies have been published for only one protein DEF[164]. It contained a short heterogeneous segment corresponding to the V region and a gap which composed almost the whole V region and the C_H1 domain. Normal synthesis resumed at a valine residue before the hinge region which may be the α chain counterpart to Glu 216 of γ chain (Figures 1.14 and 1.18). It was postulated, therefore, that protein DEF is synthesized as an internally deleted α1 heavy chain, followed by postsynthetic N-terminal proteolysis.

Deletion of the C_H3 domain appears to be present in an IgA1 monomeric myeloma protein (VO). MW studies indicated a normal L chain and an H chain with a MW of 42 000 instead of the normal 58 000. Since the molecule had an intact Fd fragment and an intact hinge, it seemed likely that the Fc fragment was smaller than normal. In fact MW determination and CNBr cleavage indicated that protein VO is missing the C_H3 domain[165,166]. Moreover, CHO analysis is consistent with this interpretation since the CHO-containing peptide associated with the C_H3 region is missing. VO existed as a monomeric molecule and it may be due to the absence of the C-terminal half-cysteine residue which has been shown to be linked to the J chain (see IgA).

1.4.1.3 μ Heavy chain disease proteins

The information on the structure of μHCD proteins is more limited. Most of them exist in the serum as pentamers similar to the $(Fc_\mu)_5$ fragment, with MW between 180 000 and 300 000, which explains the failure to find them in the urine. The mechanisms for polymer formation remain to be explained since J chain was not found in three molecules examined but appeared to be present in a fourth[167, 168]. Patients with μHCD differ from the other types of HCD in that L chains were synthesized and secreted in five out of seven patients[169]. The limited chemical studies of three proteins are consistent with immunological findings that the Fc region is present[167, 170, 171].

For reasons that are not understood alanine was found at the N-terminus in each, although their MWs are not the same. A partial amino acid sequence is available for one of the proteins[171], and its N-terminal sequence appears to correspond to that of μ chain Oμ starting with residue 338 (Figure 1.19) except for the presence of Ala instead of Val.

A larger deletion encompassing the $C_H 3$ and $C_H 4$ domains of the μ chain apparently occurred in protein KLO (Figure 1.19). Protein KLO had a MW of 130 000, contained two normal L chains and two smaller H chains (42 000 instead of 68 000 daltons) and less than 2% CHO. Based on these determinations and immunological analysis it was concluded that protein KLO

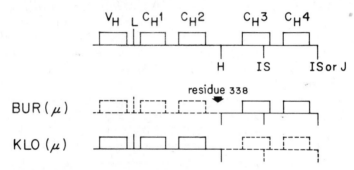

Figure 1.19 Comparison of deletion detected in variants of human μ chains. On the top are represented the domain and disulphide bridges of μ chain. IS: intersubunit; J: J chain. Dotted lines localize deletions[171,172].

is an $(Fab')_2$ μ fragment. While a synthetic origin has not been clearly documented, its presence over a long period of time in the absence of detectable proteolytic activity or intact IgM molecules suggests a synthetic origin[172].

1.4.1.4   Hybrid molecules

Studies of the genetic markers (Gm) of human IgG molecules have discovered several examples of hybrid molecules, possibly resulting from crossing over between closely related C region genes. They have been defined only by antigenic and genetic analysis. Two of them occurred in normal subjects[173, 174] and two were found in myeloma proteins[175,176]. Since no chemical data is available, they will not be described further.

1.4.1.5 Detection of variants of immunoglobulin H chains

A method, 'carboxymethylcysteine diagonal map', has been developed to detect Igs with structural defects. It is based on the comparison of all cysteine-containing peptides present in the molecule with their normal counterparts[177]. The method differs from classical diagonal maps[178] in that the proteins are subjected to mild thiol reduction and alkylated with iodo[14C]acetic acid prior to the performance of the diagonal map. Ig molecules have a high content of cysteine residues which are strategically spread along the chains and can be used as markers for different domains and intradomain regions. Since they occupy a distinct position on the map, the absence of one or more peptides defines rather accurately the nature of the defect.

1.4.2 Light chain variants—Light chain disease proteins

As mentioned before, the most encountered abnormality is the synthesis and secretion of L chain devoid of H chain. A large number of L chain sequences are now published and many of them have small gaps of one to six residues in the V regions. Their significance is unknown.

1.4.2.1 Internal deletion

The first case studied with a large internal deletion was protein Sac[179-181]. This molecule was unusual in having a sedimentation coefficient of 5.4S instead of 7S and a MW of 125 000 daltons. The L chain had an internal deletion encompassing residues 19–99 and the H chain lacked most of the V region. It appears that the prime and perhaps the sole genetic defect in this molecule is the internal deletion of the L chain, and the absence of the V_H region is the result of proteolysis[181], possibly caused by that structural change in the L chain. A similar defect exists in another IgG λ myeloma protein SM[182].

1.4.2.2 Elongated light chains

A longer L chain has been reported to be present in an IgM monomer from a continuous culture of human lymphocytes (Daudi), originally derived from a patient with Burkitt's lymphoma[183]. MW determinations indicated 330 000 daltons rather than 216 000 and suggested that κ and probably μ chains are larger than normal. The increased size in L chain is thought not to be due to extra polysaccharides. Additional studies are necessary to document this observation as was clearly done in the case of the L chain of MPC-11 which has 12 extra residues at the N-terminal[184].

1.4.2.3   Non-secretors

Plasma cell tumours unassociated with a serum or urine abnormality have been identified. While most of them have a failure of Ig synthesis[185], some have been shown to contain Igs in the cytoplasm, most often L chains which are either not secreted or rapidly degraded[186, 187]. The reason for the failure of synthesis and/or secretion remains to be determined.

1.5   DISCUSSION

The discovery, first in man and later in mouse, of tumour cells which synthesize and secrete defective immunoglobulin chains, offered an opportunity to determine whether plasma cell mutants would provide the same valuable information as those obtained from mutants in bacteria. It is assumed that in these committed cells transcription and translation have occurred faithfully so that the aberrant polypeptides can be viewed as primary gene products. Even though conclusions regarding the defects in these mutants clearly require many more chemical characterizations, at this early stage it can be said that they are not random and, at least in the mouse, the mutation rate is surprisingly high[188]. Prominent among these mutants are those affecting genes coding for H chains with deleted segments in their products. In most cases the residues deleted are outside the disulphide bridge loops. Deletions, therefore, comprise domains. A deletion can be at the C-terminal end, probably caused by a frame shift that results in a nonsense mutation and premature termination[166,172,189]. Alternatively, there can be internal deletions, and the results of chemical analyses have raised a number of interesting questions about the genetic control of Ig synthesis. The simplest explanation is that the defect is a consequence of DNA breakage with rejoining of both ends.

The fact that the majority of internal deletions observed in human γHCD involve residue 216 and that this position is homologous to the one implicated in mouse mutant IF2[190] with an internal deletion is provocative. Position 216 marks the beginning of the hinge region, a section of the H chain between the $C_H 1$ and $C_H 2$ domains which contains the inter-H chain disulphide bonds. It is unique in not having a homologous counterpart in the remainder of the molecule and its high content of proline is striking. Moreover, the hinge region can be found as a series of identical or similar repetitive sequences of small fragments (see $\gamma 3$ and $\alpha 1$ H chains). These findings indicate that the stretch of DNA coding for the hinge region is rich in poly G and appears to be the result of tandem duplications of few base pairs which have arisen by a process of mismatched intragenic crossing over. Several fundamental questions have arisen from the results of these studies. What is the origin and function of repeated sequences in eukaryotic DNA? Could highly repetitive, short nucleotide sequences constitute recognition sites for translocation mechanisms? What is the significance of position 216? While the repeated isolation of the same type of variants could be the result of the techniques used to detect them, it may also indicate a special genetic hot spot and reflect something unusual in the biochemical mechanisms of the multigene system responsible for the Ig chain synthesis.

Other variants of potential interest are those with internal deletion and reinitiation of normal synthesis at a methionine residue, position 252 (Table 1.8-III, Figure 1.18). Codon AUG functions as an initiation signal in protein biosynthesis in prokaryotes and eukaryotes[191,192]. When AUG occurs internally, it codes for insertion of methionine. Internal AUG initiation sites have been described, but only in the presence of a nearby terminator triplet[193]. Whether or not the same mechanism is operating in this type of variant remains to be elucidated.

It is interesting to point out that a urinary protein (B_2-microglobulin) present in normal individuals is related to the Fc fragment of IgG. B_2-microglobulin is part of the HL-A molecule[194-196] and it was postulated that the gene coding for it may have evolved from an Ig gene by the use of a new start signal Met 252[197], the same site for the reinitiation of the normal sequence in variant HAL (Table 1.8).

Finally, some other questions may be asked. Are the defective proteins the result of mutations in the structural genes or of derepression of normally silent genes? Taken into consideration with type III variants, the latter possibility suggests that antibody molecules may have evolved from other types of cell surface receptor molecules, and that in fact the expression of the ancestral gene for antibody chains is a 'β_2-microglobulin-like' molecule.

1.6 CONCLUDING REMARKS

Knowledge of antibody structure is now sufficient to allow investigation of problems of biological function and their relationship to structural parameter. On the basis of amino acid sequences, it has been proposed that the homology region of Igs are arranged so that each one mediates a biological function, and it has already been suggested that $C_{\gamma 2}$ and $C_{\mu 4}$ domains may play a role in complement fixation by IgG and IgM respectively[35,36,63].

Although Ig molecules of different classes and subclasses in different species have their own identity, it seems probable that rapid advances will be made in elucidating their complete structure. X-ray crystallographic studies undoubtedly will clarify details of intradomain folding and hopefully will analyse the forces that operate in generating the hypervariable segments detected in V regions.

As more amino acid sequences of V-regions have been obtained, the existence of multiple V_H and V_L genes has become more widely accepted. The presence of multiple V-genes still leaves unclear the role which a somatic generator of diversity might play. In this respect RNA/DNA hybridization studies, still in the early stages, can make an important contribution. Even if we were to know the number and arrangement of Ig genes, there are still a number of questions to be asked about regulation of gene expression. Very recently a specific interaction between Ig and H chain mRNA has been detected[198] and although this binding has been shown to control translation under certain conditions, it is conceivable that such a high affinity interaction has some other function during an immune response.

Mutations affecting Ig production opens a new era of mammalian somatic cell genetics which could lead to clarification of the arrangement of Ig genes, the mechanisms responsible for generation of antibody diversity, and the suspected translocation of V and C genes.

Acknowledgments

I wish to thank Dr. M. E. Lamm for correcting the manuscript, and Ms. Beverly Coopersmith and Ms. Marlene Chavis for their devoted secretarial assistance.

The author's experimental work presented here was supported by USPHS Grants #AM 01431 and #AM 05064.

References

1. Hood, L. and Prahl, J. (1971). *Advan. Immunol.*, **14**, 291
2. Gally, J. A. (1973). *The Antigens*, Vol. 1, p. 161 (New York: Academic Press)
3. Capra, D. J. and Kehoe, M. J. (1975). *Advan. Immunol.*, **20**, 1
4. World Health Organization. *W.H.O. Bull.*, (1964). **30**, 447; (1965) **33**, 721; (1966) **35**, 953; (1968) **38**, 151; (1969) **41**, 975; (1972) *J. Immunol.*, **108**, 1733
5. Edelman, G. M. and Gall, W. E. (1969). *Ann. Rev. Biochem.*, **38**, 415
6. Milstein, C. and Pink, J. R. L. (1970). *Prog. Biophys. Mol. Biol.*, **21**, 209
7. Jerne, N. K. (1971). *Eur. J. Immunol.*, **1**, 1
8. Edelman, G. M., Cunningham, A., Gall, W. E., Gottlieb, P. D., Rutishauser, V. and Wardal, M. J. (1969). *Proc. Nat. Acad. Sci. (USA)*, **63**, 78
9. Pitcher, S. E. and Konisberg, W. (1970). *J. Biol. Chem.*, **245**, 1267
10. Fisher, C. E., Palm, W. H. and Press, E. M. (1969). *FEBS Lett.*, **5**, 20
11. Frangione, B. and Milstein, C. (1969). *Nature (London)*, **224**, 577
12. Press, E. M. and Hogg, N. M. (1969). *Nature (London)*, **223**, 807
13. Putnam, F. W., Florent, G., Paul, C., Shinoda, T. and Shimizu, A. (1973). *Science*, **182**, 287
14. Cunningham, B. A., Pflumm, M. N., Rutishauser, V. and Edelman, G. M. (1969). *Proc. Nat. Acad. Sci. (USA)*, **64**, 997
15. Capra, J. D., Kehoe, J. M., Winchester, R. J. and Kunkel, H. G. (1971). *Ann. N.Y. Acad. Sci.*, **190**, 371
16. Ponsfingl, H., Schwartz, J., Reichel, W. and Hilsdemann, N. (1970). *Hoppe-Seyler's Z. Physiol. Chem.*, **351**, 1591

17. Pink, J. R. L. and Milstein, C. (1969). In F. Franek and D. Shugar (eds.), *Globulins: Structure and Biosynthesis*, p. 177: (New York: Academic Press)
18. Wang, A. C., Fudenberg, H. H. and Pink, J. R. L. (1971). *Proc. Nat. Acad. Sci. (USA)*, **68**, 1143
19. Terry, W. D. and Ohms, J. (1970). *Proc. Nat. Acad. Sci. (USA)*, **66**, 558
20. Capra, J. D. and Kehoe, J. M. (1973). *Proc. Nat. Acad. Sci. (USA)*, **71**, 845
21. Watanobe, S., Bernibol, H. V., Horn, J., Bertram, J. and Hilschman, N. (1973). *Hoppe-Seyler's Z. Physiol. Chem.*, **354**, 1505
22. Wolfenstein-Todel, C., Frangione, B. and Franklin, E. C. (1974). *Biochem. Biophys. Acta* (In press)
23. Porter, R. R. (1959). *Biochem J.*, **73**, 119
24. Edelman, G. M. and Poulik, M. D. (1961). *J. Exp. Med.*, **113**, 861
25. Porter, R. R. (1962). In A. Gellhorn and E. Hirschberg (eds.). *Basic Problems of Neoplastic Dis.*, p. 177 (Columbia Univ. Press)
26. Natvig, J. B. and Kunkel, H. G. (1973). *Advan. Immunol.*, **16**, 1
27. Krause, R. M. (1970). *Advan. Immunol.*, **12**, 1
28. Fleischman, J. B. (1971). *Biochemistry*, **10**, 2753
29. Apella, E., Roholt, O. A., Chersi, A., Radzimski, G. and Pressman, P. (1973). *Biochem. Biophys. Res. Commun*
30. Jaton, J. C., Brown, D. G., Strosberg, A. D., Haber, E. and Morris, J. E. (1973). *J. Immunol.*, **111**, 1838
31. Chen, K. C. S., Kindt, T. J. and Krause, R. M. (1974). *Proc. Nat. Acad. Sci. (USA)*, **71**, 1995
32. Kunkel, H. G. (1965). *Harvey Lect.*, **59**, 219
33. Ovary, Z., Kunkel, H. G. and Joslin, F. G. (1970). *J. Immunol.*, **105**, 1103
34. Ishizaka, T., Ishizaka, K., Salmon, S. and Fudenberg, H. (1967). *J. Immunol.*, **99**, 82
35. Ellerson, J. R., Yasmeen, D., Painter, R. H. and Dorrington, K. J. (1972). *FEBS Lett.*, **24**, 319
36. Kehoe, J. M. and Fougereau, M. (1969). *Nature (London)*, **224**, 1212
37. Frangione, B., Milstein, C. and Pink, J. R. L. (1969). *Nature (London)*, **221**, 145
38. Singer, S. J. and Doolittle, R. F. (1966). *Science*, **153**, 13
39. Hill, R. L., Lebovitz, H. E., Fellows, R. E. and Delaney, R. (1967). In J. Killander (ed.), *Nobel Symp.*, 3rd Ed., p. 109
40. Poljak, R. J., Amzel, L. M., Arey, H. P., Chen, B. L., Phizackerley, R. P. and Farber, S. (1973). *Proc. Nat. Acad. Sci. (USA)*, **70**, 3305
41. Frangione, B. and Milstein, C. (1968). *J. Mol. Biol.*, **33**, 893
42. Frangione, B. and Milstein, C. (1969). *Nature (London)*, **224**, 597
43. Saluk, P. H. and Clem, L. W. (1971). *J. Immunol.*, **107**, 298
44. Turner, M. W., Bennick, H. H. and Natvig, J. B. (1970). *Clin. Exp. Immunol.*, **7**, 603
45. Michaelsen, T. E. and Natvig, J. B. (1972). *FEBS Lett.*, **28**, 121
46. Michaelsen, T. E., Natvig, J. B. and Sletten, K. (1974). *Scand. J. Immunol.*, **3**, 491
47. Adlersberg, J. A., Franklin, E. C. and Frangione, B. (1975). *Proc. Nat. Acad. Sci. (USA)*, **72**, 723
48. O'Donnell, U. J., Frangione, B. and Porter, R. R. (1970). *Biochem. J.*, **116**, 261
49. DePreval, C., Pink, J. R. L. and Milstein, C. (1970). *Nature (London)*, **228**, 930
50. Oliveira, B. and Lamm, M. E. (1971). *Biochemistry*, **10**, 26
51. Frangione, B., Milstein, C. and Franklin, E. C. (1969). *Nature (London)*, **221**, 149
52. Frangione, B. and Franklin, E. C. (1972). *FEBS Lett.*, **20**, 321
53. Milstein, C. P., Steinberg, A. G., McLaughlin, C. L. and Solomon, A. (1974). *Nature (London)*, **248**, 160
54. Abel, C. A. and Despont, J. P. (1974). *J. Immuno. Genet.*, **1**, 79
55. Miller, F. and Metzger, H. (1965). *J. Biol. Chem.*, **240**, 3325

56. Halpern, M. S. and Koshland, M. E. (1970). *Nature (London)*, **228**, 1276
57. Mestecky, J., Zikan, J. and Butler, W. T. (1971). *Science*, **171**, 1163
58. Feinstein, A., Munn, E. A. and Richards, N. E. (1971). *Ann. N.Y. Acad. Sci. (USA)*, **190**, 104
59. Merler, E., Karlin, L. and Matsumoto, S. (1968). *J. Biol. Chem.*, **243**, 386
60. Ashman, R. F. and Metzger, H. (1969). *J. Biol. Chem.*, **244**, 3405
61. Oriol, R., Binagli, R. and Coltori, E. (1971). *J. Immunol.*, **106**, 932
62. Plaut, A. G., Color, S. and Tomasi, T. B. (1972). *Science*, **176**, 55
63. Hunt, M. M., Volanakis, J. E., Hester, R. B., Straud, R. M. and Bennet, J. C. (1974). *J. Exp. Med.*, **140**, 1117
64. Plaut, A. G. and Tomasi, T. P. (1970). *Proc. Nat. Acad. Sci. (USA)*, **65**, 318
65. Metzger, H. (1970). *Advan. Immunol.*, **12**, 57
66. Beale, B. and Feinstein, A. (1969). *Biochem. J.*, **112**, 187
67. Frangione, B., Prelli, F., Mihaesco, C. and Franklin, E. C. (1971). *Proc. Nat. Acad. Sci. (USA)*, **68**, 1547
68. Shimizu, A., Putnam, F. W., Paul, C., Clamp, J. R. and Johnson, I. (1971). *Nature (London) New Biol.*, **231**, 73
69. Kornfeld, R., Keller, J., Bacuzijo, F. and Kornfeld, S. (1971). *J. Biol. Chem.*, **246**, 3259
70. Chang, C. Y., Capra, D. and Kehoe, J. M. (1973). *Nature (London)*, **244**, 158
71. Moore, V. and Putnam, F. W. (1973). *Biochemistry*, **12**, 2361
72. Mendez, E., Frangione, B. and Franklin, E. C. (1973). *Biochemistry*, **12**, 5186
73. Franklin, E. C. and Frangione, B. (1968). *Biochemistry*, **7**, 4203
74. Paul, C., Shimizu, A., Kohler, H. and Putnam, F. W. (1971). *Science*, **172**, 69
75. Tomasi, T. B. and Breneastock, J. (1968). *Advan. Immunol.*, **9**, 2
76. Feinstein, D. and Franklin, E. C. (1966). *Nature (London)*, **212**, 1496
77. Kunkel, H. G. and Prendergast, R. A. (1966). *Proc. Soc. Exp. Biol. Med.*, **122**, 910
78. Vaerman, J. P. and Heremans, J. F. (1966). *Science*, **153**, 647
79. Vaerman, J. P., Heremans, J. F. and Laurell, C. B. (1968). *Immunology*, **14**, 425
80. Grey, H. M., Abel, C. A., Yount, W. J. and Kunkel, H. G. (1968). *J. Exp. Med.*, **128**, 1223
81. Kunkel, H. G., Smith, W. K., Joslin, F. G., Natvig, J. B. and Litvin, S. D. (1969). *Nature (London)*, **223**, 1247
82. Vyas, G. N. and Fudenberg, H. H. (1969). *Proc. Nat. Acad. Sci. (USA)*, **64**, 1211
83. Jerry, L. M., Kunkel, H. G. and Grey, H. M. (1970). *Proc. Nat. Acad. Sci. (USA)*, **65**, 557
84. Mihaesco, E., Seligman, M. and Frangione, B. (1971). *Nature (London), New Biology*, **232**, 220
85. Frangione, B. and Wolfenstein-Todel, C. (1972). *Proc. Nat. Acad. Sci. (USA)*, **12**, 3673
86. Putnam, F. W., Low, T., Lui, V., Huser, H., Raff, E., Wong, F. C. and Clamp, J. R. (1974). The IgA System. In J. Mesteckey and A. R. Lawton (eds). *Adv. Exp. Med. Biol.*, **45**, 177 (New York: Plenum Press)
87. Kohler, H., Shimizu, A., Paul, C., Moore, V. and Putnam, F. W. (1970). *Nature (London)*, **227**, 1318
88. Wang, A. C., Pink, J. R. L., Fudenberg, H. H. and Ohms, J. (1970). *Proc. Nat. Acad. Sci. (USA)*, **66**, 657
89. Capra, J. D., Chuang, C. Y., Kaplan, R., and Kehoe, M. (1974). The IgA System. In J. Mesteckey and A. R. Lawton (eds.). *Advan. Exp. Biol.*, **45**, 191 (New York: Plenum Press)
90. Mihaesco, E. and Migherina, R. (1974). *Advan. Exp. Med. Biol.*, **45**, 211
91. Wolfenstein-Todel, C., Prelli, F., Frangione, B. and Franklin, E. C. (1973). *Biochemistry*, **12**, 5195
92. Abel, C. A. and Grey, H. M. (1971). *Nature (London)*, **233**, 29
93. Clamp, J. R. (1972). In A. Gottschalk (ed.). *Glycoproteins*, Part A, p. 630 (Amsterdam: Elsevier Pub. Co.).
94. Baenziger, J. and Kornfeld, S. personal communication
95. Baenziger, J. and Kornfeld, S. (1974). *J. E:ol. Chem.* **249**, (I) 7260, (II) 7270

96. Mehta, S. K., Plaut, A. G., Calvanico, N. J. and Tomasi, T. P. (1973). *J. Immunol.*, **111**, 1274
97. Plaut, A. G., Genco, R. J. and Tomasi, T. B. (1974). *J. Immunol.*, **113**, 289
98. Plaut, A. G., Wister, R. and Capra, J. D. (1974). *J. Clin. Invest.*, **54**, 1295
99. O'Daly, J. A. and Cebra, J. J. (1971). *Biochemistry*, **10**, 3842
100. Schrohenloher, R. E., Mestecky, J. and Stanton, T. H. (1973). *Biochem. Biophys. Acta*, **295**, 576
101. Wilde, C. E. and Koshland, M. E. (1973). *Biochemistry*, **12**, 3218
102. Chapuis, R. M. and Koshland, M. E. (1974). *Proc. Nat. Acad. Sci. (USA)*, **71**, 657
103. Hauptman, S. P. and Tomasi, T. B. (1975). *J. Biol. Chem.*, **250**, 3891
104. Mendez, E., Frangione, B. and Franklin, E. C. (1973). *Biochem. Biophys. Res. Commun.*, **55**, 1291
105. Mestecky, J., Schrohenloher, R. E., Wright, G. P. and Tomana, M. (1974). *Proc. Nat. Acad. Sci. (USA)*, **71**, 544
106. Mestecky, J. and Schrohenloher, R. E. (1974). *Nature (London)*, **249**, 650
107. Mendez, E., Frangione, B. and Franklin, E. C. (1973). *Biochemistry*, **12**, 1119
108. Tomasi, T. B., Tan, E. M., Solomon, A. and Prendergast, R. A. (1965). *J. Exp. Med.*, **121**, 101
109. Lamm, M. E. and Greenberg, J. (1972). *Biochemistry*, **11**, 2744
110. O'Daly, J. A. and Cebra, J. J. (1971). *Biochemistry*, **10**, 3843
111. Cunningham-Rudles, C., Lamm, M. E. and Franklin, E. C. (1974). *J. Biol. Chem.*, **249**, 5649
112. Cunningham-Rudles, C. and Lamm, M. E. (1974). *J. Biol. Chem.*, **250**, 1987
113. Poger, M. E. and Lamm, M. E. (1974). *J. Exp. Med.*, **137**, 627
114. Ishizaka, K., Ishizaka, T. and Hornbrook, M. M. (1966). *J. Immunol.*, **97**, 840
115. Bennich, H., Ishizaka, K., Ishizaka, T. and Johansson, S. G. O. (1969). *J. Immunol.*, **102**, 826
116. Ogawa, M., Kochwa, S., Smith, C., Ishizaka, K. and McIntyre, O. R. (1969). *N. Eng. J. Med.*, **281**, 1217
117. Bennich, H. and Johansson, S. G. O. (1968). In K. Kilander (ed.). *Gamma Globulins*, p. 199 (New York: Wiley (Interscience))
118. Kochwa, S., Terry, W. D., Capra, J. D. and Yand, N. L. (1971). *Ann. N.Y. Acad. Sci.*, **190**, 49
119. Ishizaka, T., DeBernardo, R., Tomioka, H., Lichtenstein, L. M. and Ishizaka, K. (1972). *J. Immunol.*, **108**, 1000
120. Ishizaka, T., Sian, C. M. and Ishizaka, K. (1973). *J. Immunol.*, **111**, 500
121. Dorrington, K. and Tanford, C. (1970). *Adv. Immun.*, **12**, 333
122. Bennich, H. and Dorrington, K. (1973). In K. Ishizaka and D. H. Dayton (eds.). *Biological Role of the IgE System*, (Bethesda, Maryland: N.I. of Child Health and Human Dev.)
123. Bennich, H. and von Bahr-Lindström, H. (1974). *Progress in Immunology*, **Vol. II, 1**, 49
124. Mendez, E., Frangione, B. and Kochwa, S. (1973). *FEBS Lett.*, **33**, 4
125. Bennich, H., Milstein, C. and Secher, D. S. (1973). *FEBS Lett.*, **33**, 1
126. Rowe, D. S. and Fahey, J. L. (1965). *J. Exp. Med.*, **121**, 171
127. Rowe, D. S. and Fahey, J. L. (1965). *J. Exp. Med.*, **121**, 185
128. Fahey, J. L., Carbone, P., Rowe, D. S. and Bachman, R. (1968). *Amer. J. Med.*, **45**, 373
129. Hobbs, J. R. and Corbett, A. A. (1969). *Brit. Med. J.*, **1**, 412
130. Rowe, D. S., Dooler, F. and Welscher, H. D. (1969). *Immunochemistry*, **6**, 437
131. Spiegelberg, H. L., Prahl, J. W. and Grey, H. M. (1970). *Biochemistry*, **9**, 2115
132. Rogentine, G. N., Rowe, D. S., Bradley, J., Waldmann, T. A. and Fahey, J. L. (1966). *J. Clin. Inv.*, **45**, 1467
133. Griffiths, R. W. and Fleich, G. (1972). *J. Biol. Chem.*, **247**, 4543
134. Perry, M. B. and Milstein, C. (1970). *Nature (London)*, **228**, 934
135. Spiegelberg, H. L. (1975). *Nature (London)*, **254**, 723

136. Palmer, J. L. and Nisonoff, A. (1964). *Biochemistry*, **3**, 863
137. Rivat, C., Ropartz, C. and Rowe, D. S. (1971). *Nature (London)*, *New Biol.*, **231**, 279
138. Walzer, P. D. and Kunkel, H. G. (1974). *J. Immunol.*, **113**, 274
139. Gleich, G. J., Bieger, C. R. and Stankievic, R. (1969). *Science*, **165**, 606
140. Heiner, D. C., Saha, A. and Rose, B. (1969). *Fed. Proc.*, **28**, 766
141. Ritchie, R. F. (1968). *Arthritis Rheum.*, **11**, 506
142. Henney, C. S., Welscher, H. D., Terry, W. D. and Rowe, D. S. (1969). *Immunochemistry*, **6**, 445
143. Ovary, Z. (1969). *J. Immunol.*, **102**, 790
144. Leslie, G. A. and Swate, T. E. (1972). *J. Immunol.*, **109**, 47
145. Van Boxel, J. A., Paul, W. E., Terry, W. D. and Green, I. (1972). *J. Immunol.*, **109**, 648
146. Rowe, D. S., Hug, K., Forni, L. and Pernis, B. (1973). *J. Exp. Med.*, **138**, 965
147. Melcher, U., Vitetta, E. S., McWilliams, M., Lamm, M. E., Phillips-Quagliata, J. M. and Uhr, J. W. (1974). *J. Exp. Med.*, **141**, 206
148. Franklin, E. C., Meltzer, M., Guggenheim, F. and Lowenstein, J. (1963). *Fed. Proc.*, **22**, 619
149. Seligmann, M. (1972). *Rev. Europ. Etudes Clin. et Biol.*, **17**, 5
150. Frangione, B. and Franklin, E. C. (1973). *Seminars Hematology*, **10**, 53
151. Bloch, K. J., Lee, L., Mills, J. A. and Haber, E. (1973). *Amer. J. Med.*, **55**, 61
152. Deutsch, H. and Suzuki, T. (1971). *Ann. N.Y. Acad. Sci.*, **190**, 472
153. Fett, J. W., Deutsch, H. F. and Smithies, O. (1973). *Immunochemistry*, **10**, 115
154. Lopes, A. D. and Steiner, L. A. (1973). *Fed. Proc.*, **32**, Abstract 1003
155. Frangione, B., Lee, L., Haber, E. and Boch, K. J. (1973). *Proc. Nat. Acad. Sci. (USA)*, **70**, 1073
156. Woods, R., Blumenschein, G. and Terry, W. (1970). *Immunochemistry*, **7**, 373
157. Calvanico, B. R., Plaut, A. and Tomasi, T. B. (1972). *Fed. Proc.*, Abstract 3124
158. Smith, L. L., Barton, B. P., Garver, F. A., Lutcher, C. L. and Faguet, G. B. (1973). *Fed. Proc.*, **32**, 840
159. Terry, W. D. and Ein, D. (1972). *Ann. N.Y. Acad. Sci.*, **190**, 467
160. Adlersberg, J., Grann, V. and Franklin, E. C. (In preparation)
161. Seligmann, M., Mihaesco, E., Hurez, D., Mihaesco, C., Preud'homme, J. L. and Rambaud, J. C. (1969). *J. Clin. Invest.*, **48**, 2374
162. Seligmann, M., Mihaesco, E. and Frangione, B. (1971). *Ann. N.Y. Acad. Sci.*, **190**, 487
163. Dorrington, K. J., Mihaesco, E. and Seligmann, M. (1970). *Biochim. Biophys. Acta.* **221**, 647
164. Wolfenstein-Todel, C., Mihaesco, E. and Frangione, B. (1974). *Proc. Nat. Acad. Sci. (USA)*, **71**, 974
165. Despont, J. P. J., Abel, C. A., Grey, H. M. and Penn, G. M. (1974a). *J. Immunol.*, **112**, 1517
166. Despont, J. P. J. and Abel, C. A. (1974b). *J. Immunol.*, **112**, 1623
167. Dammacco, F., Bonomo, L. and Franklin, E. C. (1974). *Blood*, **43**, 713
168. Bonhome, M., Seligmann, M., Mihaesco, C., Clauvel, J., Danon, F., Brouet, J., Bouvry, P., Martine, J. and Clerc, M. (1974). *Blood*, **43**, 485
169. Franklin, E. C. (1974). *Arch. Int. Med.* (In press)
170. Forte, F., Prelli, F., Yount, W., Jerry, L., Kochwa, S., Franklin, E. C. and Kunkel, H. (1970). *Blood*, **36**, 137
171. Lebreton, J., Ropartz, C., Rousseaux, J., Roussel, P., Dautrevaux, M. and Bisert, G. (1974) (In press)
172. DeCoteau, W. E., Calvanico, N. J. and Tomasi, T. P. (1973). *Clin. Immunol. Immunopathol.*, **1**, 192
173. Kunkel, H. G., Natvig, J. B. and Joslin, F. G. (1969). *Proc. Nat. Acad. Sci. (USA)*, **62**, 144
174. Natvig, J. B., Michaelson, T. E., Gedde-Dahl, T. and Fischer, T. (1974). *J. Immunogen.*, **1**, 33

175. Natvig, J. B. and Kunkel, H. G. (1974). *J. Immunol.,* **112,** 1277
176. Prelli, F., Frangione, B., Franklin, E. C., Abel, C. and van Loghem, E. (1975). *FASEB Mtgs. (Atlantic City, N.J.),* Abst. 4256.
177. Frangione, B. (1973). *Biochemistry,* **12,** 3355
178. Brown, J. R. and Hartley, B. S. (1966). *Biochem. J.,* **101,** 214
179. Lewis, A. F., Bergsagel, D. E., Bruce-Roberston, A., Schachter, and Connell, G. E. (1968). *Blood,* **32,** 189
180. Smithies, O., Gibson, D., Fanning, E., Percy, M., Parr, D. and Connell, G. (1971). *Science,* **172,** 574
181. Parr, D. M., Percy, M. E. and Connell, G. E. (1972). *Immunochemistry,* **9,** 51
182. Isobe, T. and Osserman, E. F. (1974). *Blood,* **43,** 505
183. Kennel, S. J. (1974). *J. Exp. Med.,* **139,** 1031
184. Smith, G. P. (1973). *Science,* **181,** 941
185. Gach, J., Simar, L. and Salmon, J. (1971). *Amer. J. Med.,* **50,** 835
186. Hurez, D., Preud'homme, J. L. and Seligmann M. (1970), *J. Immunol.,* **104,** 263
187. Hurez, D., Flaudren, G., Preud'homme, J. L. and Seligmann, M. (1972). *Clin. Exp. Immunol.,* **10,** 223
188. Scharff, M D. (1974). *Harvey Lectures,* **69,** 125. (New York: Academic Press)
189. Secher, D. S., Cotton, R. and Milstein, C. (1973). *FEBS Lett.,* **37,** 311
190. Milstein, C., Adetugbok, K., Cowan, N. J. and Scher, D. S. (1974). *Prog. in Immunol.,* **II. Vol. 1,** 127
191. Capecchi, M. R. (1966). *Proc. Nat. Acad. Sci. (USA),* **55,** 1517
192. Lucas-Leonard, J. and Lipman, F. (1971). *Ann. Rev. Biochem.,* **40,** 409
193. Platt, T., Weber, K., Ganem, D. and Miller, J. H. (1972). *Proc. Nat. Acad. Sci. (USA),* **69,** 897
194. Nakamuro, K., Tanigaki, N. and Pressman, D. (1973). *Proc. Nat. Acad. Sci. (USA),* **70,** 2863
195. Grey, H. M., Kubo, R. T., Colon, S. M., Poulik, M. D., Cresswell, P., Springer, T., Turner, M. and Strominger, J. L. (1973). *J. Exp. Med.,* **138,** 1608
196. Paterson, P. A., Rask, L. and Lindblom, J. B. (1974). *Proc. Nat. Acad. Sci. (USA),* **71,** 35
197. Smithies, O. and Poulik, M. D. (1972). *Science,* **175,** 187
198. Stevens, R. H. and Williamson, A. R. (1973). *J. Mol. Biol.,* **78,** 517

2
Allotypes and Idiotypes

HENRY G. KUNKEL and THOMAS KINDT

2.1 INTRODUCTION

The main objective of this review is to cover the more significant points regarding immunoglobulin (Ig) allotypes and idiotypes in different species. Allotypic or inherited differences in Igs are almost entirely recognized by immunological methodology where specific amino acid interchanges produced by genetic events are detected as antigens. Most of these antigens do not involve substitutions by the acidic or basic amino acids and it has only been in the mouse system that a few electrophoretic allotypic variants have been detected. While the allotypic Ig variants are very analogous to genetic variants of other proteins, the idiotypes are entirely special to Igs. These too are detected by immunological methodology and reflect the specific amino acids of the hypervariable areas of the Ig molecule involved in the combining sites for antigen. Recently they too have been employed as genetic markers.

Primary emphasis in this review will be placed on the utilization of the allotypic and idiotypic genetic markers for answering questions in a given species where broader implications for immunology in general are most apparent. Thus far, such information has been derived primarily from work with human, rabbit and mouse studies and these will be covered in detail. The first section (Kunkel) will deal with allotypes and idiotypes in the human; the second (Kindt) will cover the rabbit and mouse information. A final section represents an attempt to bring together key information from each species and relate this material to the primary questions of immunology, particularly the problem of antibody diversity.

2.2 HUMAN ALLOTYPES AND IDIOTYPES

Much of the key initial information on the genetic control of the immunoglobulin chains stemmed from work on human Igs. Particularly significant in this respect was first the discovery that the heavy (H) and light (L) chains were under independent genetic control[1,2] and second and more important that the L chains themselves were under the control of at least two genes[3]. The principle of allelic restriction was enunciated on the basis of the occurrence of only one allelic product in myeloma proteins and certain isolated antibodies[4]. This was later established through direct analyses at the cellular level[5]. These and other major developments from human allotype studies arose primarily in conjunction with amino acid sequence studies on human myeloma proteins. The availability of large amounts of these proteins and the vast body of information on classes and subclasses of human Igs that had accumulated relatively early made the human studies more feasible. Additional important contributions of the human allotype studies included the finding of hybrid Igs, gene duplications, gene deletions and other evidence of crossover events that permitted special insight into genetic mechanisms involved in the Ig system.

Although few clues arose concerning the basic question of the origin of antibody diversity, certain constraints were imposed which ruled out various theories that had been put forward.

Idiotypic antibodies were first produced with human myeloma proteins and were shown to be specific for the myeloma protein employed in the immunization[6]. These were initially termed individually specific antibodies and also were shown to be produced by a variety of isolated human antibodies[7]. Similar findings were made in the rabbit and the term idiotypy was proposed[8]. The latter simpler term was adopted since it was clear that similar antigenic determinants involving the specific variable portion of the antibody molecule was involved. The great utility of myeloma protein and antibody idiotypic antigens as markers for studies of the hypervariable regions and the antibody combining site has become even more apparent[9,10]. Genetic studies in combination with allotypic markers have proven particularly useful primarily in the rabbit and mouse and will be discussed in the second section.

2.2.1 Heavy chain linkage group

Nine different types of heavy chains are known for the human Igs that occur in all normal individuals irrespective of population group. They determine the classes and subclasses although this is an entirely artificial subdivision. The classes show little or no antigenic cross reaction involving the constant regions of the heavy chains; the subclasses show considerable cross reactions. However, all nine types show many homologies in amino acid sequence and, although closely linked genetically, they all appear to be under independent genetic control. Table 2.1 illustrates these nine types and the dominant genetic markers characteristic of each type. Together they constitute the heavy chain linkage group. Table 2.2 lists the different individual genetic markers with the designations approved by a recent WHO nomenclature meeting. All of these are recognized primarily as antigens employing human, rabbit and subhuman primate antisera. They have been determined mainly by haemagglutination in-

Table 2.1   List of classes and subclasses
of human Igs and their genetic markers

Ig	Marker
IgG1	a, z, x–f
IgG2	n
IgG3	b0, b1, b3, b4, b5–g
IgG4	4a–4b
IgA1	
IgA2	A2(1)–A2(2)
IgM	M(1)
IgD	
IgE	

Table 2.2   List of heavy chain markers with designations determined by a WHO committee in 1974

G1m(a)	(1)*	A2m(1)
G1m(x)	(2)	A2m(2)
G1m(f)	(3)	
G1m(z)	(17)	Mm(1)
G2m(n)	(23)	
G3m*†(b0)	(11)	
G3m(b1)	(5)	
G3m(b3)	(13)	
G3m(b4)	(14)	
G3m(b5)	(10)	
G3m(g)	(21)	

* The alternate numbering system is listed and would be written as, for example, G1m(1) instead of G1m(a). In this review the always duplicated letter m will be omitted to save space

† Additional G3 markers include (C3), (C5), (t), (u)

hibition procedures utilizing anti-Rh antibodies or individual myeloma proteins as red cell coats. The details of these methods have been described in previous reviews and the readers are referred to these reviews for these and other details[11-13]. Three of the antigens also have been determined by agar gel precipitation: G2(n), G3(g) and A2(1).

Population studies have demonstrated extremely close genetic linkage; in fact this is so close that initially G1(a) and G3(b) were considered true alleles[14]. However, with the delineation of the IgG subclasses their independence became clear with G1(a) relating to the IgG1 type and G3(b) to IgG3. Extensive family studies particularly with the IgG1 and IgG3 markers have failed to show a single crossover although some evidence for an observed crossover involving Gm(n) has been obtained[12]. This is also the case for the relationship of the IgG1 and IgA2 markers although here less extensive family studies have been carried out. However, the fact that crossovers do occur between the subclass genes is clearly apparent from studies in different populations where groups of genetic markers are shifted in specific gene complexes. This is also apparent in unusual inherited gene complexes in individual populations. These points will be brought out in greater detail later in the chapter.

2.2.2   Non-markers

A special type of genetic marker which is not included in Table 2.2 has turned up among the human Igs largely because of the wide use of myeloma proteins. The subclasses of IgG cross react very strongly and sequence analyses indicate that most amino acids of the constant regions are the same. Thus, if a mutational event occurs in one subclass of cistron, it is usually antithetic to a nucleotide sequence coding for an amino acid which is common to several subclasses. These frequently are detectable as specific antigens. A rarer situation would be one where the antithetical product is an amino acid substitution and antigen that is not found in other subclasses. However, it has been found for the (z) and (f) markers of IgG1. These are products of homoalleles and both occur in the same position of the H chains. If the subclass relating to the mutated gene is isolated, then the antithetic marker serves as a true genetic marker and represents the homoallele of the marker from the new mutation. Initial peptide maps by Frangione and associates[15] showed from peptide maps that G1(a) proteins showed a new peptide while another peptide common to all proteins of the IgG2 and IgG3 subclasses as well as non-(a) proteins of the IgG1 subclass disappeared. This same distribution was found antigenically and the antigen absent in G1(a) proteins was termed non-(a) and G1(na)[16].

Many such antigens have turned up and they have proven extremely useful as genetic markers when the specific subclass is isolated or as markers in individual myeloma proteins or antibodies[12]. Two types of IgG4 are recognizable as antigens[17] and, when IgG4 is isolated from normal sera, a genetic pattern can be obtained which is similar to that of the regular genetic markers. Both of these antigens are shared with other subclasses ((4a) with all proteins of the IgG1 and IgG3 subclass; (4b) with all proteins of the IgG2 type). This distribution has broader implications and raises the possibility of these subclasses arising from the genetic variants of IgG4.

2.2.3 Multiplicity and localization of markers on single heavy chains

One of the unique characteristics observed very early for the human Igs was the multiplicity of antigenic differences between the products of allelic genes coding for the H chain constant region. The IgG1 subclass appears unique in showing for the common Caucasian types only two differences, the (z) and (a) markers on one chain and the (f) and (na) markers on the other chain. The (z) and (f) markers are both found at position 214 in the C2 region while (a) and (na) involve several substitutions at positions 355–358 of the C3 area. However, in the IgG3 subclass the two common Caucasian heavy chains, products of allelic genes, differ by many antigens. The so-called (b) chain has the separate antigens (b0), (b1), (b3), (b4) and (ng) while the (g) chain controlled by an allelic gene lacks all of these antigens and has been shown to possess (g), (nb0) and (nb1). Splitting of the H chains into the approximate C2, C3 and C4 homology regions with enzymes[18] has proven feasible and some of these genetic markers have been localized to different segments, attesting further to their individuality. Details of these localizations are described in a previous review[13]. Sequence studies are not yet available on the IgG3 chains but these differences as well as others should be apparent.

The genetic variants of the IgG2 and IgA2 classes also appear to show similar multiple substitutions although these are not as well documented as for IgG3. The general significance of these multiple differences remains of considerable significance. There is evidence that some of the mutational events that led to these genetic variants occurred among subhuman primates[19].

2.2.4 Heavy chain gene complexes in different populations

Although there is little evidence for observed crossovers among the H chain genes in family studies, studies of different populations offer strong evidence for intergenic as well as intragenic crossovers. The upper part of Figure 2.1 shows in horizontal rows the two main Caucasian complexes of genetic

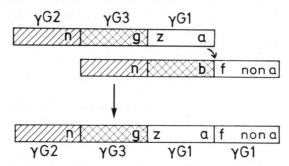

Figure 2.1 Diagram for postulated mechanism of gene duplication with mispairing of the IgG H chain genes followed by an intercistronic crossover at meiosis giving rise to two IgG1 genes, one with G1^{za} and another with G1^{fnona}. (From Natvig *et al.*, 1971.)

markers. Each horizontal row is inherited together as part of the closely linked H chain linkage group described above and the two complexes are antithetic to each other and are inherited as if controlled by two allelic gene clusters. Thus the (f) and (na) markers of IgG1 are associated with the (b) markers of IgG3; (z) and (a) of IgG1 are associated with the (g) marker of IgG3. Exactly the reverse is true in Negroid populations where the common complex has (z) and (a) of IgG1 associated with the (b) markers of IgG3. Because of the multiple markers involved it is difficult to conceive of these differences as resulting from multiple independent parent mutations. However, they are readily explained as resulting from an intergenic crossover at a position between the IgG1 and IgG3 genes. Many other examples of shifts of this type are observed in large scale surveys of different populations. In most instances the different complex is a minor one in a specific racial group and can only be traced in specific families. Certain of these are covered in previous reviews[12].

Another interesting major gene complex is found in Mongoloid populations. Here the (a) and (f) markers are found on the same H chain as has been demonstrated in myeloma proteins from these populations. In Caucasian populations they are always on separate chains (the f marker is not found in Negroid populations). This change can also best be explained on the basis of an intragenic crossover within the IgG1 gene.

It is very difficult in these situations to establish which genes are the primary ones and which resulted in recombination of the ancestral genes. Further work on subhuman primates should furnish some of the answers particularly through the use of monoclonal antibodies since myeloma proteins are not available.

2.2.5 Duplicated and hybrid genes

Considerable further evidence for recombinational events stems from a series of unusual complexes of genetic markers, inherited as a unit in families, which are readily explained as a result of gene duplication and hybrid genes. Figure 2.1 illustrates the presumed sequence of events that lead to the occurrence of two IgG1 gene products which were inherited together[20] in certain families. Detailed studies indicated that separate Ig molecules were involved and that the two common genetic types of IgG1 H chains are inherited in coupling instead of in repulsion as usual. An unequal homologous crossover event as illustrated in Figure 2.1 readily explains the formation of a duplicated IgG1 gene complex that would explain all the findings with the genetic markers.

Duplications such as these encountered in a few families are of special interest because of their relevance to the expansion of the H chain gene pool of the Igs. Another subclass of IgG might readily develop if such a duplicated gene held specific advantages. It will be of interest to study individuals that are homozygous for such complexes when they are encountered.

Two clear examples of hybrid Ig genes resembling the Lepore type observed for haemoglobins have been described and studied in considerable detail. In each case the hybrid involves the C regions of the heavy chains of IgG subclasses. In the first instance[21] the hybrid represents an IgG3–IgG1 combination which is inherited through several families and was found in the homozygous form. It was recognized initially because of the absence of expected Caucasian markers[22]. The serum of the individual homozygous for this gene showed no normal IgG1 or IgG3 molecules. The other hybrid was encountered in a myeloma protein obtained from a Negro. It was shown to represent an IgG4–IgG2 combination[23] which occurs in low incidence in Negroid populations.

The hybrid proteins have proven of special interest because they have provided information regarding the order and number of the IgG cistrons coding for the C regions of the H chains. They too can be explained readily as resulting from intragenic crossovers as a result of mispairing of the heavy chain cistrons at meiosis. They suggest the order IgG4, IgG2, IgG3, IgG1 which is also compatible with the other crossovers mentioned above[24]. However, studies of further examples are required to finally settle this sequence and to position the other heavy chain cistrons.

2.2.6 Gene deletions and immune deficiency

As might be expected in view of the many other manifestations of genetic events involving the constant region Ig genes, gene deletions also have been observed. A number of Caucasian families have been encountered who lack the expected IgG3 markers (g) and the (b) group[12]. Quantitation of IgG3 levels indicated a lowering of the IgG3 levels to approximately one half the normal in the individuals who lacked these markers. In these families this absent gene was only encountered in the heterozygous state and no symptoms of immune deficiency were apparent. Similarly in the IgG1 system which makes up the bulk of the IgG immunoglobulins an absence of expected IgG1 markers have been observed in certain members[12]. Neither the (f) (na) nor the (z) (a) markers were found associated with the IgG3 (b) group. The absence of these markers was followed and found to be inherited in a typical Mendelian fashion in a large number of individuals in these families. Quantitative studies again indicated that Ig levels of the IgG1 class were lower than normal. Again only heterozygotes were encountered but all the IgG1 present could be accounted for by the normal IgG1 gene, furnishing strong evidence for a deletion rather than a silent gene. It was of special interest that two individuals in one family with such a gene deletion had very low IgG1 levels and as a result low total Ig. These were considerably lower than expected in such heterozygous individuals and raise the possibility of interaction with another abnormal gene.

Studies similar to the above have been carried out on the families of a large group of patients with various immunodeficiency disorders. Absence of specific proteins as a result of mutational events leading to gene deletions have been described for many proteins leading to deficiency states primarily in homozygotes as a result of the specific requirement for the biological property of the protein. Similar situations would be expected to apply to the Igs and result in immune deficiency. However, here the situation is somewhat different because of the wide assortment of Igs and, since the heavy chains are under independent genetic control, only one class or subclass would be involved and the other Igs would still protect the individual. One clear case has been observed where deficiency symptoms lead to hospitalization and genetic studies demonstrated gene deletions in both parents[24]. These involved IgG1 in one parent and IgG3 in the other and both were in the asymptomatic heterozygous state. The patient inherited both abnormal genes and showed many symptoms. It is of special interest that the abnormal genes found in the parents were exactly those described above that had been observed in the general population. In the patient the IgG1 levels were very low, lower than might be expected since one normal IgG1 gene was present. However, little is known regarding the interaction of these closely linked IgG genes and the IgG3 defect may well have influenced the normal IgG1 gene. IgG3 levels were also extremely low.

The question of exactly how frequent gene defects of this type are involved in immune deficiency disease is not entirely answered. In most families studied the parents were not informative and similar gene defects could not be ruled in or out. Recently a second case has been encountered which is still under study. It would appear that these mechanisms are involved in immune deficiency but they are probably not a major cause. Another inherited gene defect encountered in families of some of these patients involves lower levels of specific genetic markers[25]. The role of these genes in immune deficiency remains unclear. A control gene defect has been postulated. It now appears more likely that the bulk of cases of immune deficiency involve other mechanisms and relate more directly to the lymphocyte.

2.2.7   Allotype, Ig level and immune response

Clear evidence has been available for a number of years in the human system that the level of a specific Ig is closely related to allotype. This was first described in the IgG3 system where normal individuals of the (b) type have twice the IgG3 level of those with the (g) allotype[26]. Similar observations have been made for IgG4 [27] and recently for IgD [28]. In the latter study it was possible to show this effect even though no genetic markers are available for IgD. However, because the Ig heavy chain genes are so closely linked it was possible to utilize the allelic markers of IgG for such a study. Marked differences were encountered.

These allotype effects on Ig levels clearly indicate an effect on the immune response and one such study involving the antigen flagellin indicates that this is indeed the case[29]. Additional evidence on this point is available in the rabbit[30].

Changes in the expression of Ig genes which appear to be hereditary also have been encountered. One family that was studied in special detail[31] showed uniquely low levels of the (g) marker over several generations. Similar findings have been seen in some parents of patients with immune deficiency involving selective genetic markers[25]. The possibility of some type of control gene defect has been postulated in these instances.

2.2.8   Unique character of heavy chain disease proteins

Although myeloma proteins were initially considered abnormal Igs, it became apparent that they really represented the normal protein products of individual clones of plasma cells. Class, subclass, genetic markers and finally amino acid sequence information demonstrated their direct relationship to individual antibodies[7]. This also proved to be the case with a hybrid myeloma protein which could be related to a minor population of normal Igs as described above. Deviations from the normal situation were seen in the relative preponderance of free L chains that were observed but their composition was not found to be unique. A very different situation has been found to hold for the H chain disease proteins. Large deletions in the H chains secreted by clones of cells from these individuals have been demonstrated[32]. However, these deletions are not the result of gene defects in the germ line of these individuals and are not inherited but are only characteristic of the single proliferating clone of cells.

Special studies have been carried out on the proteins from two individuals with this abnormality[12]. The abnormal Ig in each case was an IgG1 protein and a specific IgG1 genetic marker was absent. In the one case the (z) marker was absent while the (a) marker was present. These two markers occur together on the same H chain in Caucasian IgG1 proteins. The normal Ig pool of this individual, however, contained the usual complement of proteins with the (z) and (a) markers on the same chains. Since this was a heterozygous individual, it was clear that the abnormal protein was exceptional and did not involve a genetic defect. Family studies confirmed this interpretation.

The characterof the deletion in these proteins is also of special interest[32]. The deletion extends from inside the V region on into the C regions and is different in size in each case. However, it is of special interest that the deletion ends at position 216 in several different cases.

2.2.9 Light chain allotypes

Three genetic markers have been described for the L chains. These were initially called Inv markers but are now designated Km(1), Km(2) and Km(3) because they are all on the κ chain. They played an important role in early work on Ig genetics but their importance has decreased, partially due to the lack of availability of good reagents. The Km(1) and (2) markers frequently but not always occur together on the same kappa chain while the (3) marker is inherited as if controlled by an allelic gene.

Recent studies[33] have clarified the amino acid substitutions involved in these patterns and both positions 153 and 191 are involved in the amino acid differences between (1) and (3). It is of interest that these two positions are probably in close proximity according to recent crystallographic models. Here again multiple substitutions are found between chains controlled by allelic genes. Similar positions in the chain are also implicated in isotypic variations in the λ chains. The λ chain findings indicate that duplicated λ constant region cistrons are commonly found[34].

Thus far very few mutational defects have been observed for the L chains. If the κ chain should be involved in some type of gene deletion, the result could be very significant because all classes of Igs have predominantly κ L chains. Evidence has been obtained for one possible κ gene deletion[35] but this has only been observed in the heterozygous form and no serious deficiency was observed. L chain alterations were not encountered in the parents of immune deficiency cases[24] but these are less readily detected than those in the H chains primarily because of the poorer genetic marker systems available.

2.2.10   Idiotypic specificities

A wide variety of methods are available for the detection of idiotypic specificities. Originally these were described by precipitation analysis in agar gels or in direct precipitation. It was apparent in these early investigations that a wide variety of different antigen–antibody systems were involved in the reaction of a given myeloma protein with its specific antiserum. Precipitation curve analyses and absorption experiments indicated that a very heterogeneous system was involved[12] and the degree of heterogeneity related to the strength of the antiserum. Recent evidence indicates that the antibody combining site is directly involved in at least some of the antigenic specificities and the idiotypic antibodies were blocked by haptenes[9]. It is now clear that some of the specificities are not blocked by haptenes[36]. Recently studies in the author's laboratory indicate the reverse findings that a number of non-idiotypic antigen–antibody systems are blocked by the presence of antigen in the combining site. Antibodies specific for V region subgroups showed this to a special degree. These various studies testify to the heterogeneity of the idiotypic system which is particularly apparent when the immunization is carried out in a foreign species. Assays utilizing coated red cell agglutination and various radioimmunoassay systems involving inhibition reactions have been more widely used recently. These emphasize the extreme specificity of the idiotypic systems. In the haemagglutination inhibition system, 1 part myeloma protein could be recognized in 20 million parts of pooled γ-globulin[37]. These experiments also demonstrate the extreme diversity of immune globuin molecules because a counterpart to the myeloma proteins studied was not recognized in even such a vast pool.

Recently the idiotypic systems have proven of special use for the demonstration of similar V regions in diclonal immunoglobulins consisting of two proteins of different classes. Such double myeloma proteins had been known from earlier work to have identical L chains in a number of instances[38]. Later work with idiotypic antisera indicated that the V regions of the H chain were also identical but linked to different C regions[39,40]. This work was of considerable significance in demonstrating that the same V region with specific hypervariable areas can be linked to C regions controlled by several different genes.

Another recent use in the human system has been the demonstration of relationships between B cell membrane Igs and serum Igs. Especially interesting in this respect is the finding that IgM and IgD, the primary membrane Igs which are frequently found together on the same B cell, show identical idiotypic specificity[41]. Some evidence has also appeared suggesting that T cell receptors are blocked by idiotypic antisera[42] although most workers believe that T cell receptors are not classical Igs. Interesting observations also have appeared in the mouse system on the suppression of specific immune responses through the action of idiotypic antisera on membrane Igs[43].

2.2.11   Cross idiotypic specificities

The initial example of cross-reactions with idiotypic antisera was seen in the monoclonal IgM cold agglutinins[44]. These proteins, with combining activity for the blood group related I antigens, showed patterns of cross reactivity which were not observed with any IgM proteins lacking this activity. It was of special interest that these cross-reactions occurred with proteins of unrelated individuals and it was apparent that the antibody combining site was involved. Similar observations were made for monoclonal anti γ-globulins[45]. Despite absorption with very large amounts of pooled Igs (up to 50 mg/ml of antiserum) cross idiotypic reactions were obtained with proteins isolated from different individuals only if they possessed anti γ-globulin activity. It was possible to classify the anti-γ-globulin into several groups on the basis of similar cross idiotypic antigens. Amino acid sequence studies of both the H and L chains of these proteins substantiated these findings and indicated that the hypervariables particularly of the H chains were very similar[46]. Studies of the chains of one group of anti-γ-globulins showing such cross specificity indicated that they were all of the VK III b subgroup and that the L chain hypervariable regions were involved in the idiotypic specificities. This work suggested a relationship between the L chain V region subgroup and the hypervariable regions, a point that will be discussed further in the final section.

2.3   RABBIT AND MOUSE ALLOTYPES

In the following section allotypic markers of the rabbit and mouse will be briefly described. Structural studies that substantiate the validity of allotypes as true genetic markers will be discussed. Data relevant to linkage relationships among genes that code for antibody synthesis will be discussed, including recent data that have been obtained using idiotypes as V region markers. An attempt has been made to confine this discussion to points that relate to two basic questions: (a) How is the information for antibody synthesis encoded in the genome and (b) how is this information selectively utilized? Studies on allotypes (and idiotypes) have contributed information toward answers to both of these questions and some of these answers have involved significant departures from biological dogma.

2.4 RABBIT ALLOTYPES

Rabbit allotypes were first described by Oudin[48] who coined the name for these intraspecies antigenic determinants. The word allotype stems from the Greek words *allo* (other) and *typos* (type). At the present time the major importance of the rabbit in immunogenetic studies rests on the variety and multiplicity of allotypes which have been described for rabbit immunoglobulins[49,50]. Allotypes have been reported for the variable region of H chains (groups a, x and y), constant region of the γ chains (groups d and e), α chains (groups f and g), μ chains (group n), and for L chains of the κ (group b) and λ (group c) types. Allotypes are available for each region of the rabbit immunoglobulin molecule with the exception of the V_L region, and preliminary studies by Thunberg *et al.*[51] indicate that there may be suitable markers for this region. Table 2.3 gives a summary of the major allotypic specificities of the rabbit.

Investigations on rabbit immunoglobulin allotypes have placed the genes coding for immunoglobulin synthesis at three distinct loci. These code for the H chains, the κ and the λ L chains. The original pertinent observation was that Oudin's original two groups of allotypic markers for H chains and κ L chains[48,52,53] showed independent assortment. Genetic studies on the group c allotypes of the λ chains[54] have added the third unlinked group. The recent observation of secretory piece allotypes, which are not linked to any of the other allotypes, may add to these a fourth locus[55].

Figure 2.2 depicts the immunoglobulin genes of a single rabbit showing the

Table 2.3 Major allotypes of rabbit immunoglobulins

Molecular location	Allotypic group	Allotypes
Heavy chain		
Variable region	a	1, 2, 3
	x	32
	y	33
Constant region IgG	d	11, 12
	e	14, 15
Constant region IgA1	f	69, 70, 71, 72, 73
Constant region IgA2	g	74, 75, 76, 77
Constant region IgM	n	81, 82
κ L chains	b	4, 5, 6, 9
λ L chains	c	7, 21
Secretory piece	t	61, 62

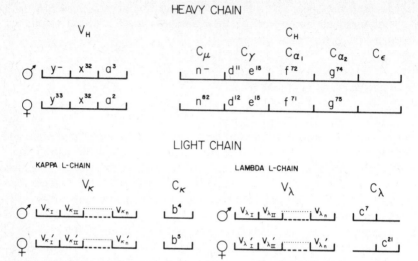

Figure 2.2 Genetic loci involved in the synthesis of rabbit immunoglobulins as determined by allotype inheritance. It is not known if V_H genes of group a, x and y exist in single or multiple copies. Observations of V_L region subgroups suggest existence of multiple V_L genes.

three unlinked loci encoding H chains, κ and λ L chains. The allotypic combinations used in this figure represent two of the observed genotypes or 'allogroups'. Although several thousand H chain allogroups are possible only 12 different ones have been observed[49]. The reasons for this restriction are not apparent.

The rabbit is unique in having allotypic markers present in the variable region of the H chain. Much of the available information concerning the nature of genes encoding antibody V regions has come from studies on rabbit V_H allotypes. For this reason the questions concerning the precise structural nature of the V_H allotypes have received considerable attention. Data that support the localization of group a allotypes to the V_H region have been recently summarized by Kindt and Mole[50].

The major amino acid substitutions that correlate with these allotypes are shown in Figure 2.3. It can be seen that the substitutions are extensive and in some instances, most notably in the peptide from residues 67–71, two of the allotypes are identical and the third different. This situation might be expected if allotypes represent mutants of a common ancestral gene[50]. Brezin and Cazenave[57] have recently observed cross-reactions between a1 and a3 H chains that were recognized only by antisera prepared in a²a² rabbits. These cross-reactions could possibly be explained by the type of substitutions observed at positions 67–71 in H chains.

In certain cases, H chains from homogeneous antibodies have been observed to carry substitutions other than those observed for the pooled H chains of a

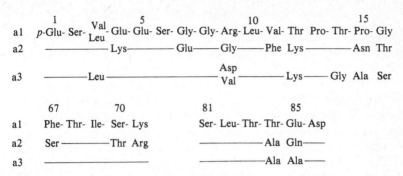

Allotype   H chain position

Figure 2.3 Peptides from rabbit H chain variable region with sequence variation that may be related to group a allotypy.

given group a allotype[58]. Similarly, it has been shown that group a allotypic specificities expressed by homogeneous antibodies are immunologically deficient with respect to those of IgG pools[59]. These findings suggest that group a allotypy may comprise a group of subspecificities in the V_H region.

2.4.1 V_H and C_H allotypes

The genetic relationships between the allotypes of the constant and variable regions of the H chain have implications beyond the field of immunology. The original observation of Todd[60] that IgM and IgG had in common a variable region allotype suggested that two or more genes interacted in some fashion prior to the synthesis of a single polypeptide chain. The presence of these V region allotypes was subsequently demonstrated for rabbit IgA by Fernstein[61] and for IgE by Kindt and Todd[62]. A more precise delineation of the genetic relationships between the hypothetical V and C region genes became open to experimental test with the discovery of rabbit H chain constant region allotypes by Mandy and Todd[63] and by Dubiski[64].

The allotypes of group e and group d were shown to be linked to group a (V region) allotypes[64,65]. Crossovers between the C and V allotypes have been documented for rabbit families[66,67] providing further support for the postulate that at least two separate genes are involved in the synthesis of a single antibody H chain. The crossover frequency for C_H and V_H genes of the rabbit based on these observed recombinations has been estimated at 0.3%[49].

By studying combinations of V and C allotypes present on the molecules from animals doubly heterozygous for these markers, it was observed that a high percentage of the H chains retained the combination of markers inherited from the parents[68]. That is, the majority of syntheses were directed by genes in the coupling phase. For example, if parents with genotypes

$$(a^2d^{12}/a^2d^{12}) \times (a^1d^{11}/a^1d^{11})$$

produced an offspring with genotype a^2d^{12}/a^1d^{11} the majority of molecules in this rabbit's circulation with allotype a1 would express d11; those with a2 would express d12 (see Figure 2.4).

The estimate of molecules with recombinant types obtained by the selective absorption experiments of Landucci-Tosi and Tosi[69] agrees well with the estimate of 1% that Pernis et al.[70] obtained by double fluorescent staining techniques. More recent experiments have measured the percentage of recombinant molecules utilizing IgA C region allotypes in combination with the allotypes of group a. The numbers obtained were slightly higher than those for IgG [71]. It is not known whether the recombinant molecules result from synthesis directed by genes in repulsion or by genes on chromosomes that result from mitotic crossovers between C_H and V_H genes.

2.4.2 Rabbit idiotypes as V region markers

Information concerning the relationships among immunoglobulin V_H and C_H genes has been recently supplemented by studies using the allotypes in conjunction with idiotypic markers. Idiotypic phenomena have been reviewed by Capra and Kehoe[72] and will not be discussed in detail here.

Studies on idiotypes of homogeneous antibodies in rabbit families[73] suggested that idiotypes were genetically transmitted. Further work on the idiotypes of rabbit antibodies showed linkage of group a allotypes to idiotypes[74,75]. The association of an idiotype to an infrequently occurring V_κ subgroup has also been demonstrated in these same rabbit families[76].

Studies on rabbit anti-streptococcal antibodies have recently given examples of idiotypically similar or identical molecules that have differences in other V region markers[77,78]. An idiotypic cross-reaction was observed between two different rabbit antibodies to streptococcal group C carbohydrate. These antibodies were isolated from the serum of an individual rabbit with allotype a^2a^3. One of the antibodies was allotype a3, while the other lacked a group a allotype and was tentatively assigned to the y group by typing carried out by S. Dray (unpublished data). Careful serological analysis failed to demonstrate any idiotypic differences between the two antibodies. The idiotypic determinants were shown to have H chain components by the fact that their expression required a specific H–L combination. Consistent with the H chain allotypic difference, preliminary amino acid sequence studies showed that the two chains differed at their amino terminals[77].

A second pair of antibodies to streptococcal carbohydrate were shown by H–L recombination experiments to have identical idiotypic determinants on their L chains[78]. In spite of this idiotypic identity, the chains differed in electrophoretic mobility and in amino terminal sequence.

2.4.3 Allelic exclusion of allotypes

It was postulated by Lyon[80] that one or the other X chromosome in somatic cells of female mammals is at some early embryonic stage rendered inactive. The inactivated X chromosome, which may be of paternal or maternal origin, will remain inactive in all progeny of the embryonic cells. The major evidences cited by Lyon[80] for this hypothesis were the occurrence of 'mottled' or 'dappled' coat colour phenotypes in heterozygous female mice and the existence of normal XO females. As a consequence of random inactivation of X chromosomes, females heterozygous for X linked traits exhibit mosaic phenotypes. Evidence in support of the hypothesis has been gathered in a variety of experiments.

A similar phenomenon was observed for the immunoglobulin allotypes, and to date this is the only example of autosomal allelic exclusion. That plasma cells from heterozygous individuals produced only one allele from each allotypic group was shown for rabbit allotypes[5] using fluorescent staining techniques, and for mouse allotypes[81] using specific enhancement of plaque formation. Immunoglobulin producing cells may therefore be said to exhibit a mosaic of phenotypes. This is depicted in Figure 2.4 using the cells of a rabbit heterozygous at three allotypes as an example.

While an individual antibody-producing cell in the rabbit exhibits only one allele of each group, any combination of paternal or maternal allotypes may be

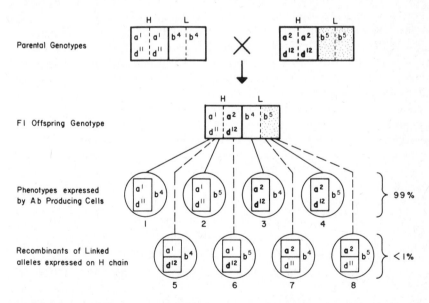

Figure 2.4 Phenotypes of Ig producing cells in a rabbit with genotype $a^1a^2/b^4b^5/d^{11}d^{12}$. Cell types numbered 5 through 8 display recombinant phenotypes of group a and d allotypes.

71

observed. Because the allotypes of group a and b are unlinked and presumably on different chromosomes, this situation necessitates the activation or inactivation of genes at two distinct loci. If the allotypes of the λ L chains and the secretory component are taken into consideration, then the activation process in certain antibody-producing cells involves four distinct loci, perhaps on four different autosomes. The fact that the synthesis of 99% of H chains utilizes information from genes in coupling must also be taken into account (Figure 2.4). The gene activation process may then have specificity for genes on the same chromosome[82]. If this were the case, the low percentage of molecules expressing non-linked markers would be synthesized by cells in which somatic crossovers have occurred.

Allelic exclusion of allotypes is more complex than the exclusion of X linked traits in that several unlinked loci are involved. Nonetheless, a strong analogy may be drawn between the two phenomena. As in the exclusion of X alleles, allotype exclusion may be random and it is permanent in that peripheral blood lymphocytes and their progeny continue to produce the same allotypes[83]. Whether the entire chromosome is involved is not known, nor is it known whether activation or inactivation is the basis of allelic selection of allotypes.

2.5 MOUSE ALLOTYPES

The mouse offers several advantages over the human and rabbit for genetic studies. These include the obvious advantages of small size and short gestation period, as well as availability of inbred and congenic strains. In addition, transplantable plasmacytomas that produce immunoglobulins in amounts sufficient for structural studies are readily induced in the mouse[84]. Mouse immunogenetic studies have been limited by the fact that allotypic markers have been identified only for the constant regions of the H chains. This shortcoming has been partially circumvented by the use of idiotypes as V_H markers in conjunction with these C_H allotypes to obtain information on organization of immunoglobulin genes in this species.

The first mouse allotypes were described by Kelus and Moor-Jankowski[85]. This work was expanded shortly thereafter and these early studies on mouse allotypes were reviewed by Potter and Lieberman[86] and by Herzenberg et al.[87] Mouse allotypes were recently reviewed in detail by Mage et al.[49] Allotypes have been described for the constant region of mouse immunoglobulin classes F (IgG1), G (IgG2a), H (IgG2b) and A (IgA); no allotypes have been described for IG1 (IgG3) or IgM. In addition, there is a group of allotypes which have not yet been assigned to any H chain class.

The mouse allotypes are often referred to by the inbred strain in which they occur. For example, the complete allotype ($G^{1,6,7,8}$, $A^{12,13,14}$, $H^{9,11,22}$, $F^{8,19}$) of the BALB/c C_H gene complex may be too cumbersome to write every time it is mentioned, and is thus often referred to as the 'BALB/c allotype'. This notation is convenient when congenic strains are being discussed. For example, the C57BL/Ka C_H allotype gene complex has been bred into the BALB/c strain to produce a congenic strain, CB-20, which may be referred to as the C57BL/Ka allotype on a BALB/c background. The formal notation for this strain would be:

$$BALB/c.C57BL/Ka, IgC_H.BC20.F3(CB-20).$$

This notation characterizes the congenic strain according to host strain, source of new gene, specific gene introduced, number of backcrosses (BC) and number of homozygous brother–sister crosses (F).

The determinants for a single class within a single strain may be also designated by a condensed notation using a number for class designation[87] with a small letter written as a superscript for the allele. The BALB/c IgG allotype ($G^{1,6,7,8}$) is written as 1^a and the C57BL/6(G^-) as 1^b. In some reports these may be written as IgG^a and IgG^b or even as G^a and G^b.

Structural correlates for mouse allotypes have not yet been described, but the recent completion of the amino acid sequence of a mouse IgG H chain[88] indicates that such data will be available in the near future.

The availability of allotypic markers for several mouse H chain classes made it possible to test the linkage among the genes encoding the different constant regions. In back crosses involving 2,371 progeny, no recombinant types were observed, indicating a very low recombination frequency among the genes that encode the C_H allotypes. The existence of allotypic combination in wild mice which do not occur in inbred strains suggests that crossovers can and have occurred among these closely linked genes[89].

2.5.1 A genetic marker for the V region of mouse κ chains

Edelman and Gottlieb[90] observed that a peptide detected by radioautography from the V_L region of certain mouse κ chains would serve as a genetic marker. This marker was found in three of 17 strains surveyed. More recently, Gottlieb[91] has shown correlation between this marker, called I_B-peptide marker, and the thymocyte cell surface antigen Ly-3.1. This finding, which represents the first report of linkage between an immunoglobulin gene and another characteristic, would place the putative V_L gene in linkage group XI on chromosome 6 of the mouse[92].

2.5.2 Mouse idiotypes

Genetic experiments on the idiotypes of the mouse have extended the original observation of idiotypic inheritance. Linkage of idiotypes to C_H allotypes has been shown for a wide selection of idiotypes. Low recombination frequencies have been observed in all instances[93-96].

Not only has linkage been observed, but also associations at the molecular level between the idiotype of a homogeneous streptococcal antibody and the allotypes of the strain in which it was induced. Eichmann[97] showed that idiotypically related antibodies produced in allotypically heterozygous mice always had the same allotype–idiotype combination. This finding indicates that the mouse idiotypes, like rabbit V_H allotypes, are usually synthesized from information present on the same chromosome as the C_H gene with which they are genetically transmitted. The bulk of genetic data obtained in mouse idiotypic studies is consistent with that obtained in studies with V_H allotypes. One of the few cases where unique information has been obtained will be described here.

One such case involved investigation of the linkage between two different mouse idiotypes (A5A and ARS), both linked to the A/J C_H allotype[98]. The observation of a crossover between the A5A idiotype and the BALB/c allotype in one male mouse provided the opportunity to test linkage between these two idiotypes. The crossover mouse was bred and the new haplotype (allogroup) was shown to be inherited without the ARS idiotype. On the basis of these data, the chromosomes of the BALB/c, A/J and recombinant might be represented:

	V_H Idiotypes		C_H Allotypes
A/J	A5A$^+$	ARS$^+$	1.e
BALB/c	A5A$^-$	ARS$^-$	1.a
Recombinant	A5A$^+$	ARS$^-$	1.a

Such observations suggest that V region genes are present in numbers large enough to observe crossovers among them and indicate that it will be possible to map V_H region genes of the mouse.

2.6 DISCUSSION AND CONCLUSIONS

The predominance of evidence from a study of the constant region genetic markers indicates that the genes involved are inherited in a typical Mendelian fashion. The heavy chain linkage group probably represents a group of sequential genes, in which case observed crossovers predictably would be extremely rare. The fact that crossovers do occur is abundantly evident from the assortment of genetic events described above which have been encountered in large scale population analyses. This is particularly clear from the two hybrid genes involving the subclasses of human IgG. Analyses of these special products of unusual genetic events have permitted partial ordering of the sequence of H chain genes and verification of portions of this order has come from widely different sources.

A few reports have appeared suggesting that the H chain genetic markers might not be the direct products of structural genes as the evidence presented above strongly implies but instead reflect some type of regulatory genes. In the human the evidence for this is very scant and stems primarily from the reported finding of Ig markers in lymphocyte cultures that were not observed in the Igs of the person from whom the lymphocytes were derived. This work has not been confirmed despite attempts in several laboratories. Recently an unexpected human marker has appeared in studies on the transfer of bone marrow into rats[99]. The recent finding of an unexpected allelic product in purified antibody from a rabbit whose whole Ig appeared to represent a different phenotype is of special interest. Members of a congenic mouse strain that has the C57BL/Ka allotype on a BALB/c background have recently been shown by Bosma and Bosma[100] to express the BALB/c (IgG^a) allotype in a transient and unpredictable manner. Similarly, Strosberg et al. recently observed that a rabbit with allotype a^{1}a^3/b^{4}b^5 produced antibodies with allotypes a2 and b6 after immunization with *Micrococcus lysodeikticus*. In addition to the rabbit that produced these antibodies, two other rabbits in the Strosberg colony were found to simultaneously express three group a allotypes. The possibility is raised that some of the polymorphisms observed in the allotype systems relate to the control of gene expression rather than simple allelism. Such a mechanism has been suggested for the HL-A system[102].

A striking feature of the Ig system has been the multiplicity of differences between polypeptide chains controlled by allelic genes. This has been apparent both from antigenic analyses as well as sequence studies showing multiple amino acid substitutions. The extreme situation is present in the IgG3 subclass of human Igs where the constant areas of the so-called (b) chain versus the (g) chain differ by at least five different antigens. Several of these have been localized in enzymatic splitting experiments to separate areas of the H chain. A similar situation appears to apply to the V region markers at the a locus in the rabbit where numerous amino acid differences are found making it unclear as to which reflects the antigenic markers. Both the antigenic and amino acid differences of the human IgG1 H chains are clearly worked out and involve three amino acid interchanges. It is of special interest that some of these markers were already present in subhuman primates. The (b) chain of the IgG3 subclass appears to be a very old type of H chain with close resemblance to earlier primate types. The immune system appears to utilize past mutational events in a special fashion in further diversification into classes and subclasses. Some evidence is available in the human that some of the other subclasses actually arose from the allelic variants of the IgG4 subclass. Clear evidence is available for gene duplications which are manifest as heritable characteristics in certain families and this mechanism of diversification is readily apparent.

The multiplicity of classes and subclasses of Igs offers a means of protecting the individual from genetic events leading to such consequences as gene deletions. As a result, immune deficiency syndromes involving all classes of Ig are unlikely to develop by such mechanisms. However, such apparent gene deletions are recognizable in the population and have been encountered in family members of a few cases of immune deficiency. If they appear in the homozygous or the doubly heterozygous state and involve the major IgG1 type of human Ig, significant symptoms may become apparent. They represent one mechanism but not apparently the common one at the basis of most forms of immune deficiency.

The H chain disease proteins have been shown to have large amino acid deletions involving both V and C regions and they hold special interest because of possible clues to joining mechanisms involving the V and C genes. In all instances the deletion begins in the V region and extends into a portion of the constant area of the heavy chain. In several cases it has been demonstrated that the deletion ends in the same place, position 216. It has been demonstrated that the genetic event leading to the deletion is not part of the germ line; normal proteins derived from the same gene have been identified and the deletion is purely a property of a specific clone. It is not inherited and stands in striking contrast to the gene deletions, hybrid genes, etc. mentioned above. The unusual H chain disease proteins bear some striking similarities to deletions that have been studied recently by Scharff and associates[103]. These have been obtained by special procedures of subcloning from mouse plasma cell tumour lines particularly after the addition of mutagenic agents.

Studies which have utilized the V region (group a) and C region (groups d and e) allotypes of the rabbit strongly support the hypothesis that separate genes encode variable and constant regions of the antibody H chains. Crossovers among these closely linked genes have allowed estimation of a recombination frequency of about 0.3%. The majority of H chains synthesized in an individual utilize genes in coupling rather than those in repulsion. Only about 1% of the H chains share markers from different parental chromosomes. More recent information obtained from studies on idiotypes and C region allotypes of the mouse have confirmed this result. It was observed that a given idiotype, shown to be inherited as a Mendelian marker, was associated with molecules that bore the C region allotype of the same parent from which the idiotype was inherited.

Studies on the inheritance of rabbit idiotypes in selectively bred rabbit families have indicated that idiotypes are linked to group a allotypes. It has, furthermore, been observed that one idiotype, at least, was associated with a given V_κ subgroup in rabbit families. Although there are interesting exceptions which will be noted below, the majority of data suggest that idiotypes are closely linked to V region markers. At the molecular level, idiotypes have been shown to be preferentially associated with the variable region markers to which they are linked.

A recent idiotypic study carried out in the mouse has shown that a crossover occurred between two different idiotypes. Such an observation argues for the presence of a relatively large number of variable region genes. It may be recalled that there are a small number of constant region genes in the mouse and these genes appear to be closely linked. Therefore, one could visualize an H chain chromosomal region comprised of a small number of very closely linked (perhaps adjacent) constant region genes, linked to a much larger number of variable region genes. There are, however, experiments that suggest that this model is an oversimplification and these data must be taken into consideration.

The clear delineation of specific hypervariable areas for the V regions of both the L and H chains has markedly altered the earlier concepts of mechanisms of antibody diversity. Probably the strongest evidence for somatic mechanisms stemmed from the rabbit V region allotypes which restricted markedly the number of V region genes. Now, however, the strong possibility has arisen that the major portion of the V region is just another C region and that the diversity of the V region results entirely from some type of insertional process by which the hypervariable areas are introduced. The rabbit allotype a markers reflect this constant portion and do not relate to the hypervariable areas. Several additional studies furnish support for such an insertional concept[104]. Particularly relevant are the findings described above for homogeneous antibodies in the rabbit system where the same hypervariable region as reflected by identical idiotypes was found in V regions with different allotypic markers. An idiotypic cross-reaction was demonstrated between two rabbit antibodies to streptococcal group C carbohydrate isolated from the serum of a rabbit with allotype a^2a^3. One antibody was typed as allotype a^3 and the other lacked a group a allotype and was tentatively assigned to the group y. Quantitative serological studies failed to demonstrate any idiotypic differences between these two antibodies. The idiotypic determinants were furthermore shown to have H chain components by the fact that their expression required a specific H and L chain combination. That a V_H allotypic difference existed between the two chains was supported by structural studies showing that the chains differed at their N terminals. The most straightforward explanation of this antibody pair involves differences in the constant parts of the variable region and identity in their hypervariable regions.

Possible evidence in the opposite direction has come from work on the human anti-γ-globulins. Here a specific cross-idiotypic pattern was only found in proteins of a single V region κ chain subgroup. These results were clear cut but involve a cross-idiotypic specificity in proteins from unrelated individuals rather than idiotypic identity in the same individual as in the rabbit study mentioned above. Other studies are also available pointing in both directions on this issue. It seems possible that both might be involved and that some types of hypervariable areas might only be inserted in a specific type of V region. This is an active area of investigation and answers to this important question should become available in the near future.

The concept of specific restriction enzymes permitting the insertion of small units of DNA into V region genes remains an appealing one to explain the hypervariable areas. The small units involved probably originate from special segments of DNA in the germ line and many of these might well be present in just a segment of the chromosome. Thus the germ line concept of antibody diversity appears most reasonable. However, somatic events must be considered involved in such an insertional process.

Although it is difficult to visualize experiments to strictly prove the existence of separate genes that interact to synthesize the total immunoglobulin chain, there are observations to support such a model. Some of these have been described above. In addition, it has been recently shown that individual cells simultaneously display on their membranes IgD and IgM molecules with identical idiotypic determinants. This demonstration could suggest that a single V_H gene may be utilized by two different C_H genes in the same cell to synthesize these H chains. The observation places constraints on the mode of utilization of the genes involved in the synthesis of these chains. For example, it is difficult to envisage in the light of this observation that there is joining of an IgM C region gene with the particular V region gene to form a DNA template because such an event precludes the joining of the IgD constant region to the same variable region gene. One might speculate that a more reasonable explanation of such events could involve the RNA messenger from the two separate genes that remain fixed in their respective positions on the H chain chromosome.

References

1. Harboe, M., Osterland, C. and Kunkel, H. G. (1962). *Science,* **136,** 979
2. Franklin, E. C., Fudenberg, H., Meltzer, M. and Stanworth, D. R. (1962). *Proc. Nat. Acad. Sci. (USA),* **48,** 914
3. Hilschmann, N. and Craig, L. C. (1965). *Proc. Nat. Acad. Sci. (USA),* **53,** 1403
4. Harboe, M., Osterland, C. K., Mannik, M. and Kunkel, H. G. (1962). *J. Exp. Med.,* **116,** 719
5. Pernis, B., Chiappino, G., Kelus, A. S. and Gell, P. G. H. (1965). *J. Exp. Med.,* **122,** 853
6. Slater, R. J., Ward, S. M. and Kunkel, H. G. (1955). *J. Exp. Med.,* **101,** 85
7. Kunkel, H. G., Mannik, M. and Williams, R. C. Jr. (1963). *Science,* **140,** 1218
8. Oudin, J. and Michael, M. (1963). *C.R. Acad. Sci.,* **257,** 805
9. Brient, B. and Nisonoff, A. (1970). *J. Exp. Med.,* **132,** 951
10. Capra, J. D., Kehoe, J. M., Winchester, R. J. and Kunkel, H. G. (1971). *Ann. N.Y. Acad. Sci.,* **190,** 371
11. Grubb, R. (1970). In A. Kleinzeller and G. F. Springer (eds.), *The Genetic Markers of Human Immunoglobulins* (New York: Springer-Verlag)
12. Natvig, J. B. and Kunkel, H. G. (1973). *Advan. Immunol.,* **16**
13. Natvig, J. B. and Kunkel, H. G. (1968). *Series Haematologica,* **1,** 66
14. Steinberg, A. G. (1966). In T. J. Greenwalt (ed.). *Symposium on Immunogenetics* (Philadelphia: J. B. Lippincott, Co.)
15. Frangione, B., Franklin, E. C., Fudenberg, H. H. and Koshland, M. E. (1966). *J. Exp. Med.,* **124,** 715
16. Natvig, J. B., Kunkel, H. G. and Joslin, F. G. (1969). *J. Immunol.,* **102,** 3
17. Kunkel, H. G., Joslin, F. G., Penn, G. M. and Natvig, J. B. (1970). *J. Exp. Med.,* **132,** 508
18. Turner, M. W., Bennich, H. and Natvig, J. B. (1972b). *Scand. J. Immunol.,* **1,** 292

19. Goldsmith, E. I. and Moor-Jankowski, J. (1969). *Ann. N.Y. Acad. Sci.,* **162**
20. Natvig, J. B., Michaelsen, T. E. and Kunkel, H. G. (1971). *J. Exp. Med.,* **133**, 1004
21. Kunkel, H. G., Natvig, J. B. and Joslin, F. G. (1969a). *Proc. Nat. Acad. Sci. (USA),* **62**, 144
22. Steinberg, A. G., Muir, W. A. and McIntire, S. A. (1968). *Amer. J. Hum. Genet.,* **20**, 258
23. Natvig, J. B. and Kunkel, H. G. (1974). *J. Immunol.,* **112**, 1277
24. Yount, W. J., Hong, R., Seligmann, M., Good, R. and Kunkel, H. G. (1970). *J. Clin. Invest.,* **49**, 1957
25. Litwin, S. D. and Fudenberg, H. H. (1972). *Proc. Nat. Acad. Sci. (USA),* **69**, 1739
26. Yount, W. J., Kunkel, H. G. and Litwin, S. D. (1967). *J. Exp. Med.,* **125**, 177
27. Steinberg, A. G., Morrell, A., Skvaril, F. and van Loghem, E. (1973). *J. Immunol.,* **110**, 1642
28. Walzer, P. D. and Kunkel, H. G. (1974). *J. Immunol.,* **113**, 274
29. Wells, J. V., Fudenberg, H. H. and MacKay, I. R. (1971). *J. Immunol.,* **107**, 1505
30. Biozzi, G., Asofsky, R., Lieberman, R., Stiffel, C., Mouton, D. and Benacerraf, B. (1970). *J. Exp. Med.,* **132**, 752
31. Gedde-Dahl, T., Natvig, J. B. and Gundersen, S. (1971). *Clin. Genet.,* **2**, 356
32. Franklin, E. C. and Frangione, B. (1971a). *J. Immunol.,* **107**, 1527
33. Milstein, C. P., Steinberg, A. G. and McLaughlin, C. L. (1974). *Nature (London),* **248**, 160
34. Ein, D. and Fahey, J. L. (1967). *Science,* **156**, 947
35. Ballieux, R. E. (Personal Comunication)
36. Clafflin, J. L., Lieberman, R. and David, J. M. (1974). *J. Immunol.;* **112**, 1747
37. Kunkel, H. G. (1970). *Fed. Proc.,* **29**, 55
38. Prendergast, R. A., Grey, H. M. and Kunkel, H. G. (1966). *J. Exp. Med.,* **124**, 185
39. Penn, G. M., Kunkel, H. G. and Grey, H. M. (1970). *Proc. Soc. Exp. Biol. Med.,* **135**, 660
40. Wang, A. C., Wilson, S. K., Hopper, J. E., Fudenberg, H. H. and Nisonoff, A. (1970a). *Proc. Nat. Acad. Sci. (USA),* **66**, 337
41. Fu, S. M., Winchester, R. J., Feizi, T., Walzer, P. D. and Kunkel, H. G. (1974). *Proc. Nat. Acad. Sci. (USA),* **71**, 4487
42. McKearn, T. J. (1974). *Science,* **183**, 94
43. Cosenza, H. and Kohler, H. (1972). *Proc. Nat. Acad. Sci. (USA),* **69**, 2701
44. Williams, R. C., Kunkel, H. G. and Capra, J. D. (1968). *Science,* **161**, 379
45. Kunkel, H. G., Agnello, V., Joslin, F. G., Winchester, R. J. and Capra, J. D. (1973). *J. Exp. Med.,* **137**, 331
46. Capra, J. D. and Kehoe, J. M. (1974). *Proc. Nat. Acad. Sci. (USA),* **71**, 4032
47. Kunkel, H. G., Winchester, R. J., Joslin, F. G. and Capra, J. D. (1974). *J. Exp. Med.,* **139**, 128
48. Oudin, J. (1956). *C.R. Acad. Sci.,* **242**, 2606
49. Mage, R., Lieberman, R., Potter, M. and Terry, W. D. (1973). In *The Antigens,* p. 300 (New York: Academic Press)
50. Kindt, T. J. (1975). *Advan. Immunol.,* **21**, 35
51. Thunberg, A. L., Lackland, H. and Kindt, T. J. (1973). *J. Immunol.* **111**, 1755
52. Dubiski, S., Rapacz, J. and Dubiska, A. (1962). *Acta Genet.,* **12**, 136
53. Oudin, J. (1966). *J. Cell. Physiol.,* **67**, 77
54. Gilman-Sachs, A., Mage, R. G., Young, G. O., Alexander, C. and Dray, S. (1969). *J. Immunol.,* **103**, 1159
55. Knight, K. L., Rosenzweig, M., Lichter, E. A. and Hanly, W. C. (1974). *J. Immunol.,* **112**, 877
56. Kindt, T. J. and Mole, L. E. (1974). *Prog. In Immunol.,* **II. vol. 1**, p. 13 (Amsterdam: North-Holland Publishing Co.)
57. Brezin, C. and Cazenave, P. A. (1975). *Immunochemistry,* **12**, 241
58. Jaton, J-C., Braun, D. G., Strosberg, A. D., Haber, E. and Morris, J. E. (1973). *J. Immunol.,* **11**, 1838

59. Kindt, T. J., Seide, R. K., Tack, B. F. and Todd, C. W. (1973). *J. Exp. Med.*, **138**, 33
60. Todd, C. W. (1963). *Biochem. Biophys. Res. Commun.*, **11**, 170
61. Feinstein, A. (1963). *Nature (London)*, **199**, 1197
62. Kindt, T. J. and Todd, C. W. (1969). *J. Exp. Med.*, **130**, 859
63. Mandy, W. J. and Todd, C. W. (1968). *Vox Sang.*, **14**, 264
64. Dubiski, S. (1969). *Proc. Colloq. Bruges*, **17**, 117
65. Zullo, D. M., Todd, C. W. and Mandy, W. J. (1968). *Proc. Con. Fed. Biol. Soc.*, **11**, 111
66. Mage, R. G., Young-Cooper, G. O. and Alexander, C. (1971). *Nature (London), New Biol.*, **230**, 63
67. Kindt, T. J. and Mandy, W. J. (1972). *J. Immunol.*, **108**, 1110
68. Kindt, T. J., Mandy, W. J. and Todd, C. W. (1970). *Biochemistry*, **9**, 2028
69. Landucci-Tosi, S. L. and Tosi, R. M. (1973). *Immunochemistry*, **10**, 65
70. Pernis, B., Forni, L., Dubiski, S., Kelus, A. S., Mandy, W. J. and Todd, C. W. (1973). *Immunochemistry*, **10**, 281
71. Knight, K. L., Malek, T. R. and Hanly, W. C. (1974). *Proc. Nat. Acad. Sci. (USA)*, **71**, 1169
72. Capra, J. D. and Kehoe, J. M. (1974). *Advan. Immunol.*, **20**, 1
73. Eichmann, K. and Kindt, T. J. (1971). *J. Exp. Med.*, **134**, 532
74. Kindt, T. J., Seide, R. K., Bokisch, V. A. and Krause, R. M. (1973). *J. Exp. Med.*, **138**, 522
75. Kindt, T. J. and Krause, R. M. (1974). *Ann. Immunol. (Inst. Pasteur)*, **125C**, 369
76. Klapper, D. G. and Kindt, T. J. (1974). *Scand. J. Immunol.*, **3**, 483
77. Kindt, T. J., Klapper, D. G. and Waterfield, M. D. (1973). *J. Exp. Med.*, **137**, 636
78. Thunberg, A. L. and Kindt, T. J. (1974). *Eur. J. Immunol.*, **4**, 478
79. Waterfield, M. D., Prahl, J. W., Hood, L. E., Kindt, T. J. and Krause, R. M. (1972). *Nature (London), New Biol.*, **240**, 215
80. Lyon, M. G. (1961). *Nature (London)*, **190**, 372
81. Weiler, E. (1965). *Proc. Nat. Acad. Sci. (USA)*, **54**, 1765
82. Tosi, R. M., Landucci-Tosi, S. and Chersi, A. (1974). *J. Immunol.*, **113**, 876
83. Jones, P. P., Cebra, J. J., and Herzenberg, L. A. (1974). *J. Exp. Med.*, **139**, 581
84. Potter, M. (1967). *Methods Cancer Res.*, **2**, 105
85. Kelus, A. and Moor-Jankowski, J. K. (1961). *Nature (London)*, **195**, 1405
86. Potter, M. and Lieberman, R. (1967). *Cold Spring Harbor Symp. Quant. Biol.*, **32**, 187
87. Herzenberg, L. A., McDevitt, H. O. and Herzenberg, L. A. (1968). *Ann. Rev. Genet.*, **2**, 209
88. Bourgois, A., Fougereau, M. and Rocca-Serra, J. (1974). *Eur. J. Biochem.*, **43**, 423
89. Lieberman, R. and Potter, M. (1969). *J. Exp. Med.*, **130**, 519
90. Edelman, G. M. and Gottlieb, P. D. (1970). *Proc. Nat. Acad. Sci. (USA)*, **67**, 1192
91. Gottlieb, P. D. (1974). *J. Exp. Med.*, **140**, 1432
92. Itakura, K., Hutton, J. J., Boyse, E. A. and Old, L. J. (1972). *Transplantation*, **13**, 239
93. Blomberg, B., Geckeler, W. R. and Weigert, M. (1972). *Science*, **177**, 178
94. Pawlak, L. L., Mushinski, E. B., Nisonoff, A. and Potter, M. (1973). *J. Exp. Med.*, **137**, 22
95. Eichmann, K. and Berek, C. (1973). *Eur. J. Immunol.*, **3**, 599
96. Lieberman, R., Potter, M., Mushinski, E. B., Humphrey, W. and Rudikoff, S. (1974). *J. Exp. Med.*, **139**, 983
97. Eichmann, K. (1973). *J. Exp. Med.*, **137**, 603
98. Eichmann, K., Tung, A. and Nisonoff, A. (1974). *Nature (London)*, **250**, 509
99. Pothier, L., Borel, H. and Adams, R. A. (1974). *J. Immunol.*, **113**, 1984
100. Bosma, M. J. and Bosma, G. C. (1974). *J. Exp. Med.*, **139**, 512
101. Strosberg, A. D., Hamers-Casterman, C., Van der Loo, W. and Hamers, R. (1974). *J. Immunol.*, **113**, 1313
102. Bodmer, W. F. (1973). *Transplant. Proc.*, 5
103. Coffino, P., Baumal, R. and Scharff, M. D. (1972). *J. Cell. Physiol.*, **79**, 429
104. Capra, J. D. and Kindt, T. J. (1975). *Immunogenetics*, **1**, 417

3
The Major Histocompatibility Complexes

J. A. FRELINGER and D. C. SHREFFLER

3.1 INTRODUCTION

In the past few years, the major histocompatibility complex of higher vertebrates has emerged as a remarkable system of multiple genes, which serve multiple, but probably related, functions and which have been maintained in close linkage in a small chromosomal segment over long evolutionary time. These gene complexes apparently have great biological significance, since they have been maintained more or less intact from species to species and class to class among the vertebrates. In man, this complex has great clinical significance, because of its roles in disease resistance and in clinical transplantation. The major histocompatibility complexes (MHCs) are also of particular interest to geneticists and immunologists because these complex systems offer useful material for investigations of fundamental mechanisms and principles in these disciplines.

Our purpose in this chapter will be to present a general overview of the features of the MHCs of various species and their particular genetic and immunological significance. We will not undertake to review any of the systems in extensive detail, since a number of recent, detailed reviews on many aspects of the MHCs are available.

To date, MHCs have been rather clearly defined in at least ten species (Table 3.1). These are all mammalian species, except the chicken. The finding of MHCs in a number of orders of mammals suggests that probably all mammals have such a complex. The occurrence of an apparently comparable system in the chicken and preliminary evidence for similar systems in amphibians[11,12] suggest that the MHC had its origins at a rather early point in vertebrate evolution. Further phylogenetic studies promise to yield useful information about the evolution of the MHC.

On the basis of information currently available, one may generalize a number of features which are probably common to all MHCs (Table 3.2). Historically, the systems have been first defined in various species by allografting or by serological methods, then have been shown to also determine MLR stimulation and immune response differences. Thus far, not all features listed have been rigorously established for all of the species listed in Table 3.1. However, it is clear that a high degree of genetic homology exists among the MHCs of various species, indicating that from species to species the various

Table 3.1 Species in which a major histocompatibility complex has been defined

Species	MHC symbol	Reference*
Man	HL-A	1
Chimpanzee	ChL-A	2
Rhesus monkey	RhL-A	3
Dog	DL-A	4
Pig	SL-A	5
Rabbit	RL-A	6
Guinea pig	GPL-A	7
Rat	AgB, H-1	8
Mouse	H-2	9
Chicken	B	10

* The references cited are to reviews or to recent publications which should provide an entrée to the relevant literature. Further references are given with the text discussion of each system

Table 3.2 Common features of major histocompatibility complexes

1. Principal transplantation barrier of species

2. Serologically detected antigens of lymphocytes — broadly distributed on other tissues

3. Major factors which stimulate mixed leukocyte reaction (MLR) and graft versus host reaction (GVHR)

4. Immune response genes; resistance to disease

5. Multiple phenotypic traits or functions controlled by tight cluster of multiple genetic loci

6. Extensive genetic polymorphism at many loci in complex

discrete genes within the complex probably carry out equivalent functions and have common evolutionary origins.

In the following sections we will review, by species, the MHCs which have been defined, emphasizing the general properties of the systems, their homologies, and the features of particular immunological and genetic interest.

3.2 THE H-2 COMPLEX OF THE MOUSE

3.2.1 Background

The first MHC to be defined was detected initially as a simple blood group antigen (antigen II) by Peter Gorer in 1936[13]. Two years later, he showed that antigen II played an important role in rejection of incompatible tumour grafts[14]. In 1948, Gorer, Lyman and Snell[15] further demonstrated the transplantation role of the antigen and mapped the H-2 'locus' to linkage group IX (now chromosome 17). Gorer and his associates subsequently developed improved serological (haemagglutination and cytotoxicity) techniques for detection of the H-2 antigens[16,17] and demonstrated the multiple serological specificities of the H-2 system[18]. In 1955, it was discovered that these specificities are occasionally recombined through genetic crossing-over[18]. Snell's development[19] of multiple *congenic resistant* inbred strains* carrying many different H-2 types demonstrated the extensive genetic polymorphism of the H-2 system and provided the material for studies which established that the H-2 system is the major transplantation barrier in the mouse.

During the 1960s, it was observed that many traits are controlled by the H-2 system in addition to the serologically detected antigens and the transplantation antigens and it was recognized that the H-2 'locus' is in fact a *complex* of multiple genes with diverse functions. Major H-2-associated traits described included serum protein variations (Ss) in 1963[20], specific thymocyte antigens (T1a) in 1964[21], susceptibility to oncogenic viruses in 1966[22], factors stimulating MLR in 1966[23], and differences in specific immune responses in 1968[24]. By 1971, the genetic map of the H-2–T1a gene complex had been resolved into five major subdivisions or regions controlling these various traits[25-27].

3.2.2 Genetic fine structure of the H-2 complex

The current view of the genetic map of the H-2 gene complex is depicted in Figure 3.1. The linear order of the discrete loci of the complex has been established by analyses of multiple crossovers inside the complex. To date more than 40 such intra-H-2 recombinants have been analysed[9]. The discrete loci, H-2K, Ir-1A, etc. are defined on the basis of two criteria: (1) determination of functions or products demonstrably different from those of other genes in the complex; (2) separation from adjacent loci by two or more intra-H-2 crossover events.

The H-2 complex controls a variety of traits, as summarized in Table 3.3. These traits are discussed in more detail below. Through analyses of appropriate intra-H-2 recombinants, it has been possible to localize most of these traits to a specific *region* of the complex[9]. A region is defined as the segment of chromosome demarcated by the intra-H-2 crossovers which have separated one specific locus from its neighbouring loci. Thus the S region is bounded by the positions of the crossovers which separated the Ss locus from the Ia-3 locus on the left and the H-2G locus on the right. Such a region *may* contain multiple genes, since we do not know whether all loci of the complex have yet been defined. In fact, there is reason to believe that the H-2 complex could encompass as many as 500 genes[25]. If this is true, an average H-2 region might contain 50 or 60 discrete loci. Therefore, the localization of several traits

---

* Congenic resistant strains are inbred strains which are genetically identical to some standard inbred strain, such as C57BL/10 (B10), except for the substitution of a distinct H-2 chromosomal segment from another strain. Thus a series of such strains may exist, all identical except that each carries a different set of H-2 genes.

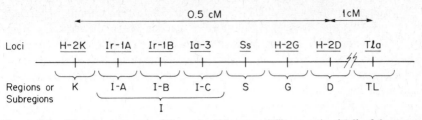

Figure 3.1 Fine structure map of the major histocompatibility complex (H-2) of the mouse and the adjacent TL region. Five major regions of the complex and three subregions of the I region are recognized. Each region or subregion is defined by a specific marker locus, H-2K, Ir-1A, etc. The boundaries of each region are defined by the crossovers which separate the marker locus for that region from the markers of adjacent regions. One centimorgan (cM) is equivalent to a 1% recombination frequency.

to the same region, e.g. of T1a thymocyte antigens and H(T1a) transplantation antigens to the TL region, does not prove that these different traits are controlled by the same gene.

As seen in Table 3.3, many diverse traits are associated with the complex. However, it may be observed that two general classes of traits predominate: (1) those involving polymorphic cell-surface structures, i.e. alloantigens; (2) those involving mechanisms of immune response or recognition. Of course, these classes need not be mutually exclusive. Many or all of the immunological traits may reflect functions of cell-membrane molecules.

Table 3.3   Genetic traits under control of the H-2 complex*

Trait	Gene symbol	Controlling region
Serologically detected H-2 alloantigens	H-2K, H-2D	K, D
Thymus-leukaemia alloantigens	T1a	TL
Erythrocyte alloantigens	H-2G	G
I region lymphocyte alloantigens	Ia	I
Transplantation antigens	H-2K, H-2D	K, D
Transplantation antigens	H(T1a)	TL
Transplantation antigens	H-2I	I
CML target antigens	H-2K, H-2D	K, D
Specific immune responses	Ir-1A, Ir-1B	I
Virus susceptibility	Rgv-1	K-I
T cell–B cell interactions	Ci	I
MLR stimulating factors	Lad	K, I, D
GVHR stimulating factors	Lad	K, I, D
Haemopoietic histocompatibility	Hh	K, D-TL
Complement receptor lymphocyte development	—	D
Serum protein variants	Ss, S1p	S
Haemolytic complement levels	—	S
Testosterone levels	Hom-1	K-I
Liver cAMP levels	—	—

* See reference 9 for detailed references to each trait

Important questions about the H-2 complex which are currently under very active investigation concern the number of discrete genes, their specific functions, the nature of their products, and whether some of the different traits which have been described may reflect different manifestations of the action of the same gene. In the following sections we will briefly consider the current state of understanding of these problems.

3.2.3 The 'classical' serologically detected H-2 alloantigens

As noted above, the H-2 system was first detected as a simple blood-group antigen. In the 1950s, serological analyses with the haemagglutination techniques by Gorer and his associates[18] and by Hoecker and his co-workers[28] established that the system determines a complex array of alloantigenic specificities. With the development of lymphocytotoxicity methods, still further serological complexity was defined[29]. It was recognized very early that a given H-2 'allele'* determines multiple antigenic specificities[18]. It must be stressed at this point that different H-2 *specificities* need not represent different H-2 *antigen molecules*. Operationally, an H-2 specificity is defined by a specific antiserum produced in mice of one H-2 type against tissues from an animal of another H-2 type. Such an antiserum recognizes a particular structural feature of a determinant group on an H-2 antigen molecule. However, different specificities may represent different facets of the same determinant group, different determinant groups on the same molecule, or different antigen molecules. Serological methods alone do not permit a distinction among these possibilities. However, the detection of genetic recombination among these specificities[18,29] and biochemical characterization of the antigens[30] led eventually to the recognition that they are determined by more than one gene[18,29].

As more specificities were defined and more recombinants were found, attempts were made to map the genetic determinants of these specificities. Through the 1960s, these analyses led to more and more complex genetic maps. Difficulties were encountered in fitting all recombination data to these complex maps[25]. Eventually, it was recognized that the data could be explained in a simpler manner, based upon two new concepts[25-27]. First, it was recognized that certain of the H-2 specificities are unique to specific haplotypes[26]. These 'private' specificities fall into two apparently allelic series, based upon strain distributions and recombination data. Furthermore, biochemical analyses of the antigens at that time indicated that a given H-2 haplotype determines two discrete H-2 antigen molecules, each carrying a

---

* The term *H-2 allele* was employed initially to denote the genetic determinants for different H-2 types. However, with the recognition that H-2 is a complex of multiple genes, each with multiple alleles, the term *haplotype* has been adopted. Haplotype refers to a specific combination of the alleles at all loci within the complex which are carried together on one chromosome. Thus, different mouse strains carry different combinations of these alleles or different H-2 haplotypes.

different private H-2 specificity[30]. Therefore, it appeared that all H-2 specificities might be controlled by only two loci, now termed H-2K and H-2D. Second, it was postulated that certain more broadly distributed, 'public' specificities, which are associated with a number of different haplotypes and which had posed the most difficult mapping problems, might be determined by either the H-2K or the H-2D genes[25,31]. A corollary to this postulate was that the H-2K and H-2D genes might have been derived by duplication of a common ancestral gene with subsequent mutational divergence (leading to different private specificities), but with retention of many structural homologies, such that certain anti-public sera could cross-react with the products of certain alleles at either locus. Thus the hypothesis was put forward that all H-2 specificities are controlled by only two genetic loci, but that these are duplicate loci whose polypeptide products have certain structural homologies[25,31].

All current data support this duplication hypothesis. These include detailed serological analyses[32], skin grafting experiments[33,34], and an extensive series of experiments to directly test the postulate of serological cross-reactivity between the products of the H-2K and H-2D genes[35]. Most importantly, further biochemical analyses of the H-2 antigens have entirely supported the hypothesis.

The biochemical properties of the H-2 antigens have been very thoroughly reviewed elsewhere[36]; we will simply summarize. By solubilization with detergent or by controlled proteolysis, two H-2 antigen molecules can be released from membranes of lymphoid or various other cells of a specific H-2 haplotype, and separated from each other. One molecule carries the H-2K private specificity and some associated public specificities, the other carries the H-2D private specificity as well as the predicted public specificities. The H-2K and H-2D detergent-solubilized molecules are both glycoproteins with apparent molecular weights of about 45 000, including two polysaccharide moieties of about 3300 daltons. Recent investigations[37] have shown that these H-2 antigen molecules are associated with molecules of an immunoglobulin-related protein, β_2-microglobulin, M.W. 11 000, both in purified antigen preparations and on the cell membrane. The functional significance of the β_2-microglobulin molecule and its association with H-2 molecules is not yet understood.

A number of lines of evidence indicate that the H-2 alloantigenic determinants of the purified glycoprotein molecules are in the polypeptide rather than the polysaccharide. The strongest evidence for this is the finding that the products of different H-2K or H-2D alleles differ in multiple tryptic peptides, indicating differences in their primary protein structure[38]. These studies also revealed common tryptic peptides in the H-2K and H-2D molecules. In fact, the numbers of peptides in common are approximately the same whether one compares products of alleles at the same locus or at the two different loci[38]. This result strongly supports the concept that H-2K and H-2D are duplicate structural genes.

One exception to the two-gene concept should be noted, involving specificity H-2.7. Stimpfling and Reichert[39] first noted that this specificity, previously considered to be determined by the H-2D locus, appeared to be separated from other H-2D-locus specificities in one intra-H-2 recombinant. Further studies in our own laboratory[40] have established that H-2.7 maps at a locus distinct from H-2D, now termed H-2G.* This antigen has also been found to be expressed very strongly on erythrocytes and weakly on lymphocytes, in contrast with other H-2 specificities. Thus, it appears that at least one of the 'classical' H-2 antigens is controlled by a new genetic locus which is discrete from H-2D and H-2K on the basis of both functional and recombinational evidence.

3.2.4   The thymus-leukaemia antigens

In 1964, Boyse et al.[21] first described a very interesting system of alloantigens which were confined in expression to thymic lymphocytes and certain leukaemias. Four specificities determined by three alleles at a single, Tla, locus were subsequently defined[41]. This locus was found to be very closely linked to, but separable from, the H-2D 'end' of the H-2 complex; the recombination frequency is about 1%. The Tla antigens have several unique and intriguing features: (1) Specificities not determined on normal thymocytes by a given Tla allele may nevertheless appear on leukaemias from strains carrying that allele, suggesting that the Tla locus may be regulatory rather than structural[41]; (2) The cell membrane expression of Tla antigens on thymocytes or leukaemias can be *modulated*, i.e. rapidly eliminated, in the presence of anti-Tla antibodies[41]; (3) The Tla antigens are expressed on thymic lymphocytes only in the environment of the thymus or in the presence of soluble thymic factors[42]; (4) The Tla and H-2D antigens exhibit an inverse relationship in level of expression on thymocytes[41]. Thus far, homologues of this very fascinating system have not been detected in the MHCs of other species.

3.2.5   Transplantation antigens and CML target antigens

The H-2 (histocompatibility-2) system was so named because differences in the serologically detected antigens were very early found to be associated with acute allograft rejections[14,15,19]. With the multiplicity of genes now defined in the H-2 complex, the question has properly been raised whether the products of the H-2K and H-2D antigens are in fact the major transplantation antigens. Although not rigorously proven, current data strongly suggest that this is the case. Skin graft experiments utilizing intra-H-2 recombinant combinations differing only in the K or D regions show strong graft rejections due to these

---

* Snell et al.[32] had previously suggested the possibility of a distinct locus, which they denoted H-2G, in the interval between Ss and H-2D.

regions[43,44]. Of course, it can not be entirely excluded that the genes controlling transplantation antigens are distinct from, but very closely linked to, the H-2K and H-2D genes, thus mapping in the same chromosomal region. Further supporting evidence comes from studies showing the capacity of purified H-2K and H-2D antigens to presensitize graft recipients to give accelerated skin graft rejections[30]. Again, it can not be entirely excluded that the preparations were contaminated with serologically undetectable transplantation antigens.

Further evidence supporting the transplantation role of H-2K and H-2D antigens comes from studies with the cell-mediated lympholysis (CML) assay, an *in vitro* correlate of the *in vivo* allograft reaction directed against MHC products. Data from a number of laboratories reveal that the target antigens are determined by the K and D regions[45-47]. Furthermore, specific antisera to the H-2K and H-2D antigens of the target cell can block the lympholytic reaction[45]. This supports the view that the serologically detected antigens are also the transplantation antigens, although it could still be argued that the antisera also contain serologically undetected antibodies to distinct transplantation antigens.

Perhaps the most compelling evidence for a transplantation role of the serologically detected antigens is the finding that mice carrying a mutant form of the $H-2^d$ haplotype, termed $H-2^{da}$, exhibit simultaneous alterations in the serologically detected H-2D antigens and transplantation incompatibility with mice of the $H-2^d$ haplotype, both in skin graft and CML tests[48,49]. Assuming that this was a point mutation in a single gene, H-2D, this evidence indicates that the product of that gene is both a serologically detected antigen and a transplantation antigen.

The evidence thus appears compelling, although not conclusive, that the H-2K and H-2D genes do play an important role in allograft compatibility. However, these are not the only histocompatibility genes in the H-2 complex. Recent data from Boyse *et al.*[50] have revealed a histocompatibility locus of moderate strength, H(Tla), closely linked to, but probably distinct from, the Tla locus. The products of this locus have not been serologically detected. Klein *et al.*[44] have also detected a histocompatibility gene, H-2I, in the I region of the complex. Incompatibility at this locus results in a relatively strong graft rejection. It is not yet resolved whether the H-2I product is related to the serologically detected I region (Ia) lymphocyte alloantigens, discussed below. In recent experiments with the CML technique in strain combinations differing only in the I region, a low level of lympholysis was observed when appropriate target cells were used[51]. In summary, the H-2–Tla complex contains at least four genes which play a major role in allograft compatibility.

3.2.6 Serum protein variants

In 1963, it was reported that a genetically determined quantitative variation in a specific serum protein, the Ss (serum serological) variant, is controlled by a locus closely linked to the H-2 complex[20]. This variation was detected by an immunodiffusion technique with a specific rabbit anti-Ss serum. Subsequently it was shown that the Ss locus maps between the H-2K and H-2D loci[52]. Later, an allotypic variant of the Ss protein was detected with an alloantiserum produced by immunizations between mouse strains of differing Ss types[53]. This allotypic variation is controlled by a locus thus far inseparable from Ss and has the unusual feature that it is sex-limited. It was therefore termed the Slp (sex-limited protein) antigen. Only males of the proper genotype normally express the antigen. Studies of this phenomenon have revealed that expression of the Slp antigen is regulated by male hormone.

It has been shown recently by Demant *et al.*[54] that differences in total serum haemolytic complement levels are controlled by the H-2 complex. Analyses of intra-H-2 recombinants showed that the gene(s) controlling this difference map(s) in the S region, along with the Ss locus. This raised the question whether the Ss–Slp proteins might be components of the complement system. Recent data[55] suggest some relationship. Within inbred strains, correlation coefficients greater than 0.8 were found between Ss levels and haemolytic complement levels. Addition to mouse serum of F(ab)$_2$ fragments of anti-Ss antibodies (lacking complement-binding sites) drastically reduces the haemolytic complement activity of the serum. These findings implicate the Ss protein in the complement system, but the precise nature of the relationship remains to be defined.

3.2.7 Traits of the immune response region

3.2.7.1 *Immune response genes*

The I (Immune response) region of the H-2 complex was initially defined by the studies of McDevitt and co-workers on the Ir-1 genes[56]. These immune response genes are reviewed in detail by Benacerraf in Chapter 4 of this volume. Therefore, we will simply summarize their principal features.

To date, H-2-associated differences in immune responses to more than 25 different antigens have been described[9,57]. In the majority of cases, these involve quantitative differences in the level of specific antibody produced in the secondary response to a given antigen. Each of these response differences has been demonstrated to be under the control of a single, major genetic determinant which is linked to the H-2 complex. Analyses of intra-H-2 recombinants have mapped most of these response differences to the interval between the H-2K and Ss loci, i.e. the I region[9,57].

These response differences do not reflect a generalized immunological deficiency of certain H-2 haplotypes. Every haplotype exhibits a different pattern of high and low responses to the various antigens. Furthermore, the pattern of high or low response by haplotype is different for every antigen. These observations suggest that multiple discrete genes are probably involved in the control of these various responses, i.e. possibly a different gene controls each response. Two crossovers at approximately the same position inside the I region have been detected which separate the determinants of these responses into two sets[58,59], corresponding to subregions I-A and I-B (Figure 3.1). Thus it may be assumed that there are at least two distinct immune response genes, Ir-1A and Ir-1B (Figure 3.1). However, it is not excluded that there may be many Ir-1 genes in the I-A and I-B subregions. Further recombination analyses and/or characterization of Ir-1 gene products will be necessary to resolve this question.

For all Ir-1-controlled responses, high response is dominant, indicating a positive functional role for the high responder allele. The Ir-1 genes appear to function, at least in most cases, at the level of the interaction between the T lymphocyte and the B lymphocyte which leads to humoral antibody production. A number of possible mechanisms have been speculated upon, but the precise function of the Ir-1 genes has not yet been resolved.

3.2.7.2 T cell–B cell interaction genes

Possibly related to mechanisms of Ir-1 gene action are the recent findings by Katz and his co-investigators[60] that effective interaction between T and B lymphocytes requires that the interacting cells express some function of the I region of the *same* H-2 haplotype. In the test system employed, allogeneic T and B cells fail to interact to produce humoral antibody, whereas semisyngeneic combinations, i.e. parental T cells with F_1 hybrid B cells or *vice versa*, do effectively interact. This indicates that allogeneic cells fail to cooperate, not because of histoincompatibility (since F_1 cells are also incompatible with parental cells), but because of lack of some essential 'interaction factors' which must be determined by the same haplotype in both cells.

By pairing of appropriate combinations of intra-H-2 recombinants, the gene(s) determining these factors (termed Ci genes) have been localized to the I region[61]. The Ir-1 genes have been implicated in this process by the observation[62] that effective interaction fails to take place between F_1 hybrid T cells and parental B cells, if the B cell is from a strain which is a nonresponder to the challenging antigen and the T-cell is from a (responder $\times$ non-responder)F_1 cross. Although not yet fully understood, these findings promise to lead to new insight into the mechanisms of action of the genes of the I region (see Chapter 4 for further discussion).

3.2.7.3 Resistance to viral oncogenesis

Another very interesting and biologically very important phenomenon associated with the H-2 complex, and probably controlled by the I region, is the difference among H-2 haplotypes in susceptibility to certain oncogenic viruses. This was first described by Lilly[22], who found that susceptibility to induction of leukaemia by the Gross virus is strongly influenced by a single gene, Rgv-1 (Resistance to Gross virus-1), which was mapped to the K or I region of the H-2 complex[63]. Subsequently, H-2-associated differences in susceptibility to a number of other viruses were found[63].

Lilly has postulated that the Rgv-1 gene may be an Ir-1 gene which controls response to virus-induced leukaemia-specific antigens[63]. Several studies have shown H-2-associated differences in level of antibody response to these antigens[63], supporting that hypothesis[63]. These findings suggest that the Ir-1 genes may play an important role in natural populations in disease resistance. The finding of an Ir-1 gene which controls level of susceptibility to autoimmune thyroiditis suggests another possible biological role for these genes, in autoimmune reactions[64].

3.2.7.4 Mixed leukocyte and graft-versus-host reactions

Another trait controlled by the I region which must be fit into the overall picture of I region gene function is the stimulation of the mixed leukocyte reaction (MLR). This reaction has become one of the hallmarks of the MHCs. Originally it was thought to detect the major transplantation antigens of the MHC, but in the past few years it has been shown in man, mouse, monkey and dog that the *major* stimulatory factors are controlled by distinct genetic loci or regions (see below).

The MLR results from a recognition of incompatibility and subsequent proliferative response when allogeneic lymphocytes are mixed in *in vitro* culture[65]. The proliferative response can be measured by uptake of [³H]thymidine into DNA. Level of uptake affords a semi-quantitative index of the 'strength' of incompatibility. A 'one-way' test is normally performed in which proliferation by lymphocytes of one donor is blocked by X-irradiation or mitomycin C, so that the proliferative response of only the second donor is assayed[65].

Initial MLR studies were done in man[65], but in 1966 Dutton[23] showed that the H-2 complex determines the principal MLR stimulation in the mouse. In 1970, using intra-H-2 recombinants, Rychlikova *et al.*[66] showed that this stimulation was principally due to genes at the 'K-end' of the complex, i.e. to the left of the Ss locus. Subsequently, through analyses of additional recombinants, it was shown that the strongest stimulation is determined by genes in the I region[67,68].

The details of the mapping of genes which stimulate the MLR, now termed Lad (Lymphocyte activating determinants), have been reviewed elsewhere[9,69]. An example of the approach taken, using mixtures of pairs of strains of different H-2 haplotypes, is shown in Figure 3.2[70]. The data from several such studies may be summarized briefly as follows: (1) The major Lad gene(s) map(s) in the I-A subregion. (2) An additional Lad gene or genes map(s) in the I-C subregion, the interval between the Ss and H-2D loci, or both. These genes

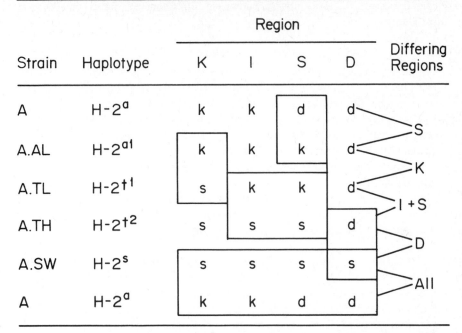

| Strain | Haplotype | Region | | | | Differing Regions |
		K	I	S	D	
A	$H-2^a$	k	k	d	d	
A.AL	$H-2^{a1}$	k	k	k	d	S
A.TL	$H-2^{t1}$	s	k	k	d	K
A.TH	$H-2^{t2}$	s	s	s	d	I + S
A.SW	$H-2^s$	s	s	s	s	D
A	$H-2^a$	k	k	d	d	All

Figure 3.2   An illustration of the method by which differences in single H-2 regions may be examined through pairwise comparisons of congenic strains carrying recombinant haplotypes. For example, an MLR assay with mixtures of cells from strains A.AL and A.TL would test for differences only in the K region, with A.TH and A.SW, for differences only in the D region, etc. Similar combinations can be employed for tests of skin graft compatibility, CML T-B interaction, etc., or for reciprocal alloimmunizations. (Modified from reference 70.)

exert a weaker stimulus than those of the I-A subregion. (3) Weak, but significant, stimulation is associated with the K and D regions, probably due to the H-2K and H-2D products themselves. (4) The S and TL regions are not associated with significant MLR stimulation. The current picture is thus that at least four different genes or sets of genes in the H-2 complex play a role in this reaction, although the roles of H-2K and H-2D are relatively minor.

Studies of factors stimulating the graft-versus-host reaction (GVHR), as measured by splenic or lymph node enlargement, by Oppltova and Demant[71] and by Klein and Park[72] have shown a very striking parallel with MLR results. It appears that the two reactions detect the same factors.

It remains to be established what, if any, relationship Lad gene functions have to Ir-1 or Ci gene functions. At one extreme, all of the I region phenotypic traits discussed could be controlled by a single functional class of genes (i.e. Ir-1 = Ci = Lad). At the opposite extreme, these genes, their products, and their functions could be entirely independent. Present data do not permit a distinction, since the I region could contain many genes, since the different phenotypic traits have not yet been clearly separated by recombination, and since nothing is known so far about the nature of the gene products.

3.2.7.5 I region associated (Ia) antigens

An attempt to detect the products of these I region genes by serological techniques led to the definition of the Ia (I region associated) system of lymphocyte alloantigens. Of critical importance to this definition was the availability of several strain pairs such as A.TL and A.TH (see Figure 3.2), which are identical in their K and D regions, but differ in the I region. (The S region also differs in these combinations, but plays no detectable role in any of the phenomena discussed.) These strains were utilized both for (1) the production of specific antibodies to I region products by alloimmunization and (2) the detection or mapping of anti-I region antibodies in complex antisera which also contained anti-H-2 antibodies. Five laboratories initially reported detection of antibodies to I region products, three using approach (1) above[73-75], two using approach (2)[76,77].

The Ia antigens have been reviewed in detail quite recently[9]. Space permits only a rather brief description here. Serologically, the antigens are detectable on lymphocytes by the cytotoxicity assay, but only 50–70% of lymphocytes are reactive, in contrast with the H-2K and H-2D antigens, which are present on 100% of lymphocytes. Through standard serological analyses, many Ia specificities have been defined. Analyses of all defined H-2 haplotypes have revealed that each haplotype determines multiple Ia specificities. Analyses of all available intra-H-2 recombinant haplotypes have indicated that the Ia specificities map in three subregions of the I region, I-A and I-B, which were previously defined by specific immune response genes, and a new subregion, I-C, defined thus far only by the Ia antigens.

Investigations of the tissue distribution of the Ia antigens reveal a much narrower tissue expression than that of the H-2 antigens. The Ia antigens are not detectable on liver, kidney, brain or red blood cells[73]. The antigens have been detected on sperm cells, epidermal cells, and macrophages[75,78]. They are apparently present on no more than 70% of lymph node or splenic lymphocytes, indicating some restriction to subpopulations of lymphocytes. Examination of the expression of Ia antigens on T and B lymphocytes indicates that they are represented relatively strongly on most B lymphocytes[75,77,79]. They are also present on some T lymphocytes, although more difficult to detect in the cytotoxic test[79]. Very probably the anti-Ia antibodies which react with B-lymphocytes are distinct from those which react with T lymphocytes. The antigens have been demonstrated by several techniques to be present on the cell membrane[9], and those on B cells, at least, are not physically associated with the H-2K and H-2D antigens[80].

The Ia antigen molecules have been identified and partially characterized by immunoprecipitation analyses[81,82]. They have an average apparent molecular weight of about 30 000, distinct from the H-2 antigens, but exhibit heterogeneity in molecular weights, with a range from 25 000 to 35 000 daltons. The molecules are glycoproteins, but, as with the H-2 antigens, the carbohydrate appears to play no role in the antigenic activity[83]. The Ia molecules can be precipitated independently of the H-2 molecules, indicating no close physical association[81]. Molecules carrying Ia specificities determined by the I-A subregion can be precipitated independently of molecules carrying Ia specificities controlled by the I-C subregion[81], strongly indicating that these particular specificities define distinct polypeptide molecules which are products of discrete genes.

Since the anti-Ia sera were initially sought for the purpose of characterizing I region gene products, a critical question concerns the relationships of the Ia antigens to other I region traits. These relationships are not yet fully understood, but several positive associations have been observed. Anti-Ia sera have been shown to inhibit MLR stimulation quite specifically and completely, when directed against the Ia antigens of the stimulating (i.e. inactivated, non-proliferating) cell in mixtures of cells differing only in the I region[84]. These results suggest that at least some Ia antigens may be Lad gene products. Anti-Ia antibodies have also been found to partially block the immune response to foreign red blood cells by splenic lymphocytes cultured *in vitro*[85]. Specific anti-H-2K and H-2D sera do not block under the same conditions. This blocking could occur at any of a number of levels in the response process, but the data indicate that at least some Ia antigens must be involved in this process. Data have also been reported which establish that anti-Ia sera can block the interaction of the B lymphocyte Fc receptor with aggregated immunoglobulin[86]. Although the precise functional significance of this observation is not yet clear, it again implicates Ia antigens in immune processes.

A point which must be strongly emphasized is that the anti-Ia sera presently available react with a heterogeneous group of discrete molecules of different molecular weights, determined by at least several discrete genes in different I subregions. Therefore, the Ia antigens cannot be regarded as a single functional class of molecules. The blocking of MLR, *in vitro* immune response and Fc receptors by anti-Ia sera need not imply any functional relationship among these traits. The blocking could be due to three different populations of antibodies directed against three different functional classes of molecules. The resolution of this question will require production of much more specific antisera and/or biochemical characterization of the molecules involved. In any event, these preliminary biochemical and functional studies of the Ia antigens have demonstrated the potential usefulness of anti-Ia antibodies as reagents for specific identification and characterization of I region gene products.

3.3 THE HL-A COMPLEX OF MAN

3.3.1 Genetic fine structure

Since the early observations of Dausset[87], Van Rood[88] and Payne[89], which led to description of the MHC of man, work has focused on the detailed serological definition of the HL-A system. Rather than the intensive analysis of a relatively few distinct haplotypes as in H-2 genetics, the HL-A geneticist was confronted with a system of equal complexity, but without the tools of in-bred and congenic recombinant lines. This forced the development of other, novel approaches. First was the study of human populations. Through the mechanism of international workshops it was found that even though different investigators could not produce identical serological reagents at will, they could at least discover and define similar reagents by exchange and testing of large numbers of reagents against large panels of lymphocytes. This approach was made feasible by the application of standardized techniques and computer-assisted analysis of the large amount of data generated.* This approach soon led to the recognition of two allelic series of antigens and the postulation of a 'two-locus' model for the structure of the HL-A complex. Extensive testing in in families and detection of recombination between the two loci, which were designated Four and LA, confirmed the two-locus hypothesis and established the map distances and gene order relative to other loci of the complex. Investigations of the MLR and other HL-A-associated traits in such families also permitted the mapping of these traits.

The current concept of the genetic map of the HL-A complex is shown in Figure 3.3. The HL-A linkage group has been assigned to chromosome 6. The gene(s) for strong stimulation in MLR is closely linked to the Four and LA

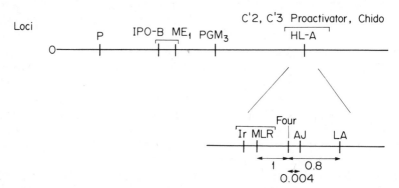

Figure 3.3   The current genetic map of human chromosome 6. The centromere is located on the left. P is an erythrocyte antigen system. IPO-B is indophenol oxidase B, ME_1 is cytoplasmic malic enzyme. PGM_3 is phosphoglucomutase. C'2, the second complement component; C'3 proactivator, factor B of the properdin pathway, and the blood group Chido are all closely linked to HL-A, and no informative recombination events have been observed. The bottom map is an expansion of the HL-A region. Ir is the immune response gene, MLR the mixed lymphocyte reaction determinant and Four, AJ and LA the classical serological determinants. This map is modified from J. Dausset, The HL-A Complex: Serology and Genetics, In G. Snell, J. Dausset, and S. Nathenson, *Immunogenetics*. (In press).

* For detailed description of the progress see *Histocompatibility Testing*, 1964, 1965, 1970, 1972.

determinants, but in contrast to the murine system it is located *outside* the region defined by the two classical serological markers, proximal to the Four locus. An Ir gene for IgE response to ragweed antigen also maps outside the complex, on the same side as MLR. A third, serologically detected locus (AJ) maps inside the complex, between Four and LA. This third locus is separable from the other two both serologically and by recombination. Closely linked to the HL-A complex are genes controlling two components of the complement system, $C'2$[90], and GBG (glycine-rich beta glycoprotein) or $C'3$ proactivator[91]. Another locus closely linked to HL-A controls the blood group antigen Chido[92], which could perhaps be analogous to the H-2G blood group locus in the mouse.

3.3.2 Serology

There are two primary sources of HL-A reagents. The first is the sera produced by intentional immunizations of volunteers. The second is the sera collected from multiparous women who have been immunized against the paternally derived antigens on their fetuses. Such sera can be characterized by the testing of large panels of cells. The results of this sort of analysis are shown in Figure 3.4.

Reagents may be classified into two general categories: (1) Those reacting with a high proportion of panel lymphocytes, which probably comprise a family of antibodies to related specificities. These are referred to as public or supertypic specificities. These 'broad' sera are believed to contain either a population of antibody molecules which truly cross-react in that the same antibodies may react with several determinants which are different, but structurally related, or antibodies which are directed at a single determinant of the antigen molecule which is common to all members of the family of related specificities. (2) Those which react with the product of a single haplotype. Such an 'operationally monospecific' serum is serologically much simpler. The specificities thus defined are called private, or subtypic.

These analyses are complicated by the possibility that the antigens which are recognized may not be structurally identical in unrelated individuals, i.e. may not have identical amino acid sequences. This raises one of the fundamental differences between H-2 and HL-A serology. H-2 serology is based on the careful and complete analysis of a relatively few independent haplotypes and of recombinants derived from them, by use of many H-2-specific sera. Analysis of HL-A antigens is based either on population analysis with relatively broad sera or on analysis of families with sera which were not raised against the identical antigens present in the families. Although the public and private terminology has been adopted by both HL-A and H-2 groups, the meanings are somewhat different. There is probably no precise HL-A equivalent to an H-2 private antigen, since the occurrence of such a specificity would probably be highly restricted. HL-A private specificities are perhaps

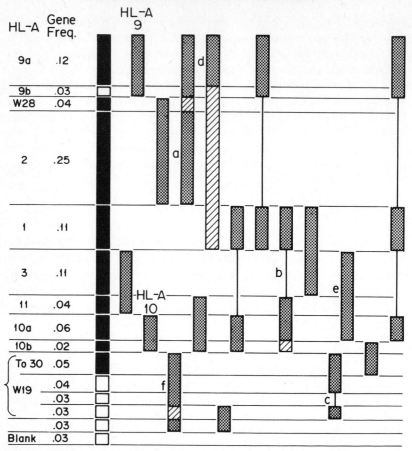

Figure 3.4 Fifteen factors (specificities) of the LA segregant series (separated by horizontal lines) with corresponding gene frequencies, as they can be recognized through the reactions with 9 'subtypic' sera represented by full blocks in the left-hand column, and also by a series of cross-reacting sera (dotted blocks). The vertical lines join the different subtypic factors recognized by the same cross-reacting serum. The striped blocks mean that the serum is CYNAP for the corresponding specificity, e.g., monospecific serum 6 is cytotoxic for factors 1, 11, 10a, but not for 10b. All activity, however, is removed by absorption with cells +10b, −1, −11, 10a. (Modified from Ceppellini, R. (1971). *Progr. in Immunol.*, Vol. I, 673.)

equivalent to the narrower H-2 public specificities, while the HL-A public specificities might be equivalent to the broadest H-2 specificities.

Initially all HL-A antigens appeared to fit into two allelic series. However, evidence for a third locus of the HL-A system was recently detected in population studies of serum AJ, and certain other sera[93]. Strong evidence that these antigens are cell surface molecules distinct from the previously defined antigens comes from capping experiments. In these experiments it was shown that the antigens of the Four and LA series cap independently of one another. When both the LA and Four antigens are capped with appropriate antisera, the

Table 3.4 HL-A antigen and gene frequencies (percentages) in Caucasoids. Blanks represent the gene frequency of unidentified antigens. Table modified from J. Dausset, *The HL-A complex: Serology and Genetics*. In G. Snell, J. Dausset and S. Nathensen, *Immunogenetics* (In press).

1st Locus, SD1			3rd Locus, SD3			2nd Locus, SD2		
Antigens	Antigen frequency	Gene frequency	Antigens	Antigen frequency	Gene frequency	Antigens	Antigen frequency	Gene frequency
HL-A1	25.1	13.4	T1 (AJ)	10.0	5.0	HL-A5	15.2	7.9
HL-A2	44.8	25.7	T2 (170)	14.9	8.0	HL-A7	18.2	9.5
HL-A3	22.6	12.0	T3 (UPS)	26.0	14.6	HL-A8	16.7	8.7
W23} HL-A9	4.3	2.2	T4 (315)	19.7	11.1	HL-A12	32.5	17.8
W24}	18.2	9.5	T5	14.0	7.4	HL-A13	5.4	2.7
W25} HL-A10	3.9	1.9	Blank		53.9	W5	15.2	7.9
W26}	8.3	4.2				W10	13.7	7.1
HL-A11	11.8	6.0				W14	8.8	4.5
W28	9.8	5.0				W15	12.3	6.3
W29	10.3	5.3				W16} W16	0.9	0.4
W30	2.4	1.2				Da31}	2.4	1.2
W31	6.8	3.5				W17	5.9	3.0
W32	9.8	5.0				W18	11.3	5.8
Fe55	1.9	0.9				W21	4.9	2.4
Blank		4.9				W22} W22	5.9	3.0
						Da30}	1.4	0.7
						W27	7.8	4.0
						Da34 (MK)	4.9	2.4
						TY	2.9	1.4
						Blank		4.4

AJ antigens are still diffusely spread over the membrane, indicating that they are distinct from the other HL-A antigens. Conversely, when AJ antigens are capped, the other HL-A determinants are unaffected[94-96].

Part of the problem in detecting the AJ antigens was the linkage disequilibrium existing between Four and AJ specificities. This led to the classification of some reagents, which in fact recognized AJ antigens, as anti-Four sera, because certain third locus specificities occur only in combination with certain second locus specificities, an 'inclusion' phenomenon which is common for HL-A specificities. Recently a recombinant has been described which unambiguously separates the Four from AJ loci and positions AJ between Four and LA[97]. In all previous recombinations within the HL-A complex, the antigens of AJ and Four segregated together, but were separated from the LA antigens, indicating very close linkage between Four and AJ.

The HL-A antigens presently defined and their gene frequencies are shown in Table 3.4. It is readily seen that in Caucasian populations almost all HL-A antigens in the LA and Four series can be serologically detected, i.e. there is only a very low frequency of blanks. Since the third locus has only recently been clearly defined, few specificities have been defined thus far and the frequency of blanks is high[98].

One of the primary features of the mouse system is the cross-reactivity between the products of the H-2D and H-2K loci, which presumably reflects the common evolutionary origin of these loci. Until recently, almost all of the emphasis on HL-A cross-reactivity was placed on cross-reactivity between antigens of the same allelic series[99]. However, evidence recently has been presented indicating that some anti-HL-A sera can cross-react with antigens determined by both loci[100].

3.3.3 Chemistry of HL-A antigens

This subject was reviewed in detail in 1971[101,102]. Recent findings have very strikingly paralleled those on the H-2 antigens. Briefly, the Four and LA antigens are carried on distinct, separable molecules. These molecules are glycoproteins with molecular weights of about 45 000[103]. The carbohydrate moiety has no apparent antigenic activity. The physical properties of the Four and LA molecules are very similar, but no peptide maps or amino acid sequence data are available thus far. No information has thus far been reported on the properties of the third locus (AJ) molecules. It has been shown in co-capping experiments[95] that the Four, LA and AJ molecules are physically independent of each other on the cell membrane.

A significant new finding with the HL-A antigens has been the molecular association of these antigens with β_2-microglobulin (β_2M), a low molecular weight (11 000 daltons) polypeptide which has strong homologies with the constant regions of the immunoglobulins[104]. The HL-A-β_2M association has been demonstrated by co-precipitation of β_2M in stoichiometric quantities upon immunoprecipitation with anti-HL-A sera[105] and by co-capping of the HL-A antigens on the cell membrane with the β_2M molecules[106]. In the latter studies, Four, LA and AJ molecules were all shown to be associated with β_2M. These studies also showed that there are additional β_2M molecules present on the membrane which are not associated with HL-A antigens. The functional significance of this association remains to be established.

3.3.4 MLR, CML and HL-A

As noted in the discussion of H-2-associated MLR, it was initially believed that the 'classical' serologically detected antigens of the MHC (H-2K and H-2D; Four and LA) are responsible for MLR stimulation[65]. However, the findings that H-2-associated stimulation is principally determined by the K-end[66] and that occasionally HL-A-identical siblings are MLR incompatible[107] led to a re-evaluation of this concept. In 1971, Yunis and Amos proposed that MLR reactivity is governed by genes separate, but closely linked, to HL-A, which code for distinct cell surface molecules[108]. Their conclusion was based on the study of recombinants between MLR and HL-A in families which showed both MLR non-stimulation among HL-A-incompatible siblings, and stimulation between sibs in spite of apparent HL-A identity. Since then, many families demonstrating recombination between MLR and HL-A have been reported[109]. It is now generally accepted that this is the correct interpretation of the data and that the strong MLR determinants map outside the Four–LA interval, proximal to the Four locus.

Originally the idea that the cell surface molecules detected by anti-HL-A antibodies and those detected by MLR are controlled by distinct genes was so striking that Bach coined the terms SD (serologically defined) for the 'classical' HL-A antigens, and LD (lymphocyte defined) for the MLR determinants[110]. He further proposed that there was an intrinsic difference between these two classes of molecules in their ability to provoke the formation of serum antibodies. However, evidence from other species, most notably the mouse[73–77] and rhesus monkey[111], has shown that with appropriate immunization combinations and assays, these antibodies can be produced and detected. Studies on inhibition of MLR by anti-HL-A sera have also revealed antibodies which can inhibit either the stimulator or responder, or both cells in MLR[112]. Those antibodies which specifically inhibit stimulator cells probably detect the molecules determined by the HL-A-associated MLR locus.

The rarity of negative MLR between unrelated individuals ($\sim 1/10^4$) suggests that, like HL-A, the MLR system has extensive polymorphism. In addition, the fact that even HL-A identical unrelated individuals regularly stimulate in MLR indicates that there is little overall linkage disequilibrium between LA, Four and MLR. However, in those haplotype combinations which show disequilibrium between LA and Four there is evidence for linkage disequilibrium between HL-A and MLR[113]. Further evidence for such linkage disequilibrium comes from the fact that there have been differences in kidney graft survival reported which depend specifically on haplotype rather than simply on the number of antigens matched[114]. It is important to remember in this connection that even a four-antigen match can be a zero-haplotype match. In populations which show strong linkage disequilibrium between HL-A and MLR, simply matching for HL-A antigens would assure a complete haplotype match including MLR. If the populations were entirely in equilibrium, matching HL-A antigens would have no effect on MLR matching. If the data on HL-A and MLR stimulation could be reassessed on the basis of haplotype matching, perhaps greater MLR–HL-A linkage disequilibrium would be apparent.

On occasion, non-reciprocal MLR reactions have been observed, i.e. reactions in which cells from A stimulate B, but B cells fail to stimulate A. The simplest explanation for such reactions is that one of the pair is homozygous for an MLR allele shared with the other cell (i.e. A is a/b while B is b/b). By using such homozygous cells as stimulator cells in MLR, it is possible to classify the MLR alleles of the responding cells by the pattern of their response to the standardized typing cells. Those cells which fail to respond to a specific homozygous stimulating cell share an allele with that cell. Such typing cells are usually obtained from the children of consanguineous marriages, in which there is a high probability of homozygosity for an MLR allele. A number of distinct MLR alleles have now been defined by this method[115,116].

MLR is believed to be the *in vitro* equivalent of early GVH reaction. (See H-2 section above). It can also be used as a procedure for generating cytotoxic ('killer') lymphocytes. Lymphocytes sensitized to allogeneic cells *in vitro* in MLR can lyse target cells from the sensitizing donor in the absence of any antibody and complement. Eijsvoogel first proposed that the antigenic determinants involved in the sensitization phase (MLR), and the effector phase of an allograft reaction (CML) are distinct[117]. His data suggested that determinants distinct from HL-A, the MLR determinants, are responsible for sensitization, while the HL-A antigens themselves are the structures which the effector cell actually recognizes as the target in the CML assay. Bach *et al.* later extended these observations in 'three cell' experiments to show that the MLR and CML specificities do not even have to be on the same cells[118]. An MLR involving antigens on one cell population can produce cytotoxic effector cells with specificity directed at the HL-A antigens carried on a different cell population present during the MLR phase. This led to the concept of a functional separation of the sensitization phase from the generation of effector cells. It has been suggested that the MLR-reactive cells and the CML killer-precursors are essentially separate subpopulations of lymphocytes, with the killer differentiating in response to signals released by the cells reacting in MLC. Such a mechanism has important implications with respect to *in vivo* allograft reactions.

3.3.5 Clinical transplantation

We do not intend this to be an extensive review of the large clinical transplantation literature, but only an overview of the relationship of HL-A and its closely associated traits to graft survival in clinical situations.

The great bulk of the clinical transplantation which has been done has involved kidney grafts for treatment of renal disease. The outcomes of transplants with living related versus cadaver kidney donors and their implications to HL-A matching are so different as to warrant separate attention. Kidney grafts between siblings who are matched for HL-A generally exhibit a very benign course, require only minimal immunosuppression, and show extremely long survival of kidney function. These donor–recipient pairs are particularly characterized by both identity for HL-A antigens and absence of MLR reactivity. Parent-child grafts are not very much, if at all, superior to grafts from cadaver donors, except where the recipient is not stimulated in MLR by the potential donor, i.e. when the parent is homozygous at the MLR locus[119].

Cadavers are now the most frequently employed source of kidneys for transplantation donors. One critical requirement for transplant matching in this situation is that the recipient should not have preformed cytotoxic antibodies directed at antigens of the donor tissue. Recently it has been observed that some recipients who have been multiply transfused do not produce cytotoxic antibodies even in the face of repeated sensitization[120]. These patients have been reported to do well after renal transplantation. These are probably individuals with a generalized hyporeactivity to HL-A antigens. In other studies, the patients who have preformed cytotoxic antibodies to a large portion of a random panel have been found also to do well, providing that they have no antibodies directed against the donor's HL-A antigens[121]. This may reflect a polymorphism of immune responsiveness similar to the H-2-linked immune response to the H-2.2 antigens[122]. The recipients who have been multiply transfused and do have antibodies to many potential donors apparently simply identify by these antibodies those potential donors to whose antigens they can respond. They thereby receive a correspondingly better match.

Of great potential importance is the ability to match donors and recipients at MLR. Eijsvoogel[117] showed that, in the absence of a strong MLR, very few cytotoxic lymphocytes developed. Now there appear to be two distinct sets of determinants to be considered. In the absence of any MLR reactivity, HL-A matching is probably of less clinical importance. However, in the presence of MLR reactivity, HL-A compatibility would be expected to have great importance[123]. Thus it would be of great practical value if serological methods of detecting MLR differences could be developed since the length of time required for an MLR test precludes MLR typing of cadaver donors. Potentially the detection of human lymphocyte alloantigens, equivalent to the mouse Ia antigens, might provide a means for such matching.

Potentially, bone marrow transplantation should offer the best possibility of long term survival for patients with aplastic anaemia or severe combined immunodeficiency disease. However, with bone marrow grafts there is not only the problem of incompatibility of the graft with the recipient, but also the problem of graft versus host reactions, in which immunocompetent cells from the graft react against antigens of the recipient. Unlike the situation with kidney grafts, in which moderate success (i.e. 50% graft survival to 2 years) is obtained, even with unrelated donors, recipients receiving marrow grafts from unrelated individuals survive poorly. These patients often die either from rejection of the grafts or from fatal graft-versus-host disease. However, it has been found that grafts between HL-A identical, MLR-negative siblings are usually manageable and this now appears to be a useful therapeutic mode[141]. It appears that MLR matching may be more important to the survival of such transplants than HL-A matching. The indications in the mouse that GVHR and MLR are stimulated by the same genetic factors tend to support this. However, to our knowledge, only a single marrow graft has been performed between MLR-negative unrelated individuals. That graft appears to be surviving and functioning, although there is evidence of some graft versus host reaction[124].

3.3.6   Ir genes and HL-A-disease associations

The discoveries of H-2-linked immune response genes and of H-2-associated differences in susceptibility to oncogenic viruses have spurred an extensive search for similar associations with the HL-A complex. Attempts to detect human Ir genes by deliberate immunizations with a variety of antigens as employed in other species are not ethically feasible. The most convincing evidence thus far for a human Ir gene has come from studies of immediate hypersensitivity to ragweed antigen[125]. In certain families, clearcut linkage between IgE-mediated ragweed sensitivity and HL-A haplotype has been demonstrated. This is *linkage* rather than *association*, because ragweed sensitivity segregates with different HL-A haplotypes in different families. The controlling locus appears to be located outside of the Four–LA interval, at the Four-end of the HL-A complex. An association of sensitivity to ragweed antigen Ra5 with the HLA-7 cross-reacting group has also been reported[126], possibly implicating linkage disequilibrium between the Ir gene and the HL-A allele(s) controlling these antigens. These analyses are complicated by the fact that ragweed sensitivity is also influenced by a gene unlinked to HL-A, which controls quantitative levels of IgE. Individuals with low serum IgE levels apparently do not develop immediate hypersensitivity regardless of their HL-A type[127]. These complexities underscore the inherent difficulties in approaching such a problem without inbred and congenic strains and without the opportunity for experimental manipulations. Nonetheless this is of such potential importance clinically that the effort must be made. Such analyses of family material, in cases in which the incidence of response is sufficiently frequent, represent one very useful approach.

Another approach to the same fundamental issue has involved the search in patient populations for associations of specific HL-A antigens with specific diseases. A group of patients with a given disease are completely typed for their HL-A antigens and the antigen frequencies are compared with those in a group of matched normal controls. Beyond the interest in detecting and defining Ir genes in man, there have been three primary motivations for such studies. First, from the evolutionary standpoint, one would like to understand the selective factors operating to maintain the extensive genetic polymorphism of the HL-A system. Second, from the practical standpoint of the physician, there is the potential for specific genetic markers which could contribute to unambiguous diagnoses and even predictions of risk of specific diseases. Third, there is the hope that strong associations might provide leads to an understanding of the underlying pathological process and thence to a more rational course of therapy.

Many laboratories have searched for involvement of Ir genes in disease susceptibility, as manifested by HL-A-disease associations. Implicit in this approach is the assumption that certain Ir alleles are in linkage disequilibrium with certain classical HL-A antigens. Otherwise, HL-A-linked Ir genes will not be detectable by this approach. If the HL-A antigen frequencies in the patient population are the same as in the controls, this does not prove that HL-A-linked Ir genes are not involved in disease resistance. It may only mean that the classical antigens are not themselves involved in resistance and that the relevant Ir genes are in linkage equilibrium, i.e. high or low response alleles are proportionately distributed with respect to alleles at the Four and LA loci. On the other hand, a positive association with an HL-A antigen could imply either that the HL-A antigen itself is causally related to the disease process or that there is an Ir gene in linkage disequilibrium with the antigen. Thus, the population approach is also subject to complexities. A combination of population and family studies will be required for clear definition of the genetic basis for any associations.

Numerous studies have been conducted with a variety of diseases in which no association with HL-A type was found. These include many types of infectious diseases and cancer[128,129], except possibly leukaemia and lymphoma. In another group of diseases, such as Hodgkins disease[130], acute lymphocytic leukaemia[131], and systemic lupus erythematosis[129], weak associations have been found which, although statistically significant, do not appear to be promising cases for detailed investigations into genetic control or causal factors. A third group of a few diseases has been found to have quite spectacular associations with a single HL-A specificity. The most notable of these is the association of antigen W27 with ankylosing spondylitis[132,133], acute anterior uveitis[134], and Reiter's disease[135]. A strikingly high frequency of the antigen has been found among patients with these conditions. In ankylosing spondylitis patients, the frequency of W27 ranges from 87–95%, compared with less than 10% in normal controls. Similar high frequencies are found in patients with Reiter's disease and acute anterior uveitis. Such a striking association of a single HL-A antigen with a particular rare disease is certainly not a chance relationship. It could be a function of the HL-A–W27 allele itself. If it reflects an HL-A-linked Ir gene function, then the linkage disequilibrium in this case must be very large. Another disease which manifests a strong association with W27 is juvenile rheumatoid arthritis[136]. In this disease there is a W27 frequency of 42%, compared to about 6% in controls. Although this is not quite as striking as the frequency in ankylosing spondylitis and Reiter's disease, the association of a single specificity, W27, with all of these diseases suggests a possible common aetiology for all. Since juvenile rheumatoid arthritis, at least, is an autoimmune disease, the question arises whether all are of autoimmune aetiology.

Some other cases of highly significant associations include coeliac disease[137] and myasthenia gravis with HL-A8[138] and psoriasis with HL-A13 and W17[139]. There are thus far no clues as to the role of the HL-A complex in the aetiology of these diseases.

One association between an MLR allele, 7a, and multiple sclerosis has been reported[140]. The frequency is about 60% in multiple sclerosis patients compared with 17% in controls. In principle, testing for association with MLR alleles might be a more sensitive approach, either because MLR reactivity may directly reflect Ir gene functions or because MLR genes may be more closely linked to Ir genes than are the Four and LA loci, and therefore might exhibit greater linkage disequilibrium. This may be a very promising future approach for detection of MHC-linked Ir genes.

It now seems rather conclusively established that HL-A-disease associations do exist. The next important question concerns the mechanisms involved. HL-A-associated disease resistance might occur in several ways. The most obvious, as implied above, is that a series of linked Ir genes control capacity to mount an immune response directed at the aetiological agent of the disease. The susceptible individual would thus carry a non-responder allele for that pathogenic agent. Alternatively, the individual carrying a responder allele for some 'self' component might be more likely to be stimulated to respond to the component under certain conditions, resulting in an autoimmune disease. Another possibility is that the HL-A antigens themselves could be molecular mimics for some infectious agents, thus causing tolerance, and non-response to those pathogens. The HL-A antigens might even serve as viral attachment sites on the cell membrane. A great deal more work will be necessary to define the basis for these associations. However, this appears at present to be biologically the most significant aspect of the MHCs. Future findings may lead to greater insight into the basis for MHC polymorphism.

3.4 THE MHC IN NON-HUMAN PRIMATES

Because of their close physiological relationship to man, primates occupy a unique place in biomedical research. As long-lived species with long generation times, they have many of the same disadvantages as man for genetic research, but their similarity to man, and the ethical limitations on human experimentation make the application of primate models necessary.

The MHC of rhesus monkeys is the best defined of the non-human primate species. Antisera have been produced in the chimpanzee and shown to define two segregant series[2,142]. The gene(s) controlling MLR stimulation is closely associated with those controlling the cellular antigens[142]. However, these traits have been studied much more extensively in the monkey. In rhesus monkeys, ten specificities of the RhL-A system have been defined at each of two loci controlling serologically detected antigens. These two loci seem to be equivalent to the Four and LA genes in man. The two genes have been separated by recombination within families in two cases[143].

Furthermore, two families have been observed in which strong MLR stimulation occurs between full sibs who are identical in RhL-A. In another family, there are sibs which mutually fail to stimulate in MLR despite an RhL-A serological difference[143]. Therefore, the MLR gene must be located outside the two loci controlling serologically detected antigens, in a position analogous to the MLR locus in man, rather than between the genes controlling these antigens, as in the mouse.

Studies similar to those now in progress in humans to develop methods of typing for specific MLR determinants have also been done in the monkey. Homozygous typing cells have been found and some preliminary typings carried out. These results indicate that, as in man, there is linkage disequilibrium between some MLR types and some RhL-A antigens.

Evidence for the existence of an Ir gene for response to an amino acid copolymer of glutamic acid and alanine (GA) has been presented. These data suggest that the gene is closely linked to RhL-A, on the same side of the complex as the MLR locus. One monkey family has been found that appears to carry a recombinant RhL-A haplotype in which the crossover occurred between the Ir gene and the MLR locus[144]. It has been shown by reciprocal immunizations between serologically identical unrelated monkeys that cytotoxic antibodies probably analogous to the anti-Ia of the mouse, can be produced[111]. There is also evidence for linkage to the RhL-A complex of a gene controlling variants of GBG (C'3 proactivator), as in man[145].

3.5 THE MHC OF DOGS

Dogs have been used extensively by surgeons as an experimental model for transplantation research. For this reason, definition of the dog MHC has become of particular importance. Since dogs, like man, are a relatively outbred species, many of the same approaches used in studies of the HL-A system have been used to study the dog MHC. As a result of the international dog immunogenetics workshop[4], the DL-A complex is relatively well defined. Two loci coding for Four- and LA-equivalent antigens have been defined and denoted SD-1 and SD-2. These two loci have been genetically separated by a number of recombinants. Each locus is defined by a set of 10 antigens, which account for about 80% of the gene frequencies in European dog populations[146].

Strong stimulation in MLR has been shown to be controlled by a gene(s) closely linked to the SD-1 and SD-2 loci, but the MLR determinants have been separated from these loci by recombination and found to map outside the DL-A complex, proximal to the SD-1 gene. In dogs, unlike man, there appear to be extremely large linkage disequilibria between the MLR and SD genes. In humans, approximately 1% of HL-A-identical, unrelated individuals are MLR-negative, while in dogs 70% of the SD-identical unrelated dogs also appear to be MLR-identical[147]. Homozygous typing cells have been used to classify MLR alleles. From these studies, the MLR system in dogs appears to be highly polymorphic; at least 10 alleles have been defined. Thus, in all respects, the dog model seems to closely resemble the genetic organization of the human system.

3.6 THE GPL-A SYSTEM OF THE GUINEA PIG

In contrast to the MHCs described for other species, which were initially defined serologically or by transplantation, the GPL-A system in the guinea pig was first detected through a gene that controls the specific immune response to the poly-L-lysine (PLL) polypeptide. In fact, this was the first clearly defined single gene control of an immune response in any species. This response was later shown to be associated with genes controlling the major serological and transplantation antigens of the guinea pig, after the discovery in the mouse that Ir genes were linked to the MHC. These MHC-linked immune responses of the guinea pig, which have been very extensively investigated by Benacerraf and co-workers are reviewed in detail in Chapter 4.

Definition of the transplantation, serological, and MLR aspects of the MHC in the guinea pig has been much less extensive than that of the immune responses. One problem is the paucity of inbred strains available. Only two strains, 2 and 13, are in general use. Antisera prepared by immunizations between these strains were shown to contain cytotoxic antibodies specific for products of genes linked to the determinant(s) of PLL response. It was also shown that genetic differences mediating graft rejection and MLR were linked to these traits, thus defining the MHC, now termed GPL-A[148].

Initially, it was assumed that the cytotoxic anti-2 and anti-13 antisera defined antigens equivalent to the H-2K and H-2D or Four and LA products. However, the '2' and '13' antigens were recently found to have a much more restricted tissue distribution than the 'classical' MHC antigens, with principal expression on lymphocytes and stronger representation on B than T lymphocytes[149]. Furthermore, anti-2 and anti-13 sera were shown to inhibit specific MHC-linked immune responses[150]. These properties appear more similar to those of the mouse Ia antigens. Sato and de Weck described a system of lymphocyte alloantigens in outbred guinea pigs which appeared to be more similar to the classical antigens[7]. Strains 2 and 13 were found to be identical with respect to these antigens, thus reciprocal immunizations between these strains fail to reveal them. Recent genetic and serological data suggest that the 2 and 13 antigens are probably Ia-equivalent, while the antigens of Sato and de Weck are H-2K-D-equivalent[151]. Thus, although no genetic map is available thus far, the guinea pig MHC shows many resemblances to the mouse MHC. A further point of homology is indicated by data which suggest that deficiency of the C′4 component of complement may also be linked to the GPL-A system[151].

3.7 MHCs IN OTHER SPECIES

The MHCs of rabbits (RL-A)[6,152], rats (AgB)[8,153 154], swine (SL-A)[5,155,156] and chickens (B)[157–160], were all initially defined by serological techniques. In all four species, extensive serological complexity and polymorphism was observed. The serologically detected alloantigens were subsequently shown to be associated with the major transplantation antigens of the species. Thus far, recombinants have not been found that separate two or more controlling genes for these antigens. In all four species, the major MLR stimulatory determinants have been found closely linked to these antigens. In rabbits and swine recombinants have been detected which separate MLR genes for the classical antigens.

In the rat, AgB-associated differences in response to a number of synthetic polypeptide and foreign protein antigens have been described[161–163]. In the chicken, the B-locus, or a linked genetic factor, has been found to control resistance to Marek's disease[164] (an avian leukosis virus-induced lymphoma), and also to autoimmune thyroiditis[10]. Differences in response to the synthetic polypeptide (T,G)-A–L have also been observed[165]. An extremely interesting observation in the chicken indicates a requirement for shared products of the same MHC haplotype in order for effective T cell–B cell cooperation to take place[166], as in the mouse.

The above data all fit, therefore, with the pattern established for the MHC in more thoroughly studied species. Definition of further points of homology may be anticipated. Of particular significance are the findings in the chicken of so many features common to mammalian MHCs, indicating an origin of these complexes at an early point in vertebrate evolution. In this connection, it is most exciting that in the clawed toad, *Xenopus laevis*, genetic determinants of MLR stimulation, graft rejection and serologically detected antigens all appear to be closely linked[11,12]. These data suggest that the MHC existed prior to the branch point of avian and mammalian classes, supporting the thesis that the MHCs of these classes had a common evolutionary origin.

3.8 FUNCTION AND SIGNIFICANCE OF THE MHC — THE UNANSWERED QUESTIONS

Although the precise extent is not yet fully defined, the homology among the MHCs of higher vertebrates that has already been revealed by research over the past ten years is truly remarkable. Not all features of the prototype H-2 and HL-A systems have so far been demonstrated for all other species examined, but it seems reasonably clear that all systems include genes controlling the 'classical' serologically detected histocompatibility (transplantation) antigens, genes controlling determinants stimulatory in MLR and GVHR, and genes controlling fundamental mechanisms in immune responses (Ir genes), that probably act at the level of cell–cell interactions. Recent data strongly imply that, at least in mammals, genes controlling components of the complement system are also included in the MHC; nothing is known so far about these genes in other vertebrate classes, however.

The existence of such very similar gene complexes in mammalian, avian and amphibian species indicates that the MHC is evolutionarily quite old. Although duplicate loci like H-2K and H-2D have not yet been demonstrated in vertebrate classes other than mammals, it may be predicted that eventually they will be found, and that gene duplication will emerge as a consistent and significant feature of MHC evolution, just as it has in immunoglobulin evolution. The tremendous genetic polymorphism associated with these complexes is a consistent feature. This suggests that the polymorphism may also be quite old and that multiple alleles at the various loci of the system may have been carried forward through many successive speciation steps. This could account for the large peptide map differences within H-2K and H-2D products, which imply an accumulation of mutational differences over long evolutionary time.

There apparently are minor differences among species in details of the genetic organization of the complexes. For example, in the mouse, the MLR stimulatory genes are localized *between* the genes for the serologically detected antigens — in man they are *outside*. Such subtle variations should probably not be surprising in view of the long evolutionary separation. What is surprising, and significant, is that these discrete genes have remained so tightly linked. Why is this so? We have no clues to this problem. It might be postulated that they have remained together purely by chance, that chromosomal rearrangements are so infrequent that in the evolutionary time from amphibian to man no such event has occurred to separate them, or at least that the species in which they have been separated have not yet been examined. We are more inclined, however, to implicate selective pressures in the preservation of the complexes. The cost to the species of such pressures would be low, since events which would separate the genes *are* infrequent; therefore every individual carrying such chromosomal rearrangements could be selected against with negligible effect on the survival of the species.

What selective forces might operate to maintain this tight clustering of genes in one complex? Two general possibilities may be suggested: (1) there may be functional requirements for close linkage, either for proper temporal expression, or for proper regulatory interrelationships among the genes (e.g. an operon-like organization); (2) there may be *co-adapted* sets of alleles at different loci that must be concurrently expressed for optimal fitness. In the latter case, close linkage would permit transmission *en bloc* of these coordinated sets of alleles, with minimal separation by recombination. Such 'supergene' constellations could be maintained because the rare recombinants would be eliminated. The conservation of the complexes suggests that they must have biologically significant functions. No MHC gene function is yet clearly defined. The Ir–Ci genes appear to be involved in cellular interactions and induction or 'triggering' of lymphocytes. Perhaps the entire complex is concerned with cell–cell recognition, interaction and/or regulation mechanisms, involving various cell types, both in immunological reactions and development. The physical proximity and certain genetic and phenotypic similarities in the mouse of the H-2 system to the t-system, which is involved in developmental processes, has raised the possibility that the MHC may play some general role in embryonic development, perhaps by mediating cell-surface recognition phenomena among different cells or tissues. However, the biological function remains an important, unsolved aspect of these gene complexes.

Likewise, the basis for the extensive genetic polymorphism of these systems is a mystery. The polymorphism could be a direct and obligatory feature of the biological activities of the MHC gene products, or it could be secondary and unrelated to the primary functions of the gene products. In either case, because the polymorphism is so extensive and is such a consistent feature of the MHCs in all species studied, it seems very likely that some rather strong selective forces must operate to maintain it. One might predict that at least one kind of selective mechanism will be found to involve immune competence and disease resistance, mediated by the Ir genes. However, the precise mechanisms by which Ir gene polymorphism might be maintained and the significance of the polymorphism of other genes of the complex are major unanswered questions — and potentially the most important questions about these systems. Tremendous progress has been made in the past 10–15 years in the genetic and phenotypic *description* of these systems, but it must be admitted that we are still very far from a thorough understanding of their *function* and *biological significance*. This promises to be one of the most challenging areas of immunogenetics for some time to come.

Acknowledgements

Original research cited from our laboratory was supported by U.S.P.H.S. Research Grants GM15419 and AI 11962. Dr. Frelinger is supported by a Jane Coffin Childs Memorial Fund for Medical Research Fellowship, Dr. Shreffler by U.S.P.H.S. Research Career Development Award K3-HL24980. We are grateful to Dr. Jacques Colombani for many helpful comments and suggestions during preparation of the manuscript.

References

1. Thorsby, E. (1974). *Transpl. Rev.,* **18**, 51
2. Ward, F. E., Seigler, H. F., Metzgar, R. S., Reid, D. M., Hill, E. D. and Guthrie (1974). *Transpl. Proc.,* **6**, 129
3. Balner, H., Gabb, B. W., Toth, E. K., Dersjant, H. and van Vreeswijk, W. (1973). *Tissue Antigens,* **3**, 257
4. Vriesendorp, H. M. *et al.* (1973). *Tissue Antigens,* **3**, 145
5. Vaiman, M., Haag, J., Arnoux, A. and Nizza, P. (1973). *Tissue Antigens,* **3**, 204
6. Tissot, R. G. and Cohen, C. (1974). *Transplantation,* **18**, 142
7. Sato, W. and deWeck, A. L. (1972). *Z. Immun.-Forsch.,* **144**, 49
8. Palm, J. and Wilson, D. B. (1973). *Transpl. Proc.,* **5**, 1573
9. Shreffler, D. C. and David, C. S. (1975). *Advan. Immunol.,* **20**, 125
10. Bacon, L. D., Kite, J. H. and Rose, N. R. (1974). *Science,* **186**, 274
11. DuPasquier, L. and Miggiano, V. C. (1973). *Transpl. Proc.,* **5**, 1457
12. DuPasquier, L., Chardonnens, X. and Miggiano, V. C. (1975). *Immunogenetics,* **1**, 482
13. Gorer, P. A. (1936). *Brit. J. Exp. Path.,* **17**, 42
14. Gorer, P. A. (1938). *J. Pathol. Bacteriol.,* **47**, 231
15. Gorer, P. A., Lyman, S. and Snell, G. D. (1948). *Proc. Roy. Soc. B,* **135**, 499
16. Gorer, P. A. and Mikulska, Z. B. (1954). *Cancer Res.,* **14**, 651
17. Gorer, P. A. and O'Gorman (1956). *Transpl. Bull.,* **3**, 142
18. Amos, D. B., Gorer, P. A. and Mikulska, Z. B. (1955). *Proc. Roy. Soc. B,* **144**, 369
19. Snell, G. D. (1958). *J. Nat. Cancer Inst.,* **21**, 843
20. Shreffler, D. C. and Owen, R. D. (1963). *Genetics,* **48**, 9
21. Boyse, E. A., Old, L. J. and Luell, S. (1964). *Nature (London),* **201**, 779
22. Lilly, F. (1966). *Genetics,* **53**, 529
23. Dutton, R. W. (1966). *J. Exp. Med.,* **123**, 665
24. McDevitt, H. O. and Tyan, M. L. (1968). *J. Exp. Med.,* **128**, 1
25. Klein, J. and Shreffler, D.C. (1971). *Transpl. Rev.,* **6**, 3
26. Snell, G. D., Cherry, M. and Demant, P. (1971). *Transpl. Proc.,* **3**, 183
27. Stimpfling, J. (1971). *Ann. Rev. Genet.,* **5**, 121
28. Hoecker, G., Counce, S. and Smith, P. (1954). *Proc. Nat. Acad. Sci. (USA),* **40**, 1040
29. Gorer, P. A. and Mikulska, Z. B. (1959). *Proc. Roy. Soc. B,* **151**, 57
30. Nathenson, S. G. (1970). *Ann. Rev. Genet.,* **4**, 69
31. Shreffler, D. C., David, C. S., Passmore, H. C. and Klein, J. (1971). *Transpl. Proc.,* **3**, 176
32. Snell, G. D., Cherry, M. and Demant, P. (1973). *Transpl. Rev.,* **15**, 1
33. Demant, P., Graff, R. J., Benesova, J. and Borovska, M. (1971). Transplantation analysis of H-2 recombinants. In *Immunogenetics of the H-2 System,* p. 148 (Basel: Karger)
34. Klein, J. and Shreffler, D. C. (1972). *J. Exp. Med.,* **135**, 924
35. Murphy, D. B. (1974). *Cross-reactivity between H-2K and H-2D products.* Ph.D. Thesis, University of Michigan
36. Nathenson, S. G. and Cullen, S. E. (1974). *Biochim. Biophys. Acta,* **344**, 1
37. Rask, L., Lindblom, J. B. and Peterson, P. A. (1974). *Nature (London),* **249**, 833
38. Brown, J. L., Kato, K., Silver, J. and Nathenson, S. G. (1974). *Biochemistry,* **13**, 3174
39. Stimpfling, J. H. and Reichert, A. E. (1970). *Transpl. Proc.,* **2**, 39
40. David, C. S., Stimpfling, J. H. and Shreffler, D. C. (1975). *Immunogenetics,* **2**, 131
41. Boyse, E. A. and Old, L. J. (1969). *Ann. Rev. Gen.,* **3**, 269
42. Scheid, M. P., Hoffman, M. K., Komuro, K., Hammerling, U., Abbot, J., Boyse, E. A., Cohen, G. H., Hooper, J. A., Schulof, R. S. and Goldstein, A. L. (1973). *J. Exp. Med.,* **138**, 350
43. Klein, J. (1972). *Tissue Antigens,* **2**, 262
44. Klein, J., Hauptfeld, M. and Hauptfeld, V. (1974). *Immunogenetics,* **1**, 45

45. Nabholz, M., Vives, J., Young, H. M., Meo, T., Miggiano, V., Rijnbeck, A. and Shreffler, D. C. (1974). *Eur. J. Immunol.,* **4**, 378

46. Alter, B. J., Schendel, D. J., Bach, M. L., Bach, F. H., Klein, J. and Stimpfling, J. H. (1973). *J. Exp. Med.,* **137**, 1303

47. Abbasi, K., Demant, P., Festenstein, H., Holmes, J., Huber, B. and Rychlikova, M. (1973). *Transpl. Proc.* **5**, 1329

48. Klein, J. and Egorov, I. K. (1973). *J. Immunol.,* **111**, 976

49. Brondz, B. D. (1972). *Transpl. Revs.,* **10**, 112

50. Boyse, E. A., Flaherty, L., Stockert, E. and Old, L. J. (1972). *Transplantation,* **13**, 431

51. Nabholz, M. (Personal communication)

52. Shreffler, D. C. (1965). The Ss system of the mouse. Quantitative serum protein difference genetically controlled by the H-2 region. In J. Palm (ed.), *Isoantigens and Cell Interactions,* p. 11 (Philadelphia: Wistar Institute Press)

53. Shreffler, D. C. and Passmore, H. C. (1971). Genetics of the H-2-associated Ss–Slp trait. In *Immunogenetics of the H-2 System,* p. 58 (Basel: Karger)

54. Demant, P., Capkova, J., Hinzova, E. and Voracova, B. (1973). *Proc. Nat. Acad. Sci. (USA),* **70**, 863

55. Hansen, T. H., Shin, H. and Shreffler, D. C. (1975). *J. Exp. Med.,* **141**, 1216

56. McDevitt, H. O., Deak, B. D., Shreffler, D. C., Klein, J., Stimpfling, J. H. and Snell, G. D. (1972). *J. Exp. Med.,* **135**, 1259

57. Benacerraf, B. and Katz, D. H. (1974). *Advan. Cancer Res.* (In press)

58. Lieberman, R., Paul, W. E., Humphrey, W. Jr. and Stimpfling, J. H. (1972). *J. Exp. Med.,* **136**, 1231

59. Dorf, M. E., Lilly, F. and Benacerraf, B. (1974). *J. Exp. Med.,* **140**, 859

60. Katz, D. H., Hamaoka, T., Dorf, M. E. and Benacerraf, B. (1973). *Proc. Nat. Acad. Sci. (USA),* **70**, 2624

61. Katz, D. H., Graves, M., Dorf, M. E., DiMuzio, H. and Benacerraf, B. (1974). *J. Exp. Med.* (In press)

62. Katz, D. H., Hamaoka, T., Dorf, M. E., Maurer, P. H. and Benacerraf, B. (1973). *J. Exp. Med.,* **138**, 734

63. Lilly, F. and Pincus, T. (1973). *Advan. Cancer Res.,* **17**, 231

64. Vladutiu, A. O. and Rose, N. R. (1971). *Science,* **174**, 1137

65. Amos, D. B. and Bach, F. H. (1968). *J. Exp. Med.,* **128**, 623

66. Rychlikova, M., Demant, P. and Ivanyi, P. (1971). *Nature (London), New Biology,* **230**, 271

67. Bach, F. H., Widmer, M. B., Bach, M. L. and Klein, J. (1972). *J. Exp. Med.,* **136**, 1430

68. Meo, T., Vives, G., Rijnbeek, A. M., Miggiano, V. C., Nabholz, M. and Shreffler, D. C. (1973). *Transpl. Proc.,* **5**, 1339

69. Demant, P. (1973). *Transpl. Rev.,* **15**, 164

70. Shreffler, D. C. (1974). Genetic fine structure of the H-2 gene complex. In G. Edelman (ed.), *Cellular Selection and Regulation in the Immune Response,* p. 83 (New York: Raven Press)

71. Oppltova, L. and Demant, P. (1973). *Transpl. Proc.,* **5**, 1367

72. Klein, J. and Park, J. M. (1973). *J. Exp. Med.,* **137**, 1213

73. David, C. S., Shreffler, D. C. and Frelinger, J. A. (1973). *Proc. Nat. Acad. Sci. (USA),* **70**, 2509

74. Hauptfeld, V., Klein, D. and Klein, J. (1973). *Science,* **181**, 167

75. Hammerling, G., Deak, B. D., Mauve, G., Hammerling, U. and McDevitt, H. O. (1974). *Immunogenetics,* **1**, 68

76. Gotze, D., Reisfeld, R. A. and Klein, J. (1973). *J. Exp. Med.,* **138**, 1003

77. Sachs, D. H. and Cone, J. L. (1973). *J. Exp. Med.,* **138**, 1289

78. Hämmerling, G. J., Mauve, G., Goldberg, E. and McDevitt, H. O. (1975). *Immunogenetics,* **1**, 428

79. Frelinger, J. A., Niederhuber, J. E., David, C. S. and Shreffler, D. C. (1974). *J. Exp. Med.,* **140**, 1273

80. Unanue, E. R., Dorf, M. E., David, C. S. and Benacerraf, B. (1974). *Proc. Nat. Acad. Sci. (USA).* (In press)

81. Cullen, S. E., David, C. S., Shreffler, D. C. and Nathenson, S. G. (1974). *Proc. Nat. Acad. Sci. (USA),* **71**, 648

82. Vitteta, E. S., Klein, J. and Uhr, J. W. (1974). *Immunogenetics,* **1**, 82

83. Cullen, S. E., Freed, J. H., Atkinson, P. H. and Nathenson, S. G. (1975). *Transpl. Proc.,* **7**, 237

84. Meo, T., David, C. S., Rijnbeek, A. M., Nabholz, M., Miggiano, V. and Shreffler, D. C. (1975). *Transpl. Proc.,* **7**, 127

85. Frelinger, J. A, Niederhuber, J. E. and Shreffler, D. C (1975). *Science,* **188**, 268

86. Dickler, H. B. and Sachs, D. H. (1974). *J. Exp. Med.,* **140**, 779

87. Dausset, J. (1958). *Acta Haematol.,* **20**, 156

88. Van Rood, J. J. and A. van Leeuwen (1963). *J. Clin. Invest.,* **42**, 1382

89. Payne, R., Tripp, M., Weigle, J., Bodmer, W. and Bodmer, J. (1964). *Cold Spring Harbor Symp. Quant. Biol.,* **29**, 285

90. Fu, S. M., Kunkel, H. G., Brusman, H. P., Allen, F. H., Jr. and Fotino, M. (1974). *J. Exp. Med.,* **140**, 1108

91. Allen, F. H. (1974). *Vox Sang.,* **27**, 382

92. Middleton, J., Crookston, M., Falk, J., Robson, E. B., Cook, P. J. L., Batchelor, J. R., Bodmer, J., Ferrara, G. B., Festenstein, H., Harris, R., Kissmeyer-Nielsen, F., Lawler, S. D., Sachs, J. A. and Wolf, E. (1974). *Tissue Antigens,* **4**, 366

93. Sanberg, L., Thorsby, E., Kissmeyer-Neilsen, F. and Lindholm, A. (1970). *Evidence of a third sub-locus within the HL-A chromosomal region.* In *Histocompatibility Testing,* p. 165. (Baltimore: Williams and Wilkins)

94. Solheim, B. G. and Thorsby, E. (1973). *Transpl. Proc.,* **5**, 1579

95. Mayr, W. R., Bernold, D., DeMarchi, M. and Ceppellini, R. (1973). *Transpl. Proc.,* **5**, 1581

96. Solheim, B. G., Bratlie, A., Sandberg, L., Staub-Neilsen, L. and Thorsby, E. (1973). *Tissue Antigens,* **3**, 439

97. Low, B., Messeter, L., Mansson, S. and Lindholm, T. (1974). *Tissue Antigens,* **4**, 405

98. Dausset, J. (Personal communication).

99. Colombani, J., Colombani, M. and Dausset, J. (1970). *Cross reactions in the HL-A system* 79. In *Histocompatibility Testing.* (Baltimore: Williams and Wilkins)

100. Tongio, M-M and Mayer, S. (1974). *Transplantation,* **18**, 163

101. Kahan, B. D. and Reisfeld, R. A. (1971). *Bacteriol. Rev.,* **35**, 59

102. Mann, D. L. and Fahey, J. L. (1971). *Ann. Rev. Microbiol.,* **25**, 679

103. Springer, T. A., Strominger, J. L. and Mann, D. L. (1974). *Proc. Nat. Acad. Sci. (USA),* **71**, 1539

104. Nakamuro, K., Tanigaki, N. and Pressman, D. (1973). *Proc. Nat. Acad. Sci. (USA),* **70**, 2863

105. Cresswell, P., Springer, T., Strominger, J. L., Turner, M. J., Grey, H. and Kubo, R. T. (1974). *Proc. Nat. Acad. Sci. (USA),* **71**, 2123

106. Solheim, B. G. and Thorsby, E. (1974). *Tissue Antigens,* **4**, 83

107. Yunis, E. J., Plate, J. M., Ward, F. E., Seigler, H. F. and Amos, D. B. (1971). *Transpl. Proc.,* **3**, 118

108. Yunis, E. J. and Amos, D. B. (1971). *Proc. Nat. Acad. Sci. (USA),* **68**, 3031

109. Eijsvoogel, V. P., Van Rood, J. J., Toit, E. D. and Schellekens, P. T. A. (1972). *Eur. J. Immunol.,* **2**, 413

110. Bach, F. H. (1973). *Transpl. Proc.,* **5**, 23

111. Balner, H. and van Vreeswijk, W. (1975). *Transpl. Proc.*, **7**, 13

112. Robert, M., Betuel, H. and Revillard, J. P. (1973). *Tissue Antigens*, **3**, 39

113. Albert, E. D., Mempel, W. and Grosse-Wilde, H. (1973. *Transpl. Proc.* **5**, 1551

114. Thompson, J. S., Bonney, W. W., Lawton, R. L., Flink, R. J. and Corry, R. J. (1974). *Transplantation*, **17**, 438

115. Jorgensen, F., Lamm, V. and Kissmeyer-Nielsen, F. (1973). *Tissue Antigens*, **3**, 323

116. Mempel, W., Grosse-Wilde, H., Baumann, P., Netzel, B., Steinbauer-Rosenthal, I., Scholz, S., Bertrams, J. and Albert, E. D. (1973). *Transpl. Proc.*, **5**, 1529

117. Eijsvoogel, V. P., duBois, R., Melief, C. J. M., Zeylemaker, W. P., Raatkoning, L. and deGroof-Kooy, L. (1973). *Transpl. Proc.*, **5**, 1301

118. Schendel, D. J., Alter, B. J. and Bach, F. H. (1973). *Transpl. Proc.*, **5**, 1651

119. Hors, J., Feingold, N., Fradelizi, D. E. and Dausset, J. (1971). *Lancet*, **i**, 609

120. Opelz, G., Mickey, M. R. and Terasaki, P. I. (1973). *Transplantation*, **16**, 649

121. Myburgh, J. A., Maier, G., Smit, J. A., Shapiro, M., Meyers, A. M., Rabkin, R., vanBlerk, P. J. P. and Jersky, J. (1974). *Transplantation*, **18**, 206

122. Lilly, F., Graham, H. and Coley, R. (1973). *Transpl. Proc.*, **5**, 193

123. Dausset, J., Hors, J., Busson, M., Festenstein, H., Oliver, R. T. D., Paris, A. M. I. and Sachs, J. A. (1974). *New Eng. J. Med.*, **290**, 979

124. Jersild, C. (1974). *Tissue Antigens*, **4**, 405

125. Blumenthal, M. N., Amos, D. B., Noreen, H., Mendell, N. R. and Yunis, E. J. (1974). *Science*, **184**, 1301

126. Marsh, D. G., Bias, W. B., Hsu, S. H. and Goodfried, L. (1973). *Science*, **179**, 691

127. Marsh, D. G., Bias, W. and Ishizaka, K. (1974). *Proc. Nat. Acad. Sci. (USA)*, **71**, 3588

128. Dausset, J., Degos, L. and Hors, J. (1974). *Clin. Immunol. Immunopath.*, **3**, 127

129. McDevitt, H. O. and Bodmer, W. F. (1974). *Lancet*, **i**, 1269

130. Bertrams, J., Kuwert, E., Bohme, U., Reis, H. E., Gallmeier, W. M., Wetter, O. and Schmidt, C. G. (1972). *Tissue Antigens*, **2**, 41

131. Rogentine, G. N., Trapani, R. J., Yankee, R. A. and Henderson, E. S. (1973). *Tissue Antigens*, **3**, 470

132. Brewerton, D. A., Hart, F. D., Nicholls, A., Caffrey, M. and James, D. C. O. (1973). *Lancet*, **i**, 904

133. Schlosstein, L., Terasaki, P. I., Bluestone, R. and Pearson, C. M. (1973). *New Engl. J. Med.*, **288**, 704

134. Brewerton, D. A., Caffrey, M., Nicholls, A., Walters, D. and James, D. C. O. (1973). *Lancet*, **ii**, 994

135. Zachariae, H., Hjortshoj, A. and Kissmeyer-Nielsen, F. (1973). *Lancet*, **ii**, 565

136. Rachelefsky, G. S., Terasaki, P. I., Katz, R. and Stiehm, E. R. (1974). *N. Engl. J. Med.*, **290**, 892

137. Katz, S. I., Falchuk, Z. M., Dahl, M. V., Rogentine, G. N. and Strober, W. (1972). *J. Clin. Invest.*, **51**, 2977

138. Fritze, D., Hermann, C. Jr., Smith, G. S. and Walford, R. L. (1973). *Lancet*, **ii**, 211

139. Seignalet, J., Clot, J., Guilhou, J. J., Duntze, F., Meynadier, J. and Robinet-Levy, M. (1974). *Tissue Antigens*, **4**, 59

140. Jersild, C., Hansen, G. S., Svejgaard, A., Fog, T., Thomsen, M. and Dupont, B. (1973). *Lancet*, **ii**, 7840

141. Storb, R., Thomas, E. D., Bruckner, C. D., Clift, R. A., Johnson, F. L., Fefer, A., Glucksberg, H., Lerner, K. G., Neiman, P. E., Weiden, P. L. and Wright, S. E. (1975). *Transpl. Proc.*, **7**, 813

142. Balner, H., D'Amaro, J. and Visser, T. P. (1974). *Transpl. Proc.*, **6**, 141

143. Balner, H., van Vreeswijk, W., de Groot, M. L. and D'Amaro, J. (1974). *Transpl. Proc.*, **6**, 111

144. Dorf, M. E., Balner, H., de Groot, M. L. and Benacerraf, B. (1974). *Transpl. Proc.*, **6**, 119

145. Ziegler, J. B., Alper, C. A. and Balner, H. (1975). *Nature (London)*, **254**, 609

146. Albert, E. D., Erickson, V. M., Graham, T. C., Parr, M., Templeton, J. W., Mickey, M. R., Thomas, E. D. and Storb, R. (1973). *Tissue Antigens,* **3,** 417

147. VandenTweel, J. G., Vriesendorp, H. M. and Westbroek, D. L. (1975). *Transpl. Proc.* (In press)

148. Ellman, L., Green, I., Martin, W. and Benacerraf, B. (1970). *Proc. Nat. Acad. Sci. (USA),* **66,** 322

149. Shevach, E., Paul, W. and Green, I. (1973). *J. Exp. Med.,* **139,** 661

150. Shevach, E., Green, I. and Paul, W. (1973). *J. Exp. Med.,* **139,** 679

151. Shevach, E. (Personal communication)

152. Cohen, C. and Tissot, R. G. (1974). *Transplantation,* **18,** 150

153. Kren, V., Stark, O., Bila, V., Frenzl, B., Krenova, D. and Krisakova, M. (1973). *Transpl. Proc.,* **5,** 1463

154. Wilson, D. B. (1967). *J. Exp. Med.,* **126,** 625

155. Vaimen, M., Renard, C., Lafage, P., Ameteau, J. and Nizza, P. (1970). *Transplantation,* **10,** 155

156. Bradley, B., White, D. and Edwards, J. (1974). *Tissue Antigens,* **4,** 283

157. Briles, W., McGibbon, W. and Irwin, M. (1950). *Genetics,* **35,** 633

158. Schierman, L. and Nordskog, A. (1961). *Science,* **134,** 1008

159. Jaffe, W. and McDermid, E. (1962). *Science,* **137,** 984

160. Miggiano, V., Birgen, I. and Pink, J. (1974). *Eur. J. Immunol.,* **4,** 397

161. Gunther, E., Rude, E. and Stark, O. (1972). *Eur. J. Immunol.,* **2,** 151

162. Gunther, E., Rude, E., Meyer-Delius, M. and Stark, O. (1973). *Transplant. Proc.,* **5,** 1467

163. Rude, E. and Gunther, E. (1975). Genetic control of the immune response to synthetic polypeptides in rats and mice. In *Proc. of the 2nd Internat. Congr. Immunol.* (In press)

164. Crittenden, L., Briles, W. and Stone, H. (1970). *Science,* **169,** 1324

165. Gunther, E., Balcarova, J., Hala, K., Rude, E. and Hraba, T. (1974). *Eur. J. Immunol.,* **4,** 548

166. Toivanen, A. and Toivanen, P. (1975). *Transpl. Proc.,* **7,** 165

4
The Nature and Function of Histocompatibility-linked Immune Response Genes

BARUJ BENACERRAF and DAVID H. KATZ

ABBREVIATIONS

AEF	= allogeneic effect factor; biologically active product of activated T cells
ASC	= extract of *Ascaris suum*
BGG	= bovine γ-globulin
BSA	= bovine serum albumin
C region	= constant region of immunoglobulins
CI gene	= Cell Interaction gene (or molecules)
D-GL	= copolymer of D-glutamic acid and D-lysine
DNP	= 2,4-dinitrophenyl
GA	= copolymer of L-glutamic acid and L-alanine
GAT	= terpolymer of L-glutamic acid, L-alanine and L-tyrosine
GEL	= gallinaceous lysozymes
GL	= copolymer of L-glutamic acid and L-lysine
GLA	= terpolymer of L-glutamic acid, L-lysine, L-alanine
GLϕ	= terpolymer of L-glutamic acid, L-lysin and L-phenylalanine
GLPro	= terpolymer of L-glutamic acid, L-lysine and L-proline
GLT	= terpolymer of L-glutamic acid, L-lysine and L-tyrosine

GPA	=	guinea pig albumin
GT	=	copolymer of L-glutamic acid and L-tyrosine
H-2	=	major histocompatibility complex of the mouse
(H,G)-A- -L	=	branched multichain synthetic polypeptide of poly-L-(histidyl, glutamyl)-poly-DL-alanyl–poly-L-lysyl
HL-A	=	major histocompatibility complex of man
H-linked	=	histocompatibility linked
I-A, I-B, I-C	=	the three defined subregions of the *I* region of *H-2*; located between *K* and *S* regions.
Ir gene	=	Immune response gene
Ir-1	=	the first identified H-linked *Ir* gene locus in the mouse; located in the *I-A* subregion of the *I* region of *H-2* gene complex
KLH	=	keyhole limpet haemocyanin
MBSA	=	methylated bovine serum albumin
NASE	=	staphylococcal nuclease
PFC	=	plaque-forming cells
(Phe,G)-A- -L	=	branched multichain synthetic polypeptide of poly-L-(phenylalanyl, glutamyl)-poly-DL-alanyl–poly-L-lysyl
PLA	=	homopolymer of poly-L-arginine
PLO	=	homopolymer of poly-L-ornithine
PLL	=	homopolymer of poly-L-lysine
PPD	=	purified protein derivative of tuberculin
RE	=	ragweed extract
RhL–A	=	major histocompatibility complex of rhesus monkeys
SRBC	=	sheep red blood cells
(T,G)-A- -L	=	branched multichain synthetic polypeptide of poly-L-(tyrosyl, glutamyl)-poly-DL-alanyl–poly-L-lysyl
V region	=	variable region of immunoglobulins

4.1 IMMUNE RESPONSES CONTROLLED BY HISTOCOMPATIBILITY-LINKED *Ir* GENES: SPECIES DISTRIBUTION

The recognition of specific antigens as immunogens by individual animals and inbred strains is governed by the products of individual dominant immune response (*Ir*) genes located in the genome in close relationship with genes of the major histocompatibility complex[1-3]. This has now been verified in mice[4], guinea pigs[5], rats[6-8] and rhesus monkeys[9,10]. These genes have been termed histocompatibility or H-linked *Ir* genes. The presence of the relevant genes permits immune responses to be formed, characterized by cellular immunity and antibody synthesis against the determinants on the antigens concerned. Three types of antigens have been most useful in the identification of H-linked *Ir* genes: (1) synthetic polypeptides with limited structural heterogeneity; (2) alloantigens which differ slightly from their autologous counterparts; and (3) complex multideterminant antigens administered in limiting immunizing doses in conditions where presumably only the most immunogenic determinants are recognized. Thus, the discovery of specific H-linked *Ir* genes has depended upon experiments wherein the immunological system is presented with a challenge of highly restricted heterogeneity and specificity. These conditions tend to limit the possibility of specific interactions between the antigens and the clones of immunocompetent cells. This approach revealed in a relatively short time that the responses of experimental animals to a wide variety of antigens are under the control of dominant H-linked *Ir* genes. All of these antigens share also an important characteristic: they are thymus-dependent antigens. No H-linked *Ir* gene control has been observed to date of a thymus-independent response, which may have considerable significance when an analysis is made of the process controlled by H-linked *Ir* genes in immune responses (Section 4.9). The dominant gene control of specific immune responses has been totally unexpected for immunologists considering the complexity of immune phenomena and the enormous range of specificities against which antibodies can be formed. These observations provide, therefore, both a challenge to the classical theory of the recognition of immunological specificity solely by pre-existing immunoglobulin receptors on immunocompetent cells, as well as powerful tools to analyse the complex interactions between antigens and the various cell types — macrophages, B and T cells — concerned collectively with the development of specific immunity.

In this section we shall address ourselves to a description of the specific immune responses which have been shown to be under the control of H-linked *Ir* genes in guinea pigs, mice, rats and rhesus monkeys.

4.1.1 Guinea pig H-linked *Ir* genes

Two inbred guinea pig strains, 2 and 13 (developed by Sewall Wright from a small closed colony), as well as random-bred lines, have been used to study the genetic control of specific immune responsiveness. The synthetic polypeptide antigens used in those studies are described in Table 4.1.

The gene which controls the response to poly-L-lysine (PLL) was the first specific immune response gene identified[11]. It controls responsiveness to the positively charged homopolymers PLL, poly-L-arginine (PLA), poly-L-ornithine (PLO), to copolymers of L-glutamic acid and L-lysine (GL), and to hapten conjugates of these polypeptides. The *PLL* gene is found in all strain 2 and some Hartley guinea pigs and is lacking in strain 13 animals.

The immune response of guinea pigs to the antigens, the recognition of which is under the control of H-linked *Ir* genes, is characterized by delayed hypersensitivity, by *in vitro* correlates of cellular immunity (such as the produc-

Table 4.1 Polypeptide antigens to which the responses are controlled by specific guinea pig *Ir* genes

(A)—Homopolymers:	
1. Poly-L-lysine	PLL
2. Poly-L-arginine	PLA
3. Poly-L-ornithine	PLO
(B)—Copolymers of:	
1. 60% L-Glutamic acid 40% L-Lysine	GL
2. 60% L-Glutamic acid 40% L-Alanine	GA
3. 50% L-Glutamic acid 50% L-Tyrosine	GT
4. 60% L-Glutamic acid 30% L-Alanine 10% L-Tyrosine	GAT
(C)—Hapten polypeptide conjugates of PLL and GL:	
1. 2,4-Dinitrophenyl–poly-L-lysine	DNP–PLL
2. Benzylpenicilloyl–poly-L-lysine	BPO–PLL
3. 2,4-Dinitrophenyl–GL	DNP–GL

tion of migration inhibitory factor or MIF, and specific blast transformation) and by the synthesis of significant levels of specific antibody[1,2]. Animals lacking the gene never develop delayed sensitivity and do not produce significant levels of antibodies under usual conditions of immunization. The activity of these immune response genes in guinea pigs is, therefore, responsible for clear-cut qualitative differences between responder and non-responder animals.

The initial breeding studies were carried out in random-bred Hartley animals previously immunized with DNP–PLL[11]. Responder and non-responder animals were mated separately. Table 4.2 shows that 82% of the offspring of eight breeding pairs of guinea pigs were responders, whereas none of 26 offspring of nine breeding pairs of non-responder parents showed a demonstrable response to DNP–PLL, indicating that responsiveness to this antigen is inherited as an autosomal Mendelian dominant trait. The experiments with inbred strain 2 and strain 13 animals confirmed this conclusion[12].

Table 4.2 Antigenicity of DNP–PLL in offspring of responder and non-responder random-bred guinea pigs

Parents	Offspring	
Responders* (8 breeding pairs)	Responders* 18; 82% (6♂, 12♀)	Non-responders† 4; 18% (1♂, 3♀)
Non-responders† (9 breeding pairs)	0	26 (14♂, 12♀)

* Responders refer to guinea pigs who showed an immune response to DNP–PLL, evidenced by skin reactivity to DNP–PLL and PCA or passive haemolysis with their sera with DNP–BSA
† Non-responders are animals which were negative to all these three tests

As shown in Table 4.3[12], the abilities of inbred guinea pigs to form immune responses to the synthetic polypeptide antigens, DNP–PLL, GA and GT and to limiting doses of native antigens and their hapten conjugates, bovine serum albumin (BSA), DNP–BSA, DNP–guinea pig albumin (DNP–GPA) are inherited according to strict Mendelian genetics, indicating that the immune responses to these antigens in the guinea pig are controlled by distinct dominant *Ir* genes. Thus, strain 2 but not strain 13 guinea pigs respond to DNP–PLL, GL, GA and to low doses of BSA and DNP–BSA, whereas strain 13, but not strain 2, respond to GT and to limiting doses of DNP–GPA. All (2 × 13) F$_1$ animals are responders to all of these antigens, illustrating the dominant character of these responses.

Table 4.3 Inheritance of specific *Ir* genes and of the major histocompatibility locus of strain 2 and strain 13 guinea pigs by (2 × 13)F$_1$ and backcross animals

Antigens	Strain		(2 × 13)F$_1$	(2 × 13)F$_1$ × 13		(2 × 13)F$_1$ × 2	
	2	13		50%*	50%	50%	50%
DNP–PLL	+†	−†	+	+	−		
GL	+	−	+	+	−		
GA	+	−	+	+	−		
GT	−	+	+			+	−
BSA 0.1 μg	+	−	+	+	−		
DNP–BSA 1 μg	+	−	+	+	−		
DNP–GPA 1 μg	−	+	+			+	−
Major H locus							
strain 2	+†		+	+	−		
strain 13		+	+			+	−

* Column identifies the same group of backcross animals
† Plus indicates responsiveness and presence of major histocompatibility specificities: minus indicates non-responsiveness and absence of major histocompatibility specificities of the inbred strains

Responsiveness to DNP–PLL, GA and to low doses of BSA and DNP–BSA segregate together in 50% of (2 × 13)F$_1$ × 13 backcross guinea pigs. On the other hand, the abilities to respond to GT and to low doses of DNP–GPA are inherited together by 50% of (2 × 13)F$_1$ × 2 backcross offspring[12].

The genetic analysis can be pursued further taking advantage of the fact that in guinea pigs, contrary to mice, the *Ir* genes detected in inbred strains are also found in a significant proportion of random-bred animals. The genes controlling immune responsiveness to GA, GT and PLL are not inherited independently. As we have seen, the *GA* gene and the *PLL* gene are linked in strain 2 and (2 × 13)F$_1$ guinea pigs. Responsiveness to GA and PLL are also linked in most Hartley responder guinea pigs. However, there is a small proportion of Hartley guinea pigs which respond to GA and not to PLL or to PLL and not to GA[12]. The existence of random-bred animals which respond to GA and not to PLL, which may result from cross-over between the *PLL* gene and the *GA* gene, may be considered evidence for the non-identity of these two genes.

Similarly, the ability to respond to GT in random-bred Hartley animals is also not independent of the PLL or GA responder status. But in this case, responsiveness to GT tends to segregate away from PLL and GA responsiveness, indicating allelism or pseudo-allelism in random-bred animals between the *GT* gene on the one hand and the *PLL* and *GA* genes on the other.

However, recent genetic studies carried out by Shevach and associates on the *GA* and *GT* genes in random-bred guinea pigs have shown that the *GT* and the *GA* genes are not alleles since they are found to be associated in some animals[13]. Responsiveness to low doses of BSA, which is found linked with both the *PLL* and *GA* genes in inbred strain 2 guinea pigs, shows no association with these genes in random-bred Hartley animals[3]. The conclusion can be drawn from the studies in outbred guinea pigs that in this species distinct non-allelic genes control responsiveness to PLL, GA, GT, low doses of BSA and low doses of DNP–GPA. In the case of certain antigens with closely related structural properties such as the homopolymers PLL, PLA, PLO and the copolymer GL, no dissociation of responsiveness could be detected in random-bred guinea pigs indicating that responsiveness to these antigens is controlled by either the same gene or very closely linked genes[14].

4.1.2 Mouse H-linked *Ir* genes

Similar to what was found in guinea pigs, specific *Ir* genes controlling responsiveness to synthetic polypeptides and to limiting doses of protein antigens have been identified in mice[1-3]. In addition, in the mouse many H-linked *Ir* genes have been discovered which control responsiveness to allo-antigens (see Figure 4.1). The mouse has truly been the most rewarding species for the study of H-linked *Ir* genes because of the availability of: (1) numerous inbred strains developed by students of tissue transplantation; (2) congenic resistant strains which differ only at the *H-2* complex; and (3) strains with documented recombinant events within the *H-2* complex, precisely in the region where the *Ir* genes are located. Whereas in the guinea pig the response to polypeptide antigens under H-linked *Ir* gene control are all-or-none responses characterized both by delayed hypersensitivity and antibody synthesis, in the mouse, a species which exhibits poor delayed hypersensitivity, the data has relied almost exclusively on the genetic control of specific antibody synthesis. Although recently, Shearer has observed that in the mouse the ability to develop delayed sensitivity to the branched copolymer (T,G)-A- -L is also under the same genetic control as the ability to form high levels of IgG antibodies to this antigen[15]. In addition, although the responder mouse strains possessing the relevant *Ir* genes always produced high levels of serum antibodies, the non-responder strains, depending upon the antigen and the strain, were often characterized as 'low-responders'. This is particularly the case for the branched

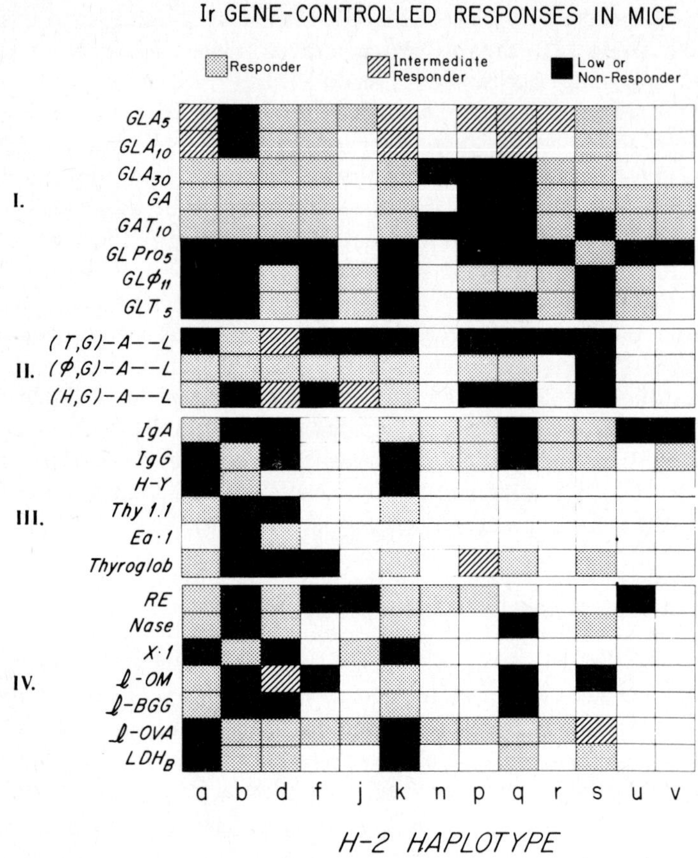

Figure 4.1 Immune responses under H-linked *Ir* gene control of mice bearing 13 different *H-2* haplotypes to four classes of antigens.

I. Random linear copolymers of L-amino acids
II. Branched copolymers of L-amino acids
III. Murine alloantigens
IV. Foreign antigens

I. *Random linear copolymers of* L-*amino acids*
   $GLA^5 = (Glu^{57}Lys^{38}Ala^5)^\eta$ (Ref. 1)
   $GLA^{30} = (Glu^{35}Lys^{35}Ala^{30})^\eta$ (Ref. 2)
   $GAT^{10} = (Glu^{60}Ala^{30}Tyr^{10})^\eta$ (Ref. 2, 4, 5)
   $GL\phi^{11} = (Glu^{53}Lys^{36}Phe^{11})^\eta$ (Ref. 2, 6)
   $GLA^{10} = (Glu^{54}Lys^{36}Ala^{10})^\eta$ (Ref. 1)
   $GA = (Glu^{60}Ala^{40})^\eta$ (Ref. 2, 3)
   $GLPro^5 = (Glu^{57}Lys^{38}Pro^5)^\eta$ (Ref. 2)
   $GLT^5 = (Glu^{57}Lys^{38}Tyr^5)^\eta$ (Ref. 2, 3)

II. *Branched copolymers of* L-*amino acids*
    (T,G)-A- -L = (Tyr,Glu)-Ala–Lys
    (H,G)-A- -L = (His,Glu)-Ala–Lys
    (ϕ,G)-A- -L = (Phe,Glu)-Ala–Lys
    (Ref. 7, 8)

III. *Murine alloantigens*
    IgA = Allotype determinants on BALB/c IgA myeloma (Ref. 9, 10)
    IgG = Allotype determinants on BALB/c IgG myeloma (Ref. 9, 10)
    H-Y = Histocompatibility antigen coded for by the Y chromosome (Ref. 11)
    Thy 1.1 = Mouse thymocyte antigen, theta (Ref. 12)
    Ea.1 = Mouse red blood cell antigen (Ref. 13)
    Thyroglob = Mouse thyroglobulin (Ref. 14)

IV. *Foreign antigens*
    RE = Ragweed extract antigens (Ref. 15)
    NASE = Staphylococcal nuclease (Ref. 16)
    X.1 = Leukaemia associated transplantation antigen (Ref. 17)
    ℓ-OM = Low dose of bovine γ-globulin
    ℓ-BGG = Low dose of bovine γ-globulin
    ℓ-OVA = Low dose of ovalbumin (Ref. 18, 19, 20)
    LDH_B = Porcine lactic dehydrogenase B (Ref. 21)

References

1. Maurer, P. H. and Merryman, C. F. (1974). *Immunogenetics,* 1, 174
2. Dorf, M. E. and Benacerraf, B. (Unpublished data)
3. Merryman, D. F. and Maurer, P. H. (1973). *Fed. Proc.,* 32, 995
4. Martin, W. J., Maurer, P. H. and Benacerraf, B. (1972). *J. Immunol.,* 107, 715
5. Merryman, C. F. and Maurer, P. H. (1972). *J. Immunol.,* 108, 135
6. Merryman, C. F., Maurer, P. H. and Bailey, D. W. (1972). *J. Immunol.,* 108, 937
7. McDevitt, H. O. and Chinitz, A. (1969). *Science,* 163, 1207
8. McDevitt, H. O. and Landy, M., (eds.). (1972). *Genetic Control of Immune Responsiveness: Relationship to Disease Susceptibility* (New York: Academic Press)
9. Lieberman, R. and Humphrey, W., Jr. (1972). *J. Exp. Med.,* 136, 1222
10. Lieberman, R., Paul, W. E., Humphrey, W., Jr. and Stimpfling, J. H. (1972). *J. Exp. Med.,* 136, 1231
11. Stimpfling, J. H. and Reichert, A. E. (1971). *Transplantation,* 12, 527
12. Fuji, H., Zaleski, M. and Milgrom, F. (1971). *Transpl. Proc.,* 3, 852
13. Gasser, D. L. (1969). *J. Immunol.,* 103, 66
14. Vladiutiu, A. O. and Rose, N. R. (1971). *Science,* 174, 1137
15. Dorf, M. E., Newburger, P. E., Hamaoka, T., Katz, D. H. and Benacerraf, B. (1974). *Eur. J. Immunol.,* 4, 346
16. Lozner, E. C., Sachs, D. H. and Shearer, G. M. (1974). *J. Exp. Med.,* 139, 1204
17. Sato, H., Boyse, E. A., Aoki, T., Iritani, C. and Old, L. J. (1973). *J. Exp. Med.,* 138, 593
18. Vaz, N. M. and Levine, B. B. (1970). *Science,* 168, 852
19. Dunham, E. K., Dorf, M. E. and Benacerraf. B. (Unpublished data)
20. Vaz, N. M. and Levine, B. B. (1970). *J. Immunol.,* 104, 1572
21. Melchers, I., Rajewsky, K. and Shreffler, D. C. (1973). *Eur. J. Immunol.,* 3, 754

multi-chain synthetic copolymers most extensively studied by McDevitt and Sela[16], (T,G)-A- -L, (H,G)-A- -L and (Phe,G)-A- -L. The response to these polypeptides was the first to be shown in mice to be under dominant H-linked *Ir* gene control at a locus designated *Ir-1*[17]. Thus, the ability of inbred mice to make antibodies in response to each of these antigens is a quantitative genetic trait. The antibody responses to other polypeptide antigens, i.e. the random copolymers of two or three of the following L-amino acids — glutamic acid, alanine, lysine, tyrosine, phenylalanine and proline — behave as all-or-none responses in most inbred strains of mice[18] as they do in guinea pigs.

In Figure 4.1 we have compiled all the available information on the responses of strains with 13 distinct *H-2* haplotypes to 24 antigens: (a) eight linear copolymers and three branched copolymers of L-amino acids; (b) six mouse allo-antigens; and (c) seven conventional native antigens. The response to each of these 24 antigens was shown to be under dominant H-linked *Ir* gene control (for references, see Figure 4.1). As will be shown in Section 4.3, many of these genes have been mapped in the *I* region within the *H-2* complex.

The relatively large number of antigens and of inbred strains which have been used to obtain the data summarized in Figure 4.1 in a chequer-board fashion makes some comparison meaningful. Analysis of the results demonstrate two important points: (1) Except for the *H-2^k* and *H-2^a* strains and the *H-2^n* and *H-2^p* strains which display identical patterns, respectively, no two strains with different *H-2* haplotypes behave alike in their response patterns when a sufficiently large panel of antigens is used. The strain bearing the *H-2^k* and *H-2^a* haplotypes should display identical response patterns as they share the left part of the *H-2* complex which comprises the *I* region where all known *Ir* genes have been mapped. Furthermore, the most recent serological analysis has raised doubts whether the strains bearing the *H-2^p* and *H-2^n* haplotypes could be distinguished[19]. (2) More significantly, most antigens for which sufficient data is available elicit different response patterns in the inbred strains bearing different *H-2* haplotypes with a few notable exceptions. These exceptions are of two types. Identical response patterns are observed for polypeptides with closely related structures such as GLA[5] and GLA[10] (which differ by only 5% L-alanine residues) and GLA[30] and G[60]A[40]. It is, therefore, very probable that the same genes control the responses to GLA[5] and GLA[10] and to GLA[30] and G[60]A[40], respectively. Identical response patterns are observed also for two couples of unrelated antigens, *i.e.* for the copolymer (H,G)-A--L and ovomucoid, and for ragweed extract (RE) and staphylococcal nuclease (NASE). The similarity in response patterns for these unrelated antigens is most probably fortuitous since, as shown in Figure 4.3, the *Ir* genes controlling the response to RE and NASE have been mapped in different segments of the *H-2* complex.

The distinctive strain distribution of responses observed for most antigens which have been studied in a sufficient number of strains with different *H-2* haplotypes may be considered a strong argument that the *Ir* genes concerned with the control of most of these responses are distinct. Additional evidence will be presented in Section 4.3 in favour of this interpretation.

The most important information which can be derived from Figure 4.1 concerns the specificity of the genetic control of the responses to synthetic polypeptides. Thus, the antigens GLT[5], GLϕ[11], GLPro[5], differ from each other only in the third amino acid which constitutes from 5 to 11% of the residues of these copolymers. The antibody responses to these antigens are so cross-reactive that responsiveness to each of these three polymers could be accurately ascertained by measuring the serum antibodies reactive with GLT[5] [20]. However, the patterns of genetic responses for GLT[5], GLϕ[11] and GLPro[5] are absolutely distinct for the different *H-2* haplotypes. Similar statements can be made with respect to the antibody responses to (T,G)-A- -L, (ϕ,G)-A- -L and (H,G)-A- -L[2] and for the antibody responses to GA and GAT[10] [18], respectively. The genetic patterns are clearly different although the specific antibodies are very cross-reactive in both cases. Taken collectively, these findings indicate that the H-linked *Ir* gene control of specific immune responsiveness is not concerned with the structural genes for immunoglobulin V regions (as will be discussed in Section 4.2) and that the specificity for individual antigens displayed by the traits controlled by the individual H-linked *Ir* genes is not contributed by conventional immunoglobulin antibodies. Another very interesting finding shown in Figure 4.1 concerns the differences observed in the responsiveness to the copolymer G[60]A[40] and GAT[10] which differ only by the presence of 10% L-tyrosine residues in GAT[10]. The pattern of responsiveness is identical for these antigens for all strains except *H-2^s* strains which are responders to GA and non-responders to GAT[10]. The significant point is that the presence of 10% L-tyrosine has destroyed responsiveness of this antigen for strains bearing the *H-2^s* haplotype. Since, as will be shown in Section 1.4, GAT is capable of stimulating the response of GAT-specific suppressor T cells in animals with the three non-responder haplotypes, including *H-2^s*, the possibility must be considered that poly-L-tyrosine sequences are particularly suited to induce suppressor T cells in *H-2^s* mice. Experiments are in progress to investigate the immunogenicity for *H-2^s* mice of poly-L-tyrosine or of GA bearing poly-L-tyrosine sequences at the C or N terminal end and the ability of these polypeptides to stimulate suppressor T cells in the *H-2^s* strain as compared to other strains. These experiments are designed to study the fine specificity of immunogenicity *versus* suppression and also the possibility that the generation of specific suppressor T cells for a given antigen is also under H-linked genetic control as is the case for the recognition of immunogenicity for thymus-dependent antigens. The finding that mice bearing the *H-2^s* haplotype are non-responders to all polypeptides containing L-tyrosine or L-phenylalanine, such as GAT[10], GLT[5], (T,G)-A- -L, GLϕ[11], (ϕ,G)-A- -L, whereas *H-2^s* is the only responder haplotype of the eleven tested for GLPro[5] is an argument for this interpretation.

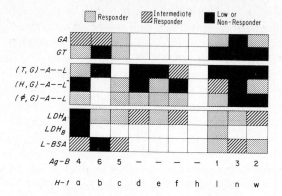

Figure 4.2 Immune responses under H-linked *Ir* gene control of rats bearing different *H-1* (*Ag-B*) haplotypes.

Antigens: Random linear copolymers of L-amino acids
GA $= (Glu^{60}A^{40})^{n}$ (Ref. 1)
GT $= (Glu^{50}Tyr^{50})^{n}$ (Ref. 1)

Branched copolymers:
(T,G)-A- -L $=$ (Tyr,Glu)-Ala- -Lys (Ref. 2)
(Phe,G)-A- -L $=$ (Phe,Glu)-Ala- -Lys (Ref. 3)
(H,G)-A- -L $=$ (His, Glu)-Ala- -Lys (Ref. 3)

Foreign antigens
LDH$_A$ $=$ Porcine lactic dehydrogenase A (Ref. 4, 5)
LDH$_B$ $=$ Porcine lactic dehydrogenase B (Ref. 6)
L-BSA $=$ Low dose bovine serum albumin (Ref. 1)

H-1, Ag-B $=$ Major histocompatibility complex in rats (Ref. 7, 8)

References

1. Armerding, D., Katz, D. H. and Benacerraf, B. (1974). *Immunogenetics*, **14**, 30
2. Gunther, R., Rude, E. and Stark, O. (1972). *Eur. J. Immunol.*, **2**, 151
3. Rude, E., Gunther, E., Liehl, E. and Wrede, J. (1972). *Eur. J. Immunol.*, **2**, 192
4. Armerding, D. and Rajewsky, K. (1970). In (H. Peeters, ed.). *Protides of Biol. Fluid. Proc. of the 17th Conf.*, p. 185 (Oxford and New York: Pergamon Press)
5. Wurzburg, V. (1971). *Eur. J. Immunol.*, **1**, 496
6. Wurzburg, V., Schutt-Gerowitt, H. and Rajewsky, K. (1973). *Eur. J. Immunol.*, **3**, 762
7. Palm, J. and Black, G. (1971). *Transplantation*, **11**, 184
8. Stark, O. and Kren, K. (1971). *Transpl. Proc.*, **3**, 165

4.1.3   Rat H-linked *Ir* genes

The same phenomenon of histocompatibility-linked gene control of specific immune responses to polypeptide and native antigens which has been demonstrated in guinea pigs and mice has also been observed in the rat (for references, see Figure 4.2). The number of antigens studied have been fewer than in the mouse but, as in other species, all the antigens for which this type of genetic control has been demonstrated are thymus-dependent antigens. The data are of considerable interest because the same results have been found in the rat and in other species and because in many cases the same antigens have been used to demonstrate the H-linked *Ir* gene control of specific immune responses in all experimental species investigated. The results available to date for the rat have been summarized in Figure 4.2. It is apparent that with the limited number of antigens studied, distinctive patterns of responsiveness have been obtained in the rat as in the mouse for (T,G)-A- -L, (H,G)-A- -L, (ϕG)-A- -L, GA and LDH$_A$. On the other hand, a similar strain distribution has been observed for the related polypeptide antigens (T,G)-A- -L and GT. The responses in the rat to antigens under H-linked *Ir* gene control are characterized as in the guinea pig by both the development of delayed hypersensitivity and the synthesis of high amounts of antibodies. On the other hand, as observed in the mouse for many antigens, rats bearing non-responder haplotypes are able to produce low amounts of antibodies. The study of H-linked *Ir* genes in different species leads to the conclusion that these genes behave in an identical manner and that they control precisely the same processes in all mammalian species in which they have been studied. These processes are essential for the development of specific immune responses to thymus-dependent antigens, are determined by different genes for structurally different antigens and presumably by the same gene or genes for structurally related antigens.

4.1.4   *Ir* Genes of the Rhesus monkey

Interest in the *Ir* genes of Rhesus monkeys stems from their phylogenetic relationship to man and the extensive data already available on the major histocompatibility complex of the monkey. At least two independent dominant H-linked *Ir* genes have been identified in the rhesus[9,10,18]. These genes control the ability of monkeys to respond to the random linear copolymer, GA, and to DNP–GL. These synthetic polymers can elicit weak delayed-type skin reactions and strong humoral responses in some monkeys. In a series of unrelated monkeys phenotyped for the serologically defined RhL–A specificity of both segregant series, there were no correlations between any RhL–A specificity and responder status to the GA or DNP–GL polymers. However, segregation analysis of 21 rhesus families sired by three fathers has established that the capacity of the offspring to form antibodies is associated with genes coded for in the RhL–A complex.

4.2 RELATIONSHIP OF H-LINKED *Ir* GENES TO ALLOTYPE-LINKED *Ir* GENES

In addition to the H-linked *Ir* genes, another class of specific *Ir* genes concerned with idiotypic specificities in immunoglobulins has been recently identified in the mouse in several laboratories. This second class of genes is not linked to histocompatibility genotype, but has been shown instead to be linked to the genes controlling immunoglobulin allotype determinants on the mouse heavy chain linkage group. These 'allotype-linked *Ir* genes' have been identified in responses of mice to antigens which stimulate the formation of antibodies with restricted specificity and heterogeneity such as $\alpha1,3$ dextran[21] and streptococcal polysaccharide[22]. Similarly, an idiotypic specificity was demonstrated by Pawlak and Nisonoff[23] to be very closely linked to heavy chain allotype markers in anti-*p*-azophenylarsonate antibodies produced by all mice of the BC9 strain possessing the heavy chain allotype of the AL/N strain on a BALB/c background. The structural genes coding for these idiotypes must, therefore, be closely linked to genes coding for the constant regions of mouse heavy chain immunoglobulins.

It is important to note that contrary to the methods used to study H-linked *Ir* genes, which rely on the identification of responder and non-responder strains and animals, the discovery of allotype-linked *Ir* genes has depended upon the characterization of the antibody produced. Allotype-linked *Ir* genes control idiotypic determinants or the fine specificity of the antibody produced. For these reasons and since the genes coding respectively for the V region and the C region of immunoglobulin chains are known to be linked, it is reasonable to conclude, and generally accepted, that allotype-linked *Ir* genes code for immunoglobulin V regions.

In contrast, there is a compelling body of evidence indicating that H-linked *Ir* genes do not code for immunoglobulin V regions. This is a crucial issue since it has been established that distinct H-linked *Ir* genes control responses to different antigens and, therefore, that the product of H-linked *Ir* genes must either directly or indirectly be concerned with specific recognition. This conclusion implies the existence of a second type of molecule and a second level concerned with immunological specificity besides immunoglobulins. The data must, therefore, be evaluated very critically in this respect. Particularly strong evidence is provided by studies on the genetics of the two systems. The immunoglobulin V regions of heavy chains are closely linked to the genes encoding the C regions. The rabbit allotype data concerning recombinants between the α and e loci is extremely convincing[24]. In addition, as stated above, the observed linkage of idiotypic specificities to H chain allotype[21-23] but not to *H-2* in inbred mice identify a new class of *Ir* genes coding for immunoglobulin V regions, as well as provide the techniques to recognize and study these genes. The objection might be raised that the evidence discussed above concerns only the H chain. However, it is clear that in man the L chain structural genes are not linked to the major histocompatibility complex, and if more precise genetic evidence is required, McDevitt observed several years ago that the response of rabbits to (T,G)-A- -L (which is under genetic control in this species as in mice) is not linked to the allotype *b* locus of the κ chain[25]. Since all current concepts of immunoglobulin structural genes postulate that the genes coding for the V and C regions are linked in both H and L chains, the genetic data discussed above establish that the H-linked *Ir* genes do not code for immunoglobulin V genes, a function which should be attributed to the increasing number of allotype-linked *Ir* genes, which are being identified in several laboratories.

The different methodologies which have permitted the detection of H-linked *Ir* genes and allotype-linked *Ir* genes support these conclusions. The ease with which H-linked *Ir* genes have been detected as determining responsiveness to antigens with limited structural heterogeneity or limited number of determinants contrasts with the sophisticated requirements to identify allotype-linked *Ir* genes which necessitate a detailed study of the fine specificity or structure of the antibody population synthesized. These differences have important implications for the two types of recognition systems coded by the two classes of *Ir* genes and indicate that the H-linked *Ir* genes are probably considerably less numerous than the range of immunoglobulin specificities that can be generated by the combination of H and L chain V regions.

Based on these considerations, the existence of another class of molecules with specificity for antigen, in addition to and distinct from immunoglobulin antibodies, was, therefore, originally proposed by Benacerraf and McDevitt[2]. Since the early data concerning the cells where the H-linked *Ir* genes are expressed (see Section 4.7) pointed to the T cells, and since the nature of the T cell receptor is still controversial, it was also proposed that this new class of antigen-specific molecule functions as the receptor for antigens on some or all T cells.

The close linkage of the H-linked *Ir* genes with genes of the major histocompatibility complex in all species investigated and the demonstration that (1) the binding of antigen by T cells[26,27] and (2) certain specific *in vitro* interactions of sensitized T cells with antigen (such as the stimulation of increased DNA synthesis by antigen[28-30]) could be inhibited by alloantisera against the products of the major histocompatibility complex motivated Benacerraf and McDevitt[2], Shevach *et al.*[29] and Katz and Benacerraf[31] to propose that this newly postulated class of antigen-specific molecule should contain polypeptide chains coded for by genes of the major histocompatibility complex. Then the demonstration by Katz, Benacerraf and associates that the essential T–B cell interactions which regulate immune responses are controlled by genes in the major histocompatibility complex located in precisely the same region as *Ir* genes[32] led to the conclusions that (1) these regulatory genes code for cell interaction (CI) molecules expressed on the surface of T and B cells, and (2) the *Ir* gene product and the CI product, if distinct, are probably expressed on the same molecular complex endowed both with specificity for antigen and with the ability to regulate immune responses[31]. These hypotheses have been given strong support by the independent demonstration by Taussig, Munro and associates[33,34], Mozes *et al.*[35] and Tada and associates[36,37] that T cells from immunized animals produce antigen-specific factors with helper or suppressor properties but which could not be absorbed by anti-immunoglobulin columns. These factors (discussed in Section 4.8) were also shown to have a molecular weight of around 50 000 daltons and to bear antigenic determinants coded for by the *I* region of the *H-2* complex, which is the very region where the H-linked *Ir* genes have been mapped (discussed in Section 4.3), and where the control of cell interactions in immune responses resides (discussed in Section 4.6). It is very possible indeed that these specific T cell factors have properties identical with the well-characterized allogeneic effect factor (AEF) studied by Armerding and Katz[38,39] produced by T cells undergoing allogeneic stimulation which is endowed with regulatory properties for both T cells and B cells (discussed in Section 4.8).

4.3 THE MAPPING OF H-LINKED *Ir* GENES OF THE MOUSE AND RHESUS MONKEY

4.3.1 Mapping of *Ir* genes of the mouse

A remarkable feature of the immune response genes is their intimate linkage in all species investigated with genes controlling histocompatibility specificities. The first evidence of such a linkage was provided in mice by the observations of McDevitt and Tyan[4] and McDevitt and Chinitz[40] that responsiveness of inbred mice to (T,G)-A- -L, (H,G)-A- -L and (Phe,G)-A- -L is determined by their *H-2* haplotype. The locus controlling these responses was termed *Ir-1*. In further studies with mice with known recombinant alleles McDevitt *et al.*[17] localized *Ir-1* in the *I* region of the *H-2* complex, a region distinct from the *K*, *D* and *S* regions.

The *I* region is located between *K* and *S* (reviewed in reference 41). Thus, as a result of the identification of *Ir-1* and of the mapping of other *Ir* genes (Table 4.4 and Figure 4.3), the *H-2* complex of the mouse has indeed been subdivided into four regions: *K*, *I*, *S* and *D*[41]. All known mouse *Ir* genes which could be precisely mapped have been localized in the *I* region and have been shown to be distinct from the genes coding for the histocompatibility

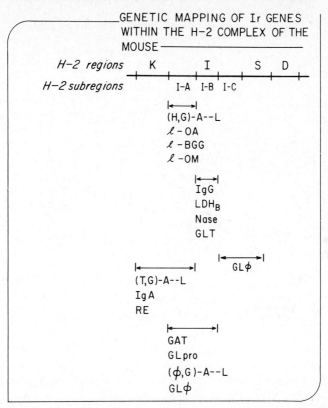

Figure 4.3 Mapping of several *Ir* genes in the *I* region of the *H-2* complex (Antigen abbreviations are explained in the legend of Figure 4.1)

References for Mapping Data

(H,G-A- -L), (Phe,G)-A- -L and (T,G)-A- -L   McDevitt, H. O., Deak, B. D., Shreffler, D. C., Klein, J., Stimpfling, J. H. and Snell, G. D. (1972). *J. Exp. Med.*, **135**, 1259

ℓ-OA   Dunham, E. K., Dorf, M. E., Shreffler, D. C. and Benacerraf, B. (1973). *J. Immunol.*, **111**, 1621

ℓ-BGG, ℓ-OM   Freed, J. H., Deak, B. D. and Bechtol, K. B. (1973). *Fed. Proc.*, **32**, 995

IgG, IgA   Lieberman, R., Paul, W. E., Humphrey, W., Jr. and Stimpfling, J. H. (1972). *J. Exp. Med.*, **136**, 1231

LDH_B   Melchers, I., Rajewsky, K. and Shreffler, D. C. (1973). *Eur. J. Immunol.*, **3**, 754

NASE   Lozner, E. C., Sachs, D. H. and Shearer, G. M. (1974). *J. Exp. Med.*, **139**, 1204

GLT, RE   Dorf, M. E., Lilly, F. and Benacerraf, B. (1974). *J. Exp. Med.*, **140**, 859

GAT, GLPro   Dorf, M. E., Plate, J. M. D., Stimpfling, J. H. and Benacerraf, B. (1975). *J. Immunol.*, **114**, 602

GLφ   Dorf, M. E., Lilly, F. and Benacerraf, B. (1974). *J. Exp. Med.*, **140**, 859

Dorf, M. E., Stimpfling, J. H. and Benacerraf, B. (1975). *J. Exp. Med.*, **41**, 1459

serological specificities which are controlled by the *K* and *D* regions. Furthermore, by the use of the few available strains with documented recombinant events in the *I* region between distinct *Ir* genes or between genes coding for serological specificities controlled by this region, the *I* region has been further subdivided into three subregions: *I-A*, *I-B* and *I-C* (see Table 4.4). To date, most *Ir* genes have been mapped in either the *I-A* and *I-B* regions; only one *Ir*

Table 4.4 Genetic fine structure of selected intra-*H-2* recombinant strains*

Strain	*H-2* haplotype	H-2 Regions†					
				I			
		K	I-A	I-B	I-C	S	D
B10.A or A/J	a	k	k	k⎮	d	d	d
B10.D2	d	d	d	d	d	d	d
A.SW	s	s	s	s	s	s	s
A.TH	t2	s	s	s	s	s⎮	d
B10.S (9R)	t4	s	s	s⎮	d	d	d
C57BL/10	b	b	b	b	b	b	b
B10.A(2R)	h2	k	k	k	d	d⎮	b
B10.A(4R)	h4	k	k⎮	b	b	b	b
B10.A(3R)	i3	b	b	b⎮	d	d	d
B10.A(5R)	i5	b	b	b⎮	d	d	d
B10.A(18R)	i18	b	b	b	b	b⎮	d
R106	i106	b	b	b	b	b⎮	da
A.AL	a1	k	k	k	k	k⎮	d
A.TL	t1	s⎮	k	k	k	k	d
D2.GD	g4	d	d⎮	b	b	b	b

* Modified from Shreffler and David[41]
† The letters under each region indicate haplotypes of origin for that region

gene has been recently localized in the *I-C* region as will be discussed later in this section. The available data is shown in Figure 4.3. The precise mapping of *Ir* genes is presently limited by the small number of *I* region recombinant strains available for study. Nevertheless, enough *Ir* genes have been shown to map in the *I* region distinct from the *K* region to permit the statement to be made that *Ir* genes are clearly distinct from the genes coding for the histocompatibility serological specificities. The crucial issues concerning the H-linked *Ir* genes are whether all genes controlling responses to different antigens can be distinguished from each other genetically and, if this is the case, how many *Ir* genes there are in the *I* region of the *H-2* complex. As illustrated in Figure 4.3, the answer to these questions has depended upon the existence of strains with documented crossing-over within the *I* region between distinct immune response genes. Two such recombinants, B10.A (4R) between *H-2^k* and *H-2^b* and D2.GD between *H-2^d* and *H-2^b* have been identified and their responses to relevant antigens have been studied. These two recombinant strains have indeed defined the two *I* subregions termed *I-A* and *I-B*. The B10.A (4R) strain was the first to be recognized by Lieberman *et al.*[42] as a recombinant in the *I* region between the *Ir* genes controlling the response to allotype determinants on IgG and IgA BALB/c myelomas, respectively. More recently, the D2.GD strain was shown by Dorf, Lilly and Benacerraf[43] to also be a recombinant between specific *Ir* genes, i.e. the gene controlling the response to ragweed extract and genes controlling the responses to the copolymers GLT[5] and GLφ[11]. It is not clear, however, whether these recombinants in the *I* region between

I-A and *I-B* were generated by cross-over events at precisely the same place in the chromosome.

The development of more recombinant strains between known specific *Ir* genes are required (1) to better resolve the *I* region, (2) to establish whether all of the other *Ir* genes located in the *I-A* and *I-B* subregions are indeed distinct genes, and (3) to arrive at an estimate of how many *Ir* loci exist. Nonetheless, on the basis of the available evidence, it is reasonable to consider that most of the specific mouse *Ir* genes controlling responsiveness to different antigens are indeed the products of distinct loci. As stated in Section 4.1, this interpretation would better account for the unique patterns of immune responsiveness to a variety of antigens characteristic of each haplotype.

Until very recently, it was generally assumed that only one H-linked *Ir* gene was required to control responsiveness to a single antigen. This conclusion was based upon (1) the finding that the mating of non-responder strains or non-responder random-bred animals yielded non-responder offspring, and (2) our success in mapping *Ir* genes specific for different antigens as shown in Figure 4.3.

There were, however, some indications that in some systems two H-linked *Ir* genes might be required for responsiveness. Rare instances had been reported where F_1 hybrids between two low responder strains gave responses higher than either parental strain[44,45]. In addition, Stimpfling and Durham[46] also obtained evidence that responses to the histocompatibility specificity *H-2.2* might be controlled by two genes.

A clear example of dual gene control of the response to an antigen $GL\phi^{11}$ has just been demonstrated in our laboratory[47]. As shown in Figure 4.1, strains bearing either the *H-2ᵃ* or the *H-2ᵇ* haplotypes behave as non-responders to the antigen $GL\phi^{11}$. However, two of the *H-2ⁱ* recombinant strains between these two haplotypes, B10.A (3R) and B10.A (5R), were found to be strong responders to $GL\phi^{11}$. These strains were the result of recombinant events between *I-B* and *I-C* and possessed the left side of *H-2ᵇ* and the right side of the *H-2ᵃ* complex (see Table 4.4). Other *H-2ⁱ* recombinants between *S* and *D* were non-responders to $GL\phi^{11}$ [47].

Several F_1 hybrids were then immunized with $GL\phi^{11}$ (see Table 4.5). All of the hybrids made between responder and non-responder strains were responders to this antigen, indicating the expected dominance of the *Ir-GLφ* gene. More interestingly, however, the (A × B10)F_1 and (A × 18R)F_1 hybrids, which were the products of the mating of two non-responder parental strains, also responded to the $GL\phi^{11}$ terpolymer. The complementary genes in the latter hybrids were localized to the *H-2* complex since the homozygous *H-2ᵃ* congenic (A × B10.A)F_1 control mice were non-responders. One of the genes responsible for responses to $GL\phi^{11}$ had been mapped in the *I* region to the left of *I-C*. The data discussed above localize the second complementary gene tentatively in the *I-C* subregion.

Four interesting conclusions can be drawn from these studies: (1) For the

Table 4.5 Immune responses to the GLϕ^{11} terpolymer

Strain	Parental haplotype*	Antigen binding† $\pm$ SE
C57BL/10	b	0
B10.D2	d	60.9 $\pm$ 4.7
B10.A	k/d (a)	3.9 $\pm$ 2.1
A/J	k/d (a)	1.9 $\pm$ 1.6
B10.A(3R)	b/a (i3)	58.5 $\pm$ 7.0
B10.A(5R)	b/a (i5)	68.3 $\pm$ 4.0
B10.A(18R)	b/a (i18)	4.7 $\pm$ 2.4
R106	b/da (i106)	0
(BALB/c $\times$ A/J)F$_1$	d $\times$ a	67.7 $\pm$ 8.5
(C57BL/6 $\times$ DBA/2)F$_1$	b $\times$ d	68.3 $\pm$ 5.6
(A $\times$ 5R)F$_1$	a $\times$ i5	55.7 $\pm$ 4.4
(A $\times$ B10.A)F$_1$	a $\times$ a	7.5 $\pm$ 2.3
(A $\times$ B10)F$_1$	a $\times$ b	62.8 $\pm$ 5.8
(A $\times$ 18R)F$_1$	a $\times$ i18	59.5 $\pm$ 6.9

* Parental *H-2* alleles are separated by slash. The designation of the recombinant haplotypes are indicated in parentheses
† Mean percentage of radio-labelled GLT ligand bound by a 1:5 dilution of antisera obtained seven days after secondary challenge with GLϕ^{11}
From Dorf *et al.*[47]

first time an *Ir* gene has been mapped in the *I-C* subregion to the right of all previously mapped *Ir* genes. (2) Evidence of the need for complementation between two *H-2* complex genes for the response to GLϕ^{11} has been presented. (3) The *Ir-GLϕ* genes can complement each other in the trans- as well as the cis-positions; and (4) Non-responder strains to GLϕ^{11} can belong to three phenotypes, i.e. they can lack both genes or only one of them.

The observation that two distinct H-linked *Ir* genes are required for the immune response to a single antigen raises several important questions.

(1) Why was the two gene requirement not detected previously, when the offspring were studied from the mating of non-responder random-bred guinea pigs or when other recombinant strains were investigated? Since most of the known *Ir* genes have been mapped to the left of *I-C*, it is probable that if the second (*I-C*) gene is always required for the response to occur, then polymorphism at the *I-C* locus or loci must be considerably less extensive, or alternatively, there are many fewer *I-C* cooperative genes than *I-A* or *I-B* genes.

(2) Do all immune responses controlled by *H-2*-linked *Ir* genes require cooperation of two distinct loci as in the case of the response to GLϕ^{11}? A systematic study of the response of F$_1$ hybrids of all non-responder *H-2* haplotypes to several antigens under the control of H-linked *Ir* genes is in progress to answer this question.

(3) Where do each of the two genes operate at the cellular level? The recent reports by Taussig *et al.*[33] and Mozes *et al.*[35] (discussed in Section 4.7), indicating that the genetic defect in non-responder strains to (T,G)-A–L is found in B cells in some strains and in both T and B cells in other strains might be ex-

plained on the basis of the two genes demonstrated to be required for the response to GLϕ[11].

(4) Lastly, the remote possibility must be entertained that both *GLϕ* genes code for variable regions of the postulated T cell receptor molecule, and that both regions are required for recognition of this antigen in responder animals.

What is the relationship of *Ir* genes to other genes of the major histocompatibility complex? Mapping data has shown conclusively that *Ir* genes are distinct from the genes coding for the transplantation antigens at the *K* and *D* loci. It has been established in both man[48] and mice[49] that the loci which control the mixed leukocyte reaction (MLR) are distinct from the loci coding for serological histocompatibility specificities. The data obtained in mice by Bach and associates[49] indicate that genetic differences at the *I* region are essential for strong MLR which suggests a close relationship between the receptors and/or the lymphocyte antigens responsible for MLR and the *Ir* gene products. This conclusion has been strengthened by the relationship in the rhesus monkey between *Ir* genes and the major MLR locus in this species[18].

4.3.2   Mapping of *Ir* genes of the Rhesus monkey

As stated in Section 4.1, segregation analysis of 21 rhesus families sired by three fathers indicated that the capacity of offspring to form antibodies to GA and DNP–GL were associated with genes coded in the RhL–A complex. In three monkeys, verified recombination within the RhL–A complex between the genes coding for the serologically defined determinants (*SD* loci) and the gene(s) controlling the lymphocyte activating determinants (*Lad* loci) responsible for mixed lymphocyte reactivity was established. In two of these monkeys the immune response gene controlling the DNP–GL response segregated with the *Lad* genes, while in the third case, the *Ir-Gl* gene segregated with the *SD* loci, tentatively localizing the *Ir-GL* gene between the *SD* and *Lad* loci. In addition, we have shown that genetically distinct genes control responsiveness to DNP–GL and GA. These genes were separated by recombination; thus one monkey inherited the *Lad, Ir-GL* and *SD* loci from one paternal haplotype and by crossing-over the gene controlling GA responsiveness from the other paternal haplotype. Therefore, the *Ir* genes of the monkey are distinct from the loci controlling the SD and Lad determinants but more closely linked to the latter. In contrast to the mouse, the genetic mapping of the rhesus major histocompatibility complex provisionally positions *Ir* and *Lad* loci approximately 5 centimorgans outside the two loci controlling the serologically defined RhL–A specificities (see Figure 4.4). The fine structure mapping of the rhesus major histocompatibility complex may provide an insight into the order of genes in the human HL-A complex. Indeed, some of the weak associations between susceptibility to disease and HL-A may be attributed to human *Ir* genes which are positioned outside the *SD* loci near the *Lad* gene(s).

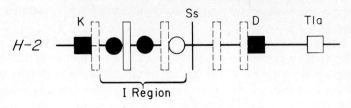

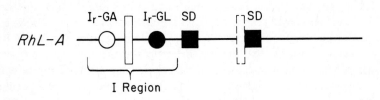

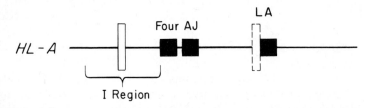

Figure 4.4 Mapping of H-linked *Ir* genes in the major histocompatibility complex of the mouse and the Rhesus monkey. The major histocompatibility complex of man, HL-A, is shown for reference

■ , Classical serologically defined tissue alloantigens characterized by broad tissue distribution; ▯ , Major lymphocyte activating determinants (Lad); minor Lad indicated with broken lines; ● , Immune response (*Ir*) genes; provisional mapping of some *Ir* genes are designated with open circles; | , Serum alloantigens related to the C system; mapping of B*ᵣ* loci is tentative.

4.4 THE SPECIFICITY OF THE PROCESS CONTROLLED BY H-LINKED *Ir* GENES

Although much has been discovered about the function of H-linked *Ir* genes, very little is known about the particular amino acid sequences responsible for triggering responses under the control of specific *Ir* genes. The polypeptide antigens, either branched or linear copolymers, which have been used to identify most of the H-linked *Ir* genes possess (with the exception of the homopolymers, PLL, PLA and PLO) a sufficiently complex structure to contain, potentially at least, a number of recognizable immunogenic determinants. Two types of approaches have been used successfully to identify the particular amino acid sequences to which responses are under the control of specific *Ir* genes. In the first case, using branched copolymers with known sequences on their side chains on the backbone of L-lysine and DL-alanine, Seaver *et al.*[50] attempted to define the exact sequences of L-tyrosine, L-glutamic acid and L-alanine recognized as immunogenic in responder animals under the control of the *Ir-1* locus.

Mice were injected with a series of (T,G)-A- -L-like compounds with side-chains of homogeneous sequences: T-A- -L, GT-A- -L, GGT-A- -L and TG-A- -L. Although T-A- -L was not immunogenic, this sequence was able to bind antibodies to (T,G)-A- -L. Furthermore, by electrostatically complexing T-A- -L to BSA, T-A- -L became immunogenic in both responder and non-responder strains of mice. Both GT-A- -L and GGT-A- -L were immunogenic and produced the same characteristic difference in C3H.SW responder mice and C3H/DiSn non-responder mice as was found with (T,G)-A- -L. TG-A- -L was also immunogenic, but there was no clear-cut difference between the titration curves for non-responder and responder mice although responder mice tended to have higher titration values for the same serum dilution. In contrast to antibodies against GGT-A- -L, antibodies against TG-A- -L bound heterologous antigens poorly[50].

Similar studies were carried out by Mozes *et al.*[51]. They also examined polypeptides of defined sequence in the A–L series: TTGG-A- -L, TGTG-A- -L and GTTG-A- -L. TTGG-A- -L was found to mimic (T,G)-A- -L in its genetic control and thus could be a sequence recognized by the *Ir-1* system. TGGT-A- -L and GTTG-A- -L behaved more liked TG-A- -L being immunogenic in both high and low responder strains.

Seaver *et al.*[50] have concluded from their own results and those of Mozes *et al.*[51] that the data are consistent with the view that the *Ir-1* gene has multiple alleles which recognize the sequences, NH_2-L-glutamyl-L-tyrosyl-poly-DL-alanyl, NH_2-di-L-tyrosyl-di-L-glutamyl-poly-DL-alanyl and NH_2-poly-L-tyrosyl-poly-DL-alanyl. The specificity of the *Ir-1* genes is therefore remarkable. The polypeptides. TG-A- -L, TGTG-A- -L, TGGT-A- -L, etc. and GTTG-A- -L are not recognized by these genes.

The other approach consisted in taking advantage of the observation that the responses of mice to various antigens of a series which differ only by a few amino acid substitutions are under the control of different *Ir* genes in an attempt to relate these amino acid differences with the process recognized by the products of the H-linked *Ir* gene studied. Hill and Sercarz investigated the fine specificity of an *Ir* gene for the gallinaceous lysozymes[52]. Because a series of gallinaceous lysozymes used in their study have known primary sequences, they provide a strong analytical tool to study the specificity of the genetic control of the immune respnse. An *H-2*-linked *Ir* locus was shown to control the ability of mice to respond to the gallinaceous lysozymes. This locus is referred to as *Ir-GEL*. $H-2^b$ mice completely fail to respond to a vigorous challenge with a group of lysozyme molecules which in responder strains elicit a heterogeneous population of antibodies. The fine specificity of the *Ir-GEL* locus was studied by ascertaining its ability to control the response to the following seven structurally related gallinaceous lysozymes: hen, bob-white, Japanese quail, guinea hen, turkey, pea fowl and ring-neck pheasant lysozymes. The first five of these lysozymes have been sequenced so that it is possible to correlate the *Ir-GEL* controlled response to each lysozyme molecule with differences in amino acid sequences. These antigens differ from each other by a small number of amino acid substitutions. The *Ir-GEL* locus is able to discriminate among these lysozymes and therefore its product must recognize fine differences in amino acid sequence. Furthermore, by analysing the small numbers of variations in the sequences of the lysozyme molecules, Hill and Sercarz have shown that the *Ir-GEL* locus probably codes for a product that recognizes a single region of these molecules, that is, those non-conservative changes found in the region from amino acids 99 to 103. Hill and Sercarz concluded that there is remarkable specificity of the control over antibody synthesis to all determinants on hen egg lysozyme in *H-2^b* mice which is apparently regulated by the recognition of a particular epitope by the *Ir* gene product[52].

Keck[53] studied the *Ir* gene control of the immunogenicity of various insulins in mice and reached similar conclusions. He compared the immunogenicity of DNP conjugates of bovine insulin and pig insulin with the DNP group in position 29 of the B chain. The only differences between the two insulins are two amino acids at position A8 and A10 in the A chain. These amino acids are located in a small loop which is formed by six amino acids (A6 to A11) and a disulphide bridge. If pig insulin is used as a carrier, the mouse strain BALB/c (*H-2^d*) produces a high titre of both anti-insulin and anti-DNP antibody, whereas the *H-2^b* and *H-2^k* strains fail to develop immune responses. In contrast, if bovine insulin is used, C57BL (*H-2^b*) is a responder, whereas C57BR (*H-2^k*) is a non-responder to both insulins. *H-2^d* mice also respond to both insulins so they apparently recognize a different determinant. On the basis of these observations, Keck concluded that the A chain loop referred to above can be regarded as a carrier determinant genetically recognized by an *Ir* gene product of *H-2^b* mice[53]. It seems very probable that the receptor which can discriminate for this loop must have a high degree of specificity.

All of these experiments emphasize the marked specificity of the process controlled by the products of H-linked *Ir* genes in the recognition of immunogenicity for both synthetic polypeptides and native antigens with known amino acid sequences.

4.5 THE DEMONSTRATION OF SUPPRESSOR T CELLS IN STRAINS BEARING NON-RESPONDER *H-2* HAPLOTYPES

It is generally recognized that T cells are concerned with the regulation of both humoral and cellular immune responses[54]. In addition to T cells capable of providing helper function for antibody responses of various classes, the administration of antigen at the appropriate time and/or in the appropriate form stimulates the generation of T lymphocytes capable of suppressing immune responses (reviewed in reference 55). These cells bear the θ antigen and lack surface immunoglobulins. In many cases, cells with suppressor activity have been found in the thymus of immune animals[55]. In some documented cases suppressor T cells appear to function by suppressing helper T cells[56] or T cells concerned with cellular immunity[57].

In view of the absence of T cell helper function in genetic non-responder animals, it appeared relevant to explore whether an antigen to which the response is under *Ir* gene control and which is unable to stimulate cellular immunity and T cell helper function in non-responder animals could nevertheless stimulate specific suppressor T cells. This possibility was first suggested by studies reported by Gershon *et al.*[58]. More recently, specific suppressor T cells have been demonstrated in our laboratory in GAT-primed non-responder mice[59,60]. We have observed that injection of GAT to mice bearing the non-responder haplotypes, $H\text{-}2^s$, $H\text{-}2^q$ or $H\text{-}2^p$, renders them unable to mount a GAT-specific plaque-forming cell (PFC) response to a subsequent challenge with GAT bound to an immunogenic carrier, methylated bovine serum albumin (MBSA), an antigen which in GAT non-responder mice can normally circumvent the genetic defect and stimulate anti-GAT antibody responses. The tolerogenic effect of GAT on GAT-specific responses to GAT–MBSA can be observed as early as 3 days following the injection of very small doses ($0.1\ \mu g$) of GAT in alum and is still detectable 5 weeks following the administration of GAT. A summary of these experiments is shown in Figure 4.5.

Treatment of non-responder DBA/1 ($H\text{-}2^q$) or SJL ($H\text{-}2^s$) mice with GAT also renders their spleen cells unable to develop a GAT-specific *in vitro* response when incubated with GAT–MBSA, although their response to sheep red blood cells (SRBC) is equivalent to that of spleen cells from normal mice (Figure 4.6).

To analyse the mechanisms of the unresponsiveness induced by GAT in non-responder mice, we have investigated: (1) the immunocompetence of T and B cells from spleens of non-responder mice previously rendered unresponsive by injection of GAT, and (2) the effects of such populations of T and B cells on the development of GAT-specific PFC responses by normal non-responder spleen cells incubated with GAT–MBSA. We have been able to show that B cells from non-responder DBA/1 mice rendered unresponsive by GAT *in vivo* can respond *in vitro* to GAT–MBSA if exogenous, MBSA-primed T cells are added to the cultures. The unresponsiveness was therefore demonstrated to be the result of impaired carrier-specific helper T cell function in the spleen cells of GAT-primed non-responder mice[60].

More importantly, spleen cells from GAT-primed non-responder DBA/1 mice specifically suppressed the GAT-specific PFC response of spleen cells from normal DBA/1 mice incubated with GAT–MBSA. This suppression was prevented by pretreatment of the GAT-primed spleen cells with anti-theta serum and complement or by X-irradiation (Figure 4.6). Identification of the suppressor cells as T cells was confirmed by the demonstration that the

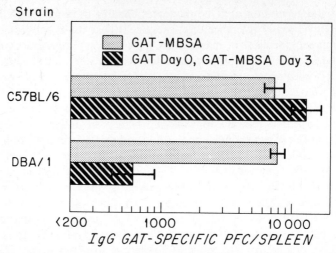

Figure 4.5 Effect of GAT on responses to GAT–MBSA by responder and non-responder mouse strains. 10 μg of GAT in Maalox and pertussis was administered i.p. on day 0 to C57BL/6 (responder) and DBA/1 (non-responder) mice. On day 3 GAT–MBSA containing 10 μg GAT in Maalox and pertussis was injected i.p. to these and control mice. Mice were sacrificed 7 days later and the IgG GAT-specific PFC/spleen determined. Values are geometric means of the responses of 8 to 12 mice. Brackets indicate standard error of the mean. (Taken from Benacerraf, B., Kapp, J. A. and Pierce, C. W. (1974). In D. H. Katz and B. Benacerraf (eds.). *Immunological Tolerance: Mechanisms and Potential Therapeutic Applications*, p. 507. (New York: Academic Press, Inc.)

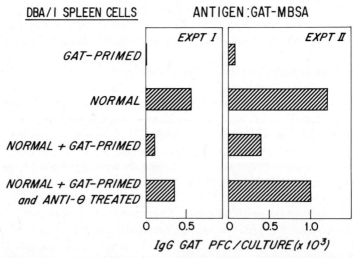

Figure 4.6 Effect of spleen cells from GAT-primed animals on the PFC response of normal DBA/1 spleen cells to GAT–MBSA *in vitro*. GAT-primed mice received 10 μg of GAT in Maalox 3 days (experiment I) or 4 days (experiment II) prior to culture initiation. (Taken from Benacerraf, B., Kapp, J. A. and Pierce, C. W. (1974). In D. H. Katz and B. Benacerraf (eds.). *Immunological Tolerance: Mechanisms and Potential Therapeutic Applications*, p. 507. (New York: Academic Press, Inc.)

142

suppressor cells were confined to the fraction of lymphocytes purified on anti-mouse immunoglobulin columns which contained theta-positive cells and only a few immunoglobulin-bearing cells (Figure 4.7).

The demonstration that non-responder mice injected with GAT, to which the response is under *Ir* gene control, do not develop an antibody response to GAT and become specifically unresponsive to a subsequent challenge with GAT–MBSA, and that this unresponsiveness is the result of an active suppressive

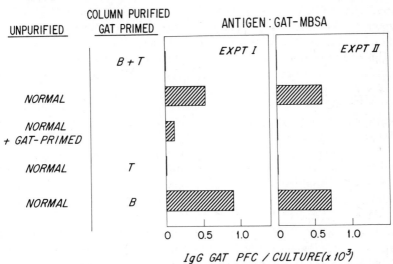

Figure 4.7 Suppressive activity of column purified T cells from GAT-primed non-responder mice. Mice were primed with 10 μg GAT in Maalox 3 days before culture initiation. Sephadex G-200 columns to which rabbit anti-mouse Fab had been conjugated were used to fractionate T and B spleen cells. (Taken from Benacerraf, B., Kapp, J. A. and Pierce, C. W. (1974). In D. H. Katz and B. Benacerraf (eds.). *Immunological Tolerance: Mechanisms and Potential Therapeutic Applications,* p. 507. (New York: Academic Press, Inc.)

process mediated by T cells, raises important questions concerning the mechanism of *Ir* gene regulation to the immune response. The first question is whether the generation of suppressor T cells in non-responder mice is unique to this system or may be generalized to other systems and species in which the response to the antigens is under the control of histocompatibility-linked *Ir* genes. Experiments are in progress to resolve this important issue. Preliminary results in our laboratory indicate that suppressor cells can be demonstrated in other, but probably not all, non-responder systems.

Furthermore we have recently demonstrated the *H-2* linked dominant genetic control of the stimulation of specific suppressor cells by immune suppressor (*Is*) genes which appear to function in a manner similar to *Ir* genes.

The possibility must also be considered that suppressor T cells in non-responder animals are not directed necessarily to the same determinants which stimulate immune responses in genetic responder animals. A random copolymer of three L-amino acids such as GAT is still a fairly complex antigen with potentially numerous determinants. The observation that the random copolymer GA is immunogenic in mice bearing the H-2^s haplotype that cannot respond to GAT is compatible with this interpretation (see Figure 4.1). GAT may be considered to contain many of the GA determinants in addition to 10% L-tyrosine residues. If indeed this hypothesis is correct, one would predict that in H-2^s mice suppressor T cells could be specifically stimulated by poly-L-tyrosine and that these suppressor T cells should be able to suppress GAT-specific responses to GAT–MBSA. Experiments are in progress to verify this hypothesis and to analyse the fine specificity of the generation of suppressor T cells in mouse strains bearing different non-responder H-2 haplotypes.

The question should also be asked whether non-responder strains which react to GAT with the development of suppressor T cells are able to develop GAT-specific helper T cells as well, and reciprocally, whether strains bearing responder H-2 haplotypes which respond to GAT immunization with the generation of radioresistant GAT-specific helper T cells are also able to produce GAT-specific suppressor T cells. We have indeed demonstrated that GAT-specific helper T cells can be elicited in DBA/1 (H-2^q) non-responder mice by immunization with GAT in the appropriate form, i.e. as GAT–MBSA or as GAT bound to macrophages in very small (nanogram) amounts[61]. In contrast, immunization of DBA/1 mice with GAT in soluble form or in alum with or without bacterial adjuvants always elicits the production of suppressor and not of helper T cells. The activity of helper T cells generated in non-responder mice immunized with GAT–MBSA or macrophage-bound GAT is clearly much less effective than that generated in responder mice, since it is capable of providing helper function *in vitro* only for responder B cells obtained from (responder × non-responder)F_1 hybrids but not for non-responder B cells exposed to macrophage-bound GAT[61]. The generation of GAT-specific helper T cells in H-2^q non-responder animals could only be demonstrated by *in vitro* culture techniques. These observations have considerable implications when we consider the cell or cells where *Ir* genes are expressed (see Section 4.7) and the process controlled by the genes (see Section 4.9).

4.6 THE ROLE OF PRODUCTS OF THE MAJOR HISTOCOMPATIBILITY LOCUS IN CELLULAR INTERACTIONS WHICH REGULATE IMMUNE RESPONSES

Over the past 2 years, observations from our own laboratories, as well as those of others, have demonstrated the involvement of histocompatibility gene products in governing the cell–cell interactions concerned with development and regulation of immune responses in several species[62–66]. These discoveries have placed the products of the major histocompatibility complex on a more complex level of biologic function than was heretofore generally considered[32].

Based on these observations, we proposed that genes in the *H-2* complex coded for products involved in the development of effective cell–cell interactions in the immune response[32,63,64].

In this section, we shall review the data that have demonstrated genetic restrictions of T–B lymphocyte interactions and of the interactions between macrophages and T lymphocytes. The conclusion we draw from these findings is that the development of functional T cells and the regulatory role of T lymphocytes in immune responses, which appears to be related to control of differentiation processes of other lymphocytes of both T and B classes, is mediated via molecules that are comprised, at least in part, of gene products of the major histocompatibility gene complex expressed on the surface membranes of such cells.

4.6.1 Evidence for genetic restrictions in cooperative T–B cell interactions

The data that will be reviewed in this section demonstrate that the participation of histocompatibility gene products in cell–cell interactions reflects a physiological control mechanism utilizing readily accessible structures that are dynamic constituents of the surface membranes of lymphoid cells. We wish to emphasize at the outset, however, that like other physiologic control mechanisms, it is not an absolute system in the sense of precluding alternate, albeit perhaps less efficient routes to the same end.

The evidence for the existence of genetic restrictions in T–B cell interactions can be succinctly summarized as follows: Under conditions in which isogeneic or syngeneic lymphoid cells interact together to develop humoral immune responses, cells lacking certain critical identities in histocompatibility genes fail to successfully interact[32,62–64,66–71]. The preceding statement must be elaborated upon to include the very important qualifications that: (1) demonstration of a 'failure' to obtain a response in the system employed in our own studies has been shown *not* to reflect a suppression phenomenon[68], and (2) the positive responses obtained are those which are elicited by interactions between antigen-specific T and B cells and not by allogeneic cell interactions. Initially, the central problem was to design an experimental scheme that specifically circumvented the possible contribution to the results of a complicating allogeneic effect. This was accomplished for *in vivo* cell transfer studies by using an F_1 hybrid as the recipient of T and B cells from the respective parental strains against which the semiallogeneic host would be genetically incapable of reacting. The intricacies of the experimental protocol employed have been described in detail elsewhere[63,64].

The protocol and data from a representative experiment using congenic-resistant mouse strains demonstrating the involvement of the *H-2* gene complex in physiological lymphocyte interactions are shown in Figure 4.8. The DNP-primed B cells were derived from congenic-resistant B10.A (*H-2ᵃ*)

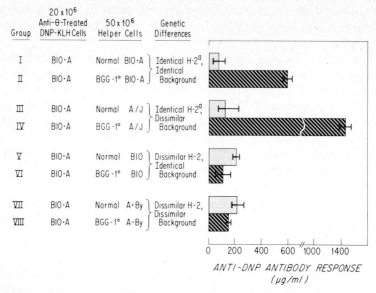

Figure 4.8   Failure of physiological cooperative interactions to occur *in vivo* between T and B lymphocytes differing at the major histocompatibility locus. The scheme followed is described in text. Recipients for all cell combinations were (A × B10)F₁ hybrids. Combinations and strain origins of T and B cells and the relevant genetic differences are indicated. Recipients in groups I–VIII were secondarily challenged with 50 μg of DNP–BGG. Mean serum anti-DNP antibody levels of groups of five mice on day 7 after secondary challenge are illustrated. Horizontal bars represent ranges of the standard error. (Taken from reference 64.)

donor mice and the relevant genetic similarities and/or differences are listed for each combination[64]. Groups I and II demonstrate the intact cooperative functional capacities of the irradiated (*in situ*) bovine γ-globulin (BGG)-primed T cells and the anti-θ-treated DNP-primed B cells of syngeneic B10.A origin within the environs of (A × B10)F₁ irradiated recipients (Group I). Similarly BGG-primed T cells derived from A/J donors, which are identical with B10.A at the major *H-2ᵃ* locus but dissimilar with respect to background genotypes are capable of exerting a clear helper effect in cooperating with B cells of B10.A origin. In sharp contrast, T cells from A.By or B10 donors, which are both *H-2ᵇ*, fail to cooperatively interact with B lymphocytes from B10.A mice. This is true irrespective of whether or not the genetic background other than *H-2* is identical such as is the case of B10 donor cells.

Among the various possible explanations for the failure of physiologic T–B cell cooperation to occur across the major histocompatibility barrier, certain possibilities which are trivial in terms of biological significance have been ruled out either by experimental design or by direct experimentation[63,64,68]. These possibilities have been described and discussed in detail elsewhere[32,63,64,68] and will not be reiterated here. These findings led us to develop the hypothesis, therefore, that the failure to observe cooperative responses when *H-2* gene differences existed reflected the necessary participation of cell surface membrane sites on B cells, which we initially termed 'acceptor' sites[63], that were reacted upon by corollary membrane sites or products from the T cells, and that these molecules were products of genes located in the *H-2* gene complex. We have recently modified the terminology of cell-interaction or CI molecules and the genes coding for such molecules as *CI* genes[31].

In our intitial studies[63], no cooperation occurred with mixtures of T and B cells from BALB/c (H-2^d) and A/J (H-2^a) donors, respectively. Since these particular strains are identical at S and the entire D end of the H–2 complex, these results indicated that gene identities only at S and D are insufficient to permit optimal cooperative interactions. Subsequent experiments were designed to determine more precisely the intra-*H-2* localization of the postulated *CI* genes. One such experiment was carried out to ask whether identities at only K and I are sufficient to allow effective cooperation. This study[69] was performed *in vitro* using lymphocytes from A/J and B10.BR mice which differ from one another at genes in the S and D regions of the H-2 complex but are identical at the K and I regions. The results were that DNP-primed B cells from A/J donors developed effective cooperative responses with keyhole limpet haemocyanin (KLH)-primed T cells from both isogeneic A/J donors and from B10.BR donors. In the reciprocal mixed cell cultures, DNP-primed B cells from B10.BR mice interacted with KLH-primed T cells from A/J as well as isogeneic T cells in response to DNP–KLH. The data did not reflect non-specific allogeneic effects as an explanation for successful cooperation between A and B10.BR lymphocytes since reciprocal controls using irradiated normal rather than KLH-primed cells failed to develop secondary responses to DNP–KLH[69]. The development of cooperative responses between A/J and B10.BR which differ for genes in S and D but are identical for K and I region genes indicates that the critical *CI* genes involved in T–B cell cooperation exist in the latter regions.

This observation has quite recently been corroborated in a totally *in vivo* double adoptive transfer scheme as well. The protocol and data from such a complementation experiment are illustrated in Figure 4.9[70]. Before discussing the data shown in Figure 4.9, it is pertinent to cite the following data from independent control experiments that are not shown in the figure: (1) All of the DNP-primed spleen cell populations were capable of developing secondary anti-DNP responses to the immunizing antigen, DNP-*Ascaris* extract (ASC), in parallel transfers utilizing spleen cells not treated with anti-θ serum; (2) Anti-θ serum treatment in the conditions employed effectively abrogated the capacity of such cells to mount an *in vivo* response in the absence of additional carrier-primed cells; and (3) The substitution of normal cells for KLH-primed cells failed to permit development of responses to DNP–KLH.

The relevant data are depicted on the right side of Figure 4.9. Groups I and VI demonstrate the capacity of syngeneic mixtures of KLH-primed T and DNP-primed B cells from DBA/2 (H-2^d) and C3H (H-2^k) mice to cooperate

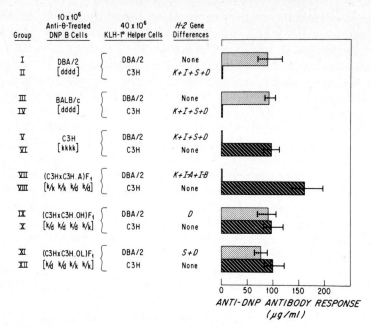

Figure 4.9 Cooperative interactions *in vivo* between T and B lymphocytes sharing *K* end genes of the *H-2* complex. Recipients for all cell combinations (C3H × DBA/2)F₁ hybrids. Combinations and strain origins of T and B cells and the relevant genetic differences are indicated. The *H-2* regions of *K, I, S* and *D* of the strains used are indicated in brackets. Mean serum levels of anti-DNP antibody of groups of four mice on day 7 after secondary challenge with 20 μg DNP–KLH are illustrated. Horizontal bars represent ranges of standard errors. Statistical comparisons between the various groups gave the following results: Groups I and II, Groups III and IV, Groups V and VI, Groups VII and VIII had *P* values less than 0.001 in all cases; Groups IX and X, Groups XI and XII had *P* values greater than 0.1 in all cases. (Taken from reference 70.)

in response to DNP–KLH within the environs of (C3H × DBA/2)F₁ irradiated recipients. Similarly, KLH-primed T cells derived from DBA/2 donors are capable of exerting a clear helper effect in cooperating with BALB/c B cells (Group III). It is important to note that DBA/2 and BALB/c strains are identical at the *H-2* locus (*H-2ᵈ*) but dissimilar with respect to numerous other genes. In sharp contrast, B cells from C3H (*H-2ᵏ*) donors fail to cooperatively interact with *H-2*-incompatible DBA/2 (*H-2ᵈ*) T lymphocytes (Group V). Likewise, physiological cooperative interactions fail to occur between T and B lymphocytes in two reciprocal combinations in which DBA/2 or BALB/c cells were mixed with *H-2*-incompatible C3H T cells (Groups II and IV).

Groups VII through XII test the ability of DBA/2 (*H-2ᵈ*) or C3H (*H-2ᵏ*) helper cells to cooperate with B cells from a series of F₁ hybrids made between C3H and selected C3H congenic mice. The C3H congenic strains carry recombinant *H-2* haplotypes derived from crossovers between the *H-2ᵈ* and *H-2ᵏ*

148

parental haplotypes. Very good cooperative responses occurred between C3H carrier-primed T cells and hapten-primed B cells derived from all of the C3H F_1 hybrids, in spite of the presence of foreign histocompatibility determinants on these F_1 hybrid cells (Groups VIII, X and XII).

As noted above, DBA/2 KLH-primed T cells failed to effectively cooperate with H-2-incompatible DNP-primed C3H B cells (Group V). Similarly, DBA/2 (H-2^d) T cells failed to effectively interact with (C3H × C3H.A)F_1 B cells, although these B cells carry the I–C, S and D regions derived from the H-2^d haplotype (Group VII). In contrast, the same pool of helper T cells from DBA/2 donors were perfectly good helpers in development of secondary anti-DNP responses with hapten-primed B cells from (C3H × C3H.OH)F_1 and (C3H × C3H.OL)F_1 hybrids (Groups IX and XI).

In this complementation experiment, we have demonstrated that one or more Ir genes that control T–B cell interactions are localized in the K end of the H-2 gene complex. Thus, DBA/2 KLH-primed T cells cooperated with (C3H × C3H.OH)F_1 and (C3H × C3H.OL)F_1 DNP-primed B cells to make a secondary response to DNP–KLH, but not with C3H or (C3H × C3H.A)F_1 DNP-primed cells. It must be emphasized that the carrier-primed DBA/2 T cells are histoincompatible with each of these B cell populations for both non-H-2 and H-2 determinants. The presence of foreign histocompatibility determinants provided by the C3H parent does not therefore prevent successful physiological T–B cell cooperation in F_1 hybrids which have at least one complement of K^d and I^d genes derived from C3H.OH or C3H.OL parents. However, complementation with D^d, S^d and I–C^d genes derived from the C3H.A parent fail to complement for successful cell interactions. Moreover, these data again argue strongly against the operation of non-specific suppression phenomena due to either H-2 or non-H-2 differences which could explain the failure to observe cooperative interactions in other cell combinations, *unless* one postulated the necessity for such differences to exist in genes located in the cis-position on the respective chromosomes in order for such suppression mechanisms to operate.

The two preceding experiments permit us to draw the conclusion that the histocompatibility genes involved in controlling optimal T–B cell interactions are located to the left of the S region of H-2 — i.e. somewhere in the K and/or I region(s). The existence of appropriate inbred and recombinant strains of mice differing at known loci of the H-2 complex makes it possible to define the relevant gene or genes. The following experiment was designed to answer this question using mixtures of T and B cells from congenic mice A.TL (H-2^{t1}), A.TH (H-2^{t2}), A.AL (H-2^{a1}), A.SW(H-2^s), inbred A/J (H-2^a) and (A × A.TH)F_1 (H-$2^{a/t2}$) in *in vitro* cooperative secondary anti-DNP antibody responses[71]. (Refer to Table 4.4 for characterization of recombinant H-2 haplotypes).

The left side of Figure 4.10 depicts the protocol and various combinations of cell mixtures analysed for cooperative responses to DNP–KLH. The gene regions of the H-2 complexes are symbolized and the gene region differences

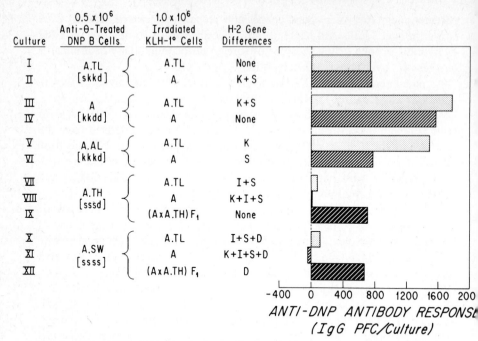

Culture	0.5 x 10⁶ Anti-θ-Treated DNP B Cells	1.0 x 10⁶ Irradiated KLH-1° Cells	H-2 Gene Differences
I	A.TL [skkd]	A.TL	None
II		A	K + S
III	A [kkdd]	A.TL	K + S
IV		A	None
V	A.AL [kkkd]	A.TL	K
VI		A	S
VII	A.TH [sssd]	A.TL	I + S
VIII		A	K + I + S
IX		(A x A.TH) F₁	None
X	A.SW [ssss]	A.TL	I + S + D
XI		A	K + I + S + D
XII		(A x A.TH) F₁	D

$$-400 \quad 0 \quad 400 \quad 800 \quad 1200 \quad 1600 \quad 2000$$

ANTI-DNP ANTIBODY RESPONSE
(IgG PFC/Culture)

Figure 4.10 DNP–ASC-primed spleen cells from A.TL, A, A.AL, A.TH and A.SW mice were depleted of T cells by *in vitro* treatment with anti-θ serum plus complement and then cultured with irradiated KLH-primed spleen cells from A.TL, A or (A × A.TH)F₁ donors in the combinations indicated. Cells were cultured with either no antigen (not shown) or DNP–KLH. The background responses of non-stimulated cultures have been subtracted from the numbers of DNP-specific PFC developed in cultures containing DNP–KLH (hence, the negative value depicted in culture XI). IgG (indirect) DNP-specific PFC responses are shown. Responses in the IgM class (not shown) were parallel. (Taken from reference 71.)

among the various combinations are summarized for convenience. The relevant data is depicted on the right side of Figure 4.10. Cultures I–IV demonstrate the capacity of syngeneic mixtures of T and B cells from A.TL and A mice to cooperate *in vitro* and reciprocal mixtures of such cells to interact together despite the existence of gene differences in both the K and S region of *H-2* in this combination. Likewise, when gene differences are restricted to only one of these respective regions (K or S), the capacity for effective T–B cell cooperation remains intact as evidenced by the ability of T cells from both A.TL and A donors to interact with B cells from A.AL donors (cultures V and VI). In marked contrast, however, is the inability of either of these primed and functionally intact T cell populations from A.TL or A donors to cooperate with B cells from either A.TH or A.SW mice (cultures VII, VIII, X and XI); in the latter combinations, gene differences exist in the I region as indicated. The failure of either A.TH or A.SW DNP-primed B cells to respond in these cultures is not a reflection of an incapacity of these B cells to function since irradiated KLH-primed cells from (A × A.TH)F₁ donors were able to provide helper function for A.TH parental cells (culture IX) and for A.SW cells which differ only at genes in the D region (culture XII). Moreover, the capacity of A.TH primed cells to develop effective syngeneic cooperative interactions was not inhibited or diminished by the addition of irradiated KLH-primed spleen cells from A.TL donors thereby ruling out a possible suppression mechanism due to, e.g. an allogeneic effect as an explanation for these findings. Thus, in a syngeneic cooperative control culture response, A.TH cells developed 1253 IgG anti-DNP PFC in the absence of A.TL cells and 1486 anti-DNP PFC in the presence of 1.0×10^6 irradiated KLH-primed A.TL cells[71].

The results of this experiment provide compelling evidence for the existence of the CI gene or genes controlling optimal T–B cell cooperative interactions in the designated I region of the H-2 gene complex. This point is particularly emphasized by the inability of A.TL to provide helper T cell function for A.TH or A.SW B cells in which combinations there are gene identities in the K region but differences in I region genes.

The precise genetic mapping of these genes will require experiments using mixtures of T and B cells from strain combinations with differences and identities at one or more subregions, I–A, I–B and I–C, on the basis of documented cross-overs between definable Ir genes and also Ia serological specificities[41]. The data presented here indicate that the genes responsible for control of T–B cell interactions in this system are located in the I–A and/or I–B subregions. This follows from the fact that the A↔B10.BR, A↔A.TL and A↔A.AL combinations, all of which are identical for all genes in I–A and I–B, were capable of effectively interacting despite the existence of gene differences in the I–C subregion. However, despite the fact that the I–C subregions of these strains are derived from different paternal haplotypes, they may nevertheless conceivably share genes coded for in the I–C subregion which permit effective T–B cell cooperation. Further definition of these possibilities should be forthcoming.

It is relevant to point out that the I–A and I–B subregions where the CI genes appear to be mapped by our studies (Figure 4.10) are precisely the subregions where the majority of all known immune response or Ir genes have been mapped[72]. However, as discussed at length elsewhere[31], while this suggests an association between Ir and CI gene products in lymphocyte function, it does not imply that these are necessarily products of the same gene(s).

The close functional association between Ir and CI gene products in T–B cell cooperative interactions is perhaps most strikingly illustrated by the following experiment. By taking advantage of our previous demonstration of highly effective cooperation between reciprocal combinations of parental and F_1 hybrid T and B lymphocytes when the carrier molecule employed is one to which both parental strains are genetic responders[63], an experiment was designed to determine whether F_1 carrier-primed T cells can serve as helper cells for either or both parental B cells when: (a) the response to the carrier molecule employed is under genetic control such that one parental strain is a responder and the other is a non-responder, and (b) the determinant specificity of the parental B cells being assessed is not under genetic control and bears no relationship to the specificity of the carrier molecule[67]. The experimental system utilized an immune response gene controlling responses to the ter-polymer L-glutamic acid-L-lysine-L-tyrosine (GLT) to which A strain mice (H-2^a) are non-responders whereas BALB/c (H-2^d) and (BALB/c × A)F$_1$ hybrids (CAF$_1$) are responders.

As shown in Figure 4.11, BALB/c (Group II) and A/J (Group VIII) DNP-specific B cells are effectively 'helped' by KLH-specific F$_1$ T cells in responses to DNP–KLH. Similarly, GLT-primed CAF$_1$ T cells cooperate very well with B cells from BALB/c donors in response to either soluble or macrophage-bound DNP–GLT (Groups IV and VI). In marked contrast, however, these same GLT-specific F$_1$ T cells fail to serve as helper cells for DNP-specific B cells from A/J donor mice irrespective of whether soluble or macrophage-

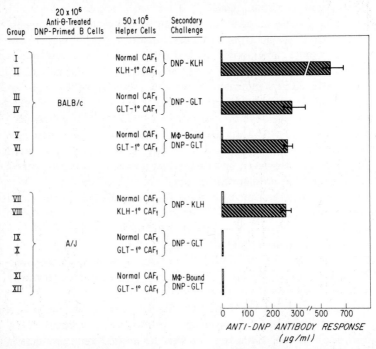

Figure 4.11 Involvement of *Ir* gene in control of T and B lymphocyte interactions *in vivo*. Recipients for all cell combinations were CAF$_1$ hybrids. The transfer scheme is the same as in Figures 4.8 and 4.9. Combinations, strain origins and specificities of T and B cells are indicated. Secondary challenge was performed intraperitoneally with either 20 μg of soluble DNP–KLH or 100 μg of soluble DNP–GLT or intravenously with 10^7 F$_1$ macrophages (Mϕ) containing 2.4 μg DNP–GLT per mouse as indicated. Mean serum anti-DNP antibody levels of groups of five mice on day 7 after secondary challenge are illustrated. Horizontal bars represent ranges of the standard errors. (Taken from references 67 and 32.)

bound DNP–GLT is employed for secondary challenge (Groups X and XII). These results demonstrate, therefore, that GLT-primed CAF_1 T cells can provide for responder BALB/c but not for non-responder A/J, the required stimulus for the anti-DNP responses of DNP-specific B cells of these respective parental strains to the DNP conjugate of GLT[67].

As discussed in the preceding sections above, the number of specific H-linked *Ir* genes that have been identified and the specific manner in which they permit immune responses to distinct antigens to take place, particularly at the T cell level, has suggested that they are somehow involved in either the specificity or the function of the T cell antigen receptors and may, therefore, be clonally expressed in this class of lymphocytes.

The implications of our experiments on the F_1-parent cooperative response to DNP–GLT described above have been discussed by us[31,32,67] to mean either: (1) that *Ir* genes may also be expressed, and non-clonally, in B cells of responder animals (as discussed in Section 4.7), and/or (2) that the activation of the *Ir* gene product determines the activation in turn of the molecules involved in T–B cell interactions coded for by the same haplotype. According to the latter alternative, there would be no requirement for the *functional* expression of the *Ir* gene product in the B cell but only a requirement for the *Ir* gene product or associated *I* region gene product(s) from the T cell to govern the interaction with the B cell at the histocompatibility 'acceptor' or CI site on the B cell surface.

4.6.2 Evidence for the participation of histocompatibility gene products in macrophage–T cell interactions

The participation of histocompatibility molecules in macrophage–lymphocyte interactions was first discovered by Rosenthal and Shevach[73]. In their studies, a very sensitive system was employed in which purified peritoneal exudate lymphocytes and lymph node lymphocytes, both consisting of highly enriched populations of antigen-reactive T lymphocytes, from previously immunized inbred guinea pigs were assessed for induction of DNA synthesis following exposure to antigen-bearing macrophages. Thus, lymphocytes from strain 2 and strain 13 guinea pigs sensitized to purified protein derivative of tuberculin (PPD) were induced to undergo a high degree of DNA synthesis by PPD-bearing macrophages from respective syngeneic donors, but failed to respond or responded poorly to PPD-macrophages from respective allogeneic donors. This failure of antigen-bearing allogeneic macrophages to stimulate T cells was clearly shown *not* to reflect inhibitory effects due to the presence of allogeneic macrophages in the cultures or due to the development of conflicting mixed lymphocyte interactions[73]. Moreover, in reciprocal mixtures of antigen-bearing macrophages and T lymphocytes from $(2 \times 13)F_1$ hybrid and parental donors, it was found that the level of stimulation was only about 50% of that observed in totally syngeneic mixtures[73]. The conclusion of Rosenthal and Shevach that optimal interaction between macrophages and T cells is mediated via histocompatibility molecules or closely-associated membrane structures was further substantiated by their finding that alloantisera directed against such molecules were effective in blocking such interactions particularly when such alloantisera were directed against H-antigen determinants of both the macrophage and the lymphocyte[73].

Further studies by Shevach and Rosenthal[74] using responses to antigen under unigenic *Ir* gene control demonstrated that (responder and nonresponder)F_1 lymphocytes were poorly or not at all stimulated by nonresponder parental macrophages pulsed with the antigen under *Ir* gene control; macrophages from the responder parent pulsed with same antigen were considerably better stimulators of such F_1 cells. Moreover, alloantisera-inhibition studies demonstrated that in mixtures of parental antigen-pulsed macrophages and F_1 T lymphocytes alloantisera directed against H-determinants present solely on the T cell only inhibited the recognition of antigens controlled by the *Ir* gene linked to the histocompatibility determinants against which they are directed[74].

In a recent series of experiments, the basic observation of genetic restrictions in macrophage-T cell interactions have been extended to the mouse. Thus, Erb and Feldmann have employed an *in vitro* system for the development of carrier-specific helper T lymphocytes in which they have found that the presence of histocompatible macrophages or supernatants from antigen-pulsed histocompatible macrophages were necessary for the development of such T cells[75]. Allogeneic macrophages or supernatants from antigen-pulsed allogeneic macrophages were ineffective in the induction of helper T cells *in vitro*[75].

It appears, therefore, that in two systems analysed using guinea pigs and mice, the interaction between macrophages and T cells in the induction of certain T cell functions involves participation of histocompatibility molecules[73-75]. Before closing this issue, it is pertinent to note that in studies performed in our own laboratories using different assay systems, such genetic restrictions were not observed. Thus, Katz and Unanue using antigen-pulsed macrophages for stimulation of *secondary* anti-DNP responses *in vitro* to DNP-protein conjugates found that allogeneic macrophages were as effective as syngeneic macrophages in this regard[76]. It must be emphasized, however, that in those studies, the T cells were previously primed and, indeed, were capable of exerting a helper function without undergoing a proliferative response in order to perform in this manner and, moreover, that the absolute requirement for macrophages in such secondary *in vitro* responses was found to be substantially less than appears to be true for primary responses[76]. These data do not, therefore, pose a contradiction to the guinea pig or mouse studies described above since in the latter studies responses involved DNA synthesis and/or proliferation and differentiation[73-75]. Other experiments by Kapp *et al.*[77] demonstrating the capacity of histoincompatible GAT-bound macrophages to stimulate primary *in vitro* anti-GAT responses may reflect the existence of certain *I* region gene compatibilities between the particular macrophages and lymphocytes employed.

4.6.3 Evidence for the relationship of histocompatibility gene products to each other in nature and function

In order to develop a better understanding of the relationship of histocompatibility antigens, *Ir* genes and immune recognition, studies have been carried out in several laboratories in the past several years on the functional effects of certain specific alloantisera on lymphocyte responses to antigen. The first studies of this type were made in guinea pigs by Shevach *et al.*[28], who examined the effect of specific alloantisera on lymphocyte stimulation induced by antigens under *Ir* gene control. Their experiments demonstrated that the *in vitro* proliferative response of lymphocytes from strain 2 or strain 13 animals both to antigens under *Ir* gene control (DNP–GL in strain 2 and GT in strain 13) and to PPD which is not known to be under genetic control were inhibited by the appropriate alloantiserum to a similar degree. However, when cells from $(2 \times 13)F_1$ animals were used, only the response linked to the histocompatibility antigens against which the serum was directed could be inhibited by a given alloantiserum. Thus, anti-2 serum inhibited the response of F_1 cells to DNP–GL but not to GT, whereas the anti-13 serum inhibited the response to GT but not to DNP–GL. The authors concluded from these data that the alloantisera were inhibiting T lymphocyte antigen recognition through interference with the activity of *Ir* gene products on the cell surface. Studies in the mouse by Lonai and McDevitt[78], which have demonstrated that anti-*H-2* sera block the induction of tritiated thymidine uptake from responder mice immunized with (H,G)-A- -L and (Phe,G)-A- -L, have been similarly interpreted.

Subsequent studies in the guinea pig performed more recently were designed to delineate whether the inhibitory antibodies in the alloantisera were directed against associated H specificities or against the products of the *Ir* genes[29,30] by examining the capacity of anti-2 serum to inhibit the response under the control of the *Ir–GA* gene, which in most outbred Hartley guinea pigs is linked to genes bearing strain 2 specificities, when the *GA* gene occurs in an outbred animal lacking strain 2 H genes. In this situation, anti-2 serum which effectively inhibited the *in vitro* proliferative response to GA of T cells derived from animals that were GA^+ and 2^+, had little or no effect on such responses of T cells from GA^+ 2^- guinea pigs. Moreover, an antiserum prepared in strain 13 animals against lymphoid cells of a GA^+ 2^- outbred animal failed to exhibit any inhibitory activity, whereas a strain 13 anti-GA^+ 2^+ antiserum specifically inhibited the response to GA of cells from $(2 \times 13)F_1$ guinea pigs. These data indicate that the inhibitory activity of anti-2 serum on GA responses is mediated via antibodies directed toward strain 2 H antigens rather than antibodies specific for the product of the *Ir-GA* gene, leading the authors to speculate on the possible covalent linkage of *Ir* gene products with H antigens[29].

In a recent series of experiments, Pierce *et al.*[79] have analysed the effects of alloantisera on Mishell-Dutton *in vitro* primary antibody responses in the mouse. These studies have shown that antisera directed against *H-2* antigens markedly inhibit (up to 90%) the primary antibody response to sheep erythrocytes (SRBC); both IgM and IgG antibody classes are so affected with whole anti-*H-2* sera. The inhibitory activity can be absorbed with lymphoid cells bearing the appropriate haplotype but cannot be absorbed by mouse immunoglobulins. When F_1 cells are tested, anti-*H-2* sera directed against either parental haplotype will effectively inhibit the primary *in vitro* response.

The specificity characteristics of the inhibition of *in vitro* antibody responses can be summarized as follows[79]: (1) Antisera directed against the entire *H-2* complex will block both IgM and IgG responses; (2) Antisera tested in congenic strains against non-*H-2* gene products will also inhibit in certain cases, thus indicating the involvement of other specificities in these phenomena; (3) Antisera directed against unique *K* specificities — i.e. private specificity *H-2.19* — will inhibit both IgM and IgG responses; (4) Antisera directed against specificities in the *K* end of the *H-2* block the whole response, whereas anti-*D* sera fail to inhibit at all; and (5) Finally, antisera directed against *I* specificities inhibit selectively responses of the IgG antibody class.

The cellular locus of action of these antisera is of particular interest in view of the above discussion concerning histocompatibility requirements for cell interactions. Thus, it appears that the antisera act at two levels: First, on macrophages in exerting their inhibitory effects; when this occurs, both IgM and IgG responses are blocked[79]. Nonetheless, macrophages that have been exposed to the appropriate alloantiserum are not deficient in their capacity to bind and handle antigen. It is clear therefore that the mechanism of inhibition at the level of the macrophage involves events other than simple antigen uptake by these cells and probably indicates a block in macrophage–lymphocyte interactions. In addition, the alloantisera can also be shown to inhibit at the level of the lymphocyte populations; however, only IgG responses are inhibited in the latter circumstances implying the probable action of antibodies directed against *I* region antigens when inhibition is operative at the level of the lymphocytes. These data corroborate, therefore, the previous studies of Rosenthal and Shevach[73,74] discussed above in which stimulation of T lymphocyte responses by antigen-pulsed macrophages could be inhibited by alloantisera only when the determinants against such sera were present on both T cells and macrophages[73].

4.6.4 Conclusion

The observations discussed in this section have pointed out the involvement of the histocompatibility gene complex in the various cell interactions that normally transpire in the development and regulation of immune responses. This has been shown for interactions between T cells and B cells and between macrophages and T cells by (1) analysis of interactions between such cells derived from donors with appropriate identities and/or differences in genes located in the major histocompatibility complex, and by (2) inhibition studies employing alloantisera of appropriate specificities. Notably absent from this discussion has been any evidence for genetic restrictions in T–T cell interactions, but suitable analysis of this point is considerably more difficult to perform than in the case of T–B cell interactions.

The evidence to date indicates that the cell-interaction genes involved in T–B cell interactions map in the *I* region, more specifically in the *I–A* and/or *I–B* subregions. The location of *CI* genes involved in macrophage–T cell interactions and those possibly involved in T–T interactions are not as clearly mapped as yet.

In closing this section, we would like to emphasize the following point. It is apparent to us that the involvement of histocompatibility gene products in the most effective cell interactions was not an evolutionary design to *prevent* interactions from occurring between histoincompatible cells but rather to optimize and control successful interactions between isogeneic cells which share the relevant genes. As such, the failure to obtain cooperative interactions in cell combinations lacking the relevant gene identities has to be viewed as a fortuitous circumstance that permitted us to *recognize* the critical role of *H-2* gene products in such interactions and, by extension of this reasoning, should not be considered to reflect an *absolute* restriction to cell interactions. Hence, one might expect to observe certain situations in which cells lacking *H-2* gene identities may undergo successful cooperative interactions, perhaps via alternative or less efficient mechanisms. This may explain the capacity of T and B cells in mice, which lack certain critical *H-2* gene identities, to manifest cooperative interactions in some circumstances[80].

Moreover, it should also be stated that the high degree of polymorphism in the *H-2* gene complex indicates that there would likely be sharing of some of the various *CI* genes among different inbred lines that would permit, under appropriate circumstances (i.e. longer duration of interaction) the development of successful interactions between cells derived from seemingly disparate genetic origins.

4.7   THE CELL TYPE WHERE HISTOCOMPATIBILITY-LINKED *Ir* GENES ARE EXPRESSED

Let us consider now the cells where the H-linked *Ir* genes are expressed. In the two systems most extensively studied, the *PLL* gene in guinea pigs and genes at the *Ir-1* locus (*I–A* subregion) in mice, responsiveness can be passively transferred to irradiated non-responder recipient strains with immunocompetent cells from animals possessing the *Ir* genes, demonstrating that the genes are indeed expressed in cells which participate in the immune response[1]. It should be noted that in these chimeras, the responding cells have been found to be of donor origin[81]. Thus, the *Ir* genes are expressed in immunocompetent cells. This conclusion is further supported by studies on the immune response of mouse spleen cells in culture to the terpolymer GAT[10]. As described in Section 4.1, mice bearing the *a, b, d, f, k, r, u,* or *v H-2* haplotypes respond to GAT with high levels of IgG antibodies whereas mice of the *H-2*^{n,p,q,s} types do not respond to this antigen.

In vitro cultures of spleen cells from inbred and congenic-resistant strains in the presence of 1 or 10 μg of soluble GAT[10] have shown identical results as those observed *in vivo*[82]. Soluble GAT in these concentrations stimulates the development of IgG GAT-specific PFC responses in cultures of spleen cells from responder C57BL/6 (*H-2*^{b}), F$_1$(C57 × SJL) (*H-2*$^{b/s}$) and A/J (*H-2*^{a}) mice. Soluble GAT did not stimulate the development of GAT-specific PFC responses in cultures of spleen cells from non-responder *H-2*^{s} mice (SJL, B10.S, A.SW) or *H-2* mice (DBA/1). It is of interest to note that GAT did not stimulate antibody production of the IgM class by responder or non-responder strains either *in vivo* or *in vitro*. The GAT[10] terpolymer differs, therefore, markedly in this respect from the branched polymers such as (T,G)-A- -L which stimulate the synthesis of IgM antibodies in both responder and non-responder strains.

The next question to be considered is the type of cell of the immune system, macrophages, T cells or B cells, where the product of histocompatibility-linked *Ir* genes are necessarily expressed for immune responses to develop. The data concerning the function of H-linked *Ir* genes obtained in different species have not revealed any important species differences. In many cases, the very same antigens were used in different species to detect H-linked genetic control of immune responses, which led to the conclusion that H-linked *Ir* genes control the same processes in all the experimental species where they have been identified (mouse, rat, guinea pig and monkey), and that all conclusions with respect to gene function or expression reached with distinct systems in different species can be generalized to the behaviour of all H-linked *Ir* genes. The finding that H-linked *Ir* gene control of immune responsiveness is, without any exception, limited to thymus-dependent antigens and that in the guinea pig particularly, but also in the mouse, the relevant *Ir* genes are required for the development of cellular immunity, led to the initial conclusion that in these systems the non-responder strains had a defect in their T cells. Considerable data was then brought forth indicating the expression in T cells of many H-linked *Ir* genes in both guinea pigs and mice. We propose first to summarize the evidence in favour of this interpretation and then to discuss the recent findings which localize H-linked *Ir* gene defects also in B cells in selected systems and mouse strains.

Supporting the expression of H-linked *Ir* genes in T cells, we can list the following observations:

(1) As stated above, the presence of the *Ir* gene is absolutely required for

the development of cellular immunity, a characteristic T cell function. In guinea pigs those functions of 'thymus-derived' cells, such as delayed sensitivity, MIF production and antigen-stimulated *in vitro* blast transformation, depend exclusively upon the presence of the relevant *Ir* gene. The reactions of cellular immunity to PLL, DNP–PLL, GA and GT are totally under the control of corresponding specific *Ir* genes. They are never observed in animals lacking the genes (reviewed in reference 2).

(2) H-linked *Ir* genes are concerned with the recognition of responses to the carrier molecules of hapten-carrier conjugates and not to the haptens they bear (reviewed in reference 2). Thus, guinea pigs possessing the *PLL* gene and therefore capable of responding to DNP–PLL with the synthesis of anti-DNP antibodies, respond similarly to immunization with PLL conjugates of other non-cross-reacting haptens with vigorous anti-hapten antibody synthesis. Guinea pigs lacking the *PLL* gene and therefore incapable of responding to DNP–PLL are also incapable of forming anti-benzylpenicilloyl antibodies in response to benzylpenicilloyl-PLL[83]. This experiment indicates that the *PLL* gene is concerned with the specific recognition of the immunogenic carrier molecule, a function of thymus-derived cells. Similar conclusions can also be made for *Ir* genes which control the anti-DNP antibody responses to limiting doses of DNP_7–BSA or DNP_6–GPA. As mentioned earlier (Table 4.3), strain 2 but not strain 13 guinea pigs synthesize anti-DNP antibodies when immunized with 1 μg of DNP_7–BSA, whereas strain 13 but not strain 2 guinea pigs produce anti-DNP antibodies in response to 1 μg DNP_6–GPA[84]. The capacity to form anti-DNP antibody exists equally in both inbred strains, but for these antigens the anti-DNP response is determined by the genetically-controlled recognition of the carrier, again a function of thymus-derived cells.

(3) An animal unable to respond to an antigen because it lacks the required *Ir* gene may nevertheless be stimulated to form antibodies against determinants on that antigen, when immunized with the antigen bound to an immunogenic carrier to which its helper T cells are able to respond. Thus, when a genetically non-immunogenic molecule such as DNP–PLL[85] or GAT[82] is administered to a non-responder animal complexed with an immunogenic carrier which is able to stimulate thymus-derived helper cells, an antibody response is induced against DNP–PLL or GAT and the antibody produced cannot be distinguished from those produced by responder animals with respect to amount, class or specificity. These observations support the conclusion that the genetic defect in non-responder animals is not a result of the inability to synthesize antibodies to determinants on the molecule. As would be expected, non-responder animals possess B cells capable of binding antigens to which they are genetically unable to respond in numbers comparable to those found in responder animals[86].

(4) The genetic differences between responder and non-responder mouse strains in the response to (T,G)-A- -L (i.e. the production of IgG antibodies and the development of specific memory by the responder strains) are abolished by

neonatal thymectomy of responder animals[87]. This illustrates directly the required role of T cells in the capacity of responder mice to develop IgG responses to (T,G)-A- -L.

The demonstration that non-specific T cell stimulation of B cells by the 'allogeneic effect' can stimulate strong antibody responses by genetic non-responder strains[88] and the finding that tetraparental mice generated from responder and non-responder strains behave as responders to (T,G)-A- -L and synthesize antibody of non-responder allotype[80] may be considered further evidence for the lack of expression of H-linked *Ir* gene function in B cells in this system.

Other experiments, however, have led to the conclusion that in some systems H-linked *Ir* genes are expressed in B cells, and are concerned with the control in these cells of the process by which T cell regulation of B cell responses is expressed.

The first indication that in some systems B cell defects may explain non-responder status was obtained by Shearer, Mozes and Sela[89] in studies of the transfer of limited number of bone marrow cells and thymocytes to irradiated recipients to reconstitute their responses. Using this approach, they found that the defect in the response of SJL mice to (Phe,G)-A- -L could be attributed to both thymocytes and bone marrow cells, whereas with the antigen (Phe,G)-Pro- -L, the defect in SJL and DBA/1 mice was located only in bone marrow cells[89].

More recently, Taussig, Mozes and Isac[33] have reported that they could obtain from thymocytes educated *in vivo* to (T,G)-A- -L a factor which provided specific help for bone marrow cells in their response to this antigen in irradiated syngeneic recipients (see Section 4.8). This factor was obtained from thymocytes of responder strains as well as of selected non-responder strains such as C3H/HeJ (*H-2^k*) strain. This factor was only active, however, for bone marrow cells from responder strains and not from non-responder strains, indicating that the inability of *H-2* mice to respond to (T,G)-A- -L may reside in their bone marrow B cells rather than in their T cells, and that it is caused by their unresponsiveness to the helper factor from T cells. In more recent experiments, Mozes, Isac and Taussig[35] noted that thymocytes from non-responder strains to (T,G)-A- -L differ in their ability to produce the helper factor active on responder bone marrow cells. For instance, thymocytes from SJL (*H-2^s*) mice educated to (T,G)-A- -L are unable to produce a (T,G)-A- -L specific helper factor although they could when educated with (T,G)-Pro- -L (an antigen to which they are able to respond) produce a (T,G)-Pro- -L-specific factor capable of providing help for SJL bone marrow cells challenged with (T,G)-Pro- -L.

Experiments in our laboratory have also indicated the possible expression of H-linked *Ir* genes in B cells in selected systems. Thus, in the course of our studies on the genetic control of T–B cell cooperation (see Section 4.7), we observed that carrier-primed F_1 T cells could cooperate equally well with B cells bearing either parental *H-2* haplotype in responses to conventional antigens[63]. In contrast, when we employed an antigen to which the response is under the control of an H-linked *Ir* gene such as GLT[5], GLT[5]-primed T cells from (responder × non-responder)F_1 mice were able to provide helper function for responder, but not for non-responder, DNP-primed parental B cells challenged with DNP–GLT[5] [67]. This result could be interpreted as indicating an *Ir* gene defect in non-responder B cells restricting their ability to respond to the helper signal from activated T cells. This is discussed at greater length in Section 4.6.

Lastly, we should therefore consider the possible expression of H-linked *Ir* genes in macrophages. The possible role of macrophages in responses controlled by an H-linked *Ir* gene was investigated by studying the cellular requirements for the response of mice to GAT[10] *in vitro*[77]. Macrophages were shown to be required for development of responses to GAT[10] and GAT–MBSA in cultures of spleen cells from responder mice and for responses to GAT–MBSA in cultures of spleen cells from non-responder mice. Macrophages from non-responder mice supported the development of responses to GAT[10] by non-adherent responder spleen cells, indicating that the failure of non-responder mice to respond to GAT[10] is not due to a macrophage defect.

The following conclusions can be made concerning the cell type where *Ir* genes are expressed:

(1) The process controlled by H-linked *Ir* genes is probably intimately concerned with the regulation of T–B cell interactions, and the gene codes for the molecule or part of the molecular complex responsible for this process.

(2) The non-responder phenotype may result from a T cell defect, from a B cell defect or from defects in both cell types.

(3) If the molecules on T and B cells which are responsible for the interactions of these cells are different, they are probably controlled by two closely linked genes subject to considerable linkage disequilibrium due to strong selective pressures. The two-gene hypothesis is given support by the demonstration of the need for two *Ir* genes in the control of responsiveness to $GL\phi^{11}$ (see Section 4.2).

(4) In certain cases the defect in T cells may result in the production of suppressor *versus* helper T cells. The generation of suppressor cells is probably also under H-linked *Ir* gene control.

(5) In some species, and for immune responses such as cellular immunity in guinea pigs, an *Ir* gene defect can only be detected in T cells as these are the only cells other than macrophages concerned with the response.

4.8 PROPERTIES OF BIOLOGICALLY ACTIVE PRODUCTS OF ACTIVATED T CELLS MEDIATING HELPER OR SUPPRESSOR ACTIVITIES

A major effort in studies on the mechanism of T–B cell interactions has been focused on the identification and characterization of various biologically active substances capable of influencing lymphocyte function in antibody responses to different antigens elicited in *in vitro* systems. The demonstration by Dutton *et al.*[90] that supernatants obtained from short-term cultures of histoincompatible mouse spleen cells contained a non-antigen-specific biologically active mediator capable of markedly affecting *in vitro* antibody responses to thymus-dependent antigens provided evidence for the existence of such a possible mediator. In the subsequent 4 years, a number of different factors which appear to have biological activity have been described by various investigators. Since a comprehensive review of all of these factors is beyond the scope of this chapter, we will confine the present discussion to consideration of those factors which have been found to have certain distinctive physicochemical and immunological properties in common with one another and, most importantly, with other molecules known to be products of genes in the major histocompatibility complex. Certain of these factors have been shown to be antigen-specific, others non-specific, and to be endowed with either helper or suppressor activity depending on the experimental conditions employed. Major properties shared in common by these factors are their molecular size (around 40 000 to 50 000 daltons), their failure to react with anti-immunoglobulin reagents and the presence on them of determinants of gene products of the major histocompatibility complex.

4.8.1 Properties of antigen-specific biologically active T cell products

4.8.1.1 *Factors with suppressive properties*

One of the first antigen-specific T cell factors of the molecular size noted above and that was not reactive with anti-immunoglobulin reagents was the factor discovered by Tada and co-workers (reviewed in references 36 and 37). The initial experiments demonstrated two different antigen-specific factors, extractable from mechanically disrupted thymocytes or spleen cells from primed animals, capable of regulating IgE antibody responses in the rat[91-93]. One of these factors, capable of enhancing IgE responses, was of MW between 100 000 and 200 000 daltons and reacted with anti-Fab and anti-μ chain antisera, thus resembling the IgT specific factor described by Feldmann and colleagues[94,95]. The other factor, and the one upon which we will focus in this section, was endowed with suppressor activity, contained no immunoglobulin determinants as revealed by absorption studies with various anti-immunoglobulin reagents and was found to be of molecular weight less than 100 000.

Subsequently, Tada and associates developed a similar model of antigen-specific suppression by primed T cells and factors from such cells on IgM and IgG antibody responses in the mouse[36,37,96,97]. Studies in the mouse system have been performed both *in vivo* and *in vitro* thus permitting a more extensive analysis of the suppressor factor, Briefly, the factor obtained by sonication of thymuses and/or spleens from KLH-primed donors was found to be capable of suppressing primary responses to DNP–KLH either *in vivo* or *in vitro*. The specificity of the factor was shown by (1) its failure to suppress responses to an unrelated DNP-carrier, i.e. DNP–BGG, and (2) by specific adsorption onto an immunoadsorbent column containing the antigen, KLH. The molecular size has been approximated to be in the range of around 50 000 daltons[98]. The factor does not react with anti-immunoglobulin reagents but very recently has been shown to react with anti-*H-2* antisera[37], more specifically with anti-*H-2* sera reactive with determinants coded for by genes in the *K* and/or *I* regions of *H-2*[98]. The biological activity of this factor appears to be directed to supressing the function of helper T lymphocytes since suppression of anti-DNP–KLH responses could be circumvented by co-culturing cells with a population of OVA-primed T cells in the presence of DNP–OVA[37]. In this regard the suppressor factor of Tada and associates appears to function in a manner analogous to the antigen-specific factor described recently by Zembala *et al.*[99] which is capable of suppressing contact hypersensitivity reactions in mice. The latter factor has also been found to be around 50 000 daltons, but it is not yet known whether it possesses *H-2* determinants.

4.8.1.2 Factors with enhancing properties

Another type of antigen-specific T cell factor with similar physicochemical and immunochemical properties has been described and studied by Taussig, Mozes and Munro and co-workers[33,34]. These investigators have elicited a factor from T cells activated to the antigen (T,G)-A- -L, to which the response is controlled by the *Ir-1* gene in mice, by short-term culture of such T cells with the antigen *in vitro*. This factor has been shown to replace the requirement for T cells in the development of anti-(T,G)-A- -L primary IgM responses of bone marrow cells *in vivo*. The specificity of the factor for (T,G)-A- -L was demonstrated by (1) its failure to facilitate responses of bone marrow cells to SRBC, and (2) its specific removal by an immunoadsorbent column containing the antigen, (T,G)-A- -L. The factor does not react with anti-immunoglobulin reagents but is very clearly reactive with anti-*H-2* antisera[34]. More recently, these investigators have found that this factor can be adsorbed by immunoadsorbents prepared from antisera reactive with Ia antigens of the relevant *H-2* haplotype from which the factor was derived[100].

The functional target cell of action of the (T,G)-A- -L factor is of considerable importance to discuss in view of the provocative nature of the findings to date. Thus, in their studies Taussig *et al.*[33] found that the factor could be obtained from activated T cells of both responder (C3H.SW, *H-2^b*) and non-responder (C3H/HeJ, *H-2^k*) origin. Moreover, although the bone marrow cells of donors of responder haplotype were comparably enhanced by factors obtained from either responder or non-responder activated T cells, neither factor could enhance the response of non-responder bone marrow cells to (T,G)-A- -L. This finding led the authors to conclude that in these non-responder mice, the *Ir* gene defect was expressed in B cells[33]. This interpretation has been strengthened by the more recent observations of Mozes *et al.*[35] demonstrating that in another non-responder strain, i.e. SJL (*H-2*^{s}) both T and B cells appear to be defective in the response to (T,G)-A- -L.

In fact, however, it must be pointed out that as yet the precise cellular locus of action of the antigen-specific T cell factor of Taussig and colleagues has not been defined and must be considered to be open at the moment. The fact that the latter factor works with bone marrow cells does not mean that its effect is directly on B cells since bone marrow is known to contain variable numbers of T cells and T cell precursors. Thus, the effect of the factor could be to facilitate maturation of precursor T cells to functional helper cells which would in turn cooperate with B cells. Moreover, it is possible that if the factor does indeed work directly on B cells, that this may be peculiar to immature B cells of bone marrow and not as much so in the case of more mature peripheral B lymphocytes. Further analysis is required to distinguish between these possibilities.

Thus, two functionally distinct types of antigen-specific T cell factors have been described, one exerting suppressor and the other helper activity. Although manifesting distinct functional properties, however, these two factors appear to be remarkably similar in terms of their physicochemical and immunochemical properties. In the following section, we will describe a non-specific T cell factor which has been studied more extensively and which shares many of the above-mentioned properties in common with the antigen-specific factors.

4.8.2 Properties of a non-specific biologically active T cell product

As mentioned above, prior to the discovery of antigen-specific T cell factors, the demonstration was made by Dutton and colleagues[90], and shortly thereafter by Schimpl and Wecker[101,102], that a non-antigen-specific biologically active mediator could be obtained from short-term cultures of histoincompatible mouse spleen cells. In this section, we will briefly review published observations from our own laboratory[38,39,103−106] and then present our most recent data on the biological, biochemical and immunological properties of such an active moiety produced in supernatants of short-term (24 hours) *in vitro* reactions between T cells specifically activated to foreign alloantigens and the corresponding target cell population. We have termed the factor that we have been studying 'allogeneic effect factor' (AEF) since its biological action on *in vitro* antibody responses appears to be identical to the *in vivo* phenomenon known as the allogeneic effect[107].

4.8.2.1 Biological properties of AEF

The AEF preparations that are the focus of this discussion have been prepared by culturing DBA/2 (*H-2*^{d}) T cells (which had been activated for six days against (C3H × DBA/2)F$_1$ (*H-2*$^{k/d}$) target lymphocytes in irradiated DBA/2 hosts) for 24 hours with irradiated (C3H × DBA/2)F$_1$ target spleen cells[38]. The culture supernatants from such allogeneic cell mixtures are biologically active in enhancing *in vitro* immune responses when such supernatants are obtained as early as 12 hours after culture initiation of allogeneic cell cultures, display peak activity at 24 hours and thereafter become progressively more suppressive. We have prepared numerous AEF from various genetic mixtures of effector and target cell populations and all appear to behave in analogous fashion biologically. The AEF are active as unfractionated (crude) supernatants or, as will be discussed below, as relatively purified fractions obtained by gel and/or ion exchange chromatography.

The principal biological activity of AEF that has been studied in depth is the capacity of this material to functionally replace the requirement for helper T cells in *in vitro* antibody responses. The earlier work of Dutton *et al.*[90] and Schimpl and Wecker[101,102] made it clear that such factors were active in this regard insofar as *in vitro* responses to particulate erythrocyte antigens or haptenated erythrocytes were concerned. Our own studies extended these observations to soluble DNP-protein conjugates in which case AEF can reconstitute helper cell function in responses of T cell-depleted primed spleen cells[38]. The strongest evidence that our active AEF acts directly on B cells stems from the capacity of AEF to stimulate B cells exposed to DNP conjugated to the D-glutamic acid, D-lysine (D–GL) copolymer[38]. This compound has been demonstrated to be highly tolerogenic for DNP-specific B cells both *in vivo* or *in vitro* under normal circumstances (reviewed in references 108 and 109). However, when administered to appropriately-primed animals during a critical time period after induction of an *in vivo* allogeneic effect, DNP–D–GL can provide a definite inductive stimulus for primary or secondary anti-DNP antibody responses[107,110,111]. Since no demonstrable T cell function specific for the D–GL carrier has been demonstrated, these observations provided the strongest indirect proof that the *in vivo* allogeneic effect is mediated by a direct interaction on the responding B cells. The capacity of AEF to permit *in vitro* responses to DNP–D–GL constitutes conclusive evidence, therefore, that the active moiety involved is acting directly on B lymphocytes[38].

4.8.2.2 *Biochemical properties to AEF*

The experiments performed thus far on the physicochemical features of AEF indicate that the active component(s) consists of protein and/or glycoprotein which is heat-labile (56 °C, 1 hour), thereby indicating the importance of tertiary structure to activity, and is in the molecular weight range of 30 000 to 45 000[38,105]. Moreover, the active moiety appears to consist of two components associated non-covalently[39,104,105].

Initially, crude allogeneic supernatants were fractionated first on Sephadex G-200 yielding multiple peaks of which only one contained active enhancing AEF[38]. This active peak from G-200 was then subjected to chromatography on Sephadex G-100 yielding two fractions of which only one eluting in the range of an insulin marker (MW 36 000) was biologically active in triggering B lymphocyte responses to SRBC[38]. On this basis we have estimated the MW of AEF to be in the range of 30 000 to 45 000. Ion exchange chromatography on DEAE cellulose indicates that AEF is homogeneous with regard to charge and that it could be either positive or nearly neutral[39,104,105]. Electrophoresis of the active fraction of AEF radio-labelled with ^{125}I on 10% SDS-polyacrylamide gel yielded a pattern that consisted of a large molecular peak which coincided with molecular weight of around 47 000 and a smaller peak in the molecular weight range of 11 500[105]. Moreover, the large molecular weight band stains positively with periodic acid Schiff's reagent indicating that it is probably a glycoprotein[105].

It was of great interest to determine the biological activity of the two definable molecular species observed on SDS-polyacrylamide. Since the likelihood of recovering biologically active material by elution from SDS–acrylamide gel is extremely low, comparable dissociation of AEF into sub-fractions was attempted by chromatography on Sepharose-6B in 6 M guanidine HC1. The elution pattern obtained by such chromatography is depicted on the far left panel of Figure 4.12[39,104,105]. The corresponding biological activities of the tested fractions (after removal of guanidine HC1 by dialysis) are shown on the middle and right panels of Figure 4.12. Six peaks (II–VII) of u.v.-absorbing material were demarcated as indicated by the dotted lines. Two heavier molecular weight fractions eluting after the void volume

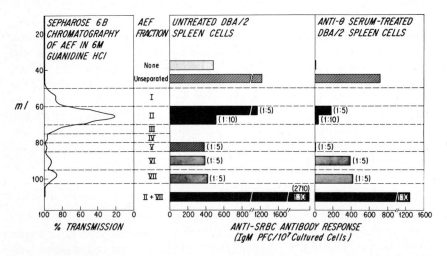

Figure 4.12 Activities of AEF fractions obtained by chromatography on Sepharose 6B in guanidine-HC1. Biologically active AEF purified by gel chromatography on Sephadex G-100 was chromatographed on Sepharose-6B in guanidine-HC1. The elution patterns of this supernatant are shown on the far left panel. The corresponding biological activities of unseparated AEF, the tested fractions (after removal of guanidine-HC1 by dialysis) and combinations of fractions II and VII on primary IgM anti-SRBC responses of untreated (middle panel) and anti-θ serum-treated DBA/2 spleen cells (right panel) are shown. (Taken from references 39 and 104.)

(fractions II and V) and two lighter molecular weight fractions (VI and VII) were tested for activity on *in vitro* primary anti-SRBC antibody responses of untreated (middle panel) and anti-θ serum-treated (far right panel) spleen cells from DBA/2 mice.

As shown in Figure 4.12, the addition of unfractionated AEF enhanced the response of untreated spleen cells and fully reconstituted the response of spleen cells depleted of T cells by anti-θ serum treatment. Fraction II from the column substantially enhanced the response of untreated spleen cells at the 1:5 concentration (around 3-fold) but exerted only a partial effect on anti-θ-treated cells. The 1:10 concentration of fraction II and 1:5 of fraction V had no significant effect on responses of either the intact or depleted cell population. The lighter molecular weight materials in fractions VI and VII exerted no detectable effect on the response of untreated spleen cells but did manifest some activity in reconstituting the responses of the anti-θ-treated cells which was approximately 50% of the activity exhibited by the unfractionated AEF. The striking observation, however, is the effect obtained when fraction II and fraction VII were mixed together prior to addition to the cultures. This mixture exerted a marked enhancing effect on the response of untreated spleen cells (around 5-fold over the normal response) and displayed the highest reconstituting activity on the response of anti-θ-treated cells, which was almost 50% greater than that obtained with unfractionated AEF. It should be noted that: (1) the final concentration of the fraction II and VII components of the mixture was 1:10 (c.f. the low activity of the 1:10 concentration of fraction II), and (2) the observed activity of the mixture is substantially greater than the additive effects expected from the biological activity of the individual components themselves[39,104,105]. This finding strongly indicates, therefore, that the active moiety of AEF may consist of a bicomponent complex — one heavy and one light — which are associated noncovalently.

4.8.2.3 Immunological properties of AEF

Thus far, we have analysed the immunological properties of AEF by various immunochemical and functional techniques. Immunochemical analysis has shown that AEF purified on Sephadex G-100 does not react or cross-react with any heterologous antisera directed against immunoglobulin determinants[105]. In our initial studies on the activity of AEF, we found that although it did not manifest any specificity for antigens against which the *in vitro* antibody responses were directed, AEF did exhibit some strain-specific properties suggesting a relationship to antigens or gene products coded in the major histocompatibility gene complex[38].

The aforementioned observations prompted us to explore the relationship of AEF to histocompatibility antigens by functional analysis. Thus, experiments were designed to determine whether immunoadsorbents prepared with antisera reactive with *H-2* determinants would specifically remove the biologically active moiety of AEF. In the first experiments we found that antisera directed against either the entire $H-2^d$ haplotype or the K end of $H-2^d$ would indeed remove the activity of AEF derived from DBA/2 T cells; in contrast, antisera directed against specificities coded by genes in the D end of $H-2^d$ failed to absorb AEF activity[106]. Recently, investigations in several laboratories using anti-lymphoid cell antisera prepared between recombinant mice differing at genes present in the I region of the $H-2$ complex identified a new antigen system, which has been termed Ia, coded for by genes in the I region; the Ia antigens have been found to exist predominantly on B cells and macrophages and to varying extents on T cells[41,112-116]. Accordingly, we considered the possibility that gene products in this region may be involved in regulatory cell interactions in immune responses. The experiment presented in Figure 4.13 demonstrates that the active enhancing factor(s) in AEF can be removed by an immunoadsorbent prepared with an anti-Ia antiserum indicating that, indeed, the biologically active moieties responsible for T–B cell interactions are probably products of genes in the I region of the $H-2$ gene complex[103]. The following antisera were used: (1) B10.A anti-B10 — this antiserum contains antibodies reactive with antigens coded by genes in the I region of $H-2^d$ (Ia.8) but not with antigens coded by genes in either K or D regions of $H-2^d$; (2) (B6A)F$_1$ anti-B10.D2 — this antiserum contains predominantly antibodies reactive with specificity $H-2.31$ present on cells from animals with the $H-2^d$ allele; recent analyses have demonstrated the presence in this antiserum also of antibodies reactive with a new Ia specificity (Ia.11) present in $H-2^d$ [117].

In the experiment shown in Figure 4.13, three different concentrations of AEF were directly absorbed independently by immunoadsorbents prepared from (B6A)F$_1$ anti-B10.D2 and B10.A anti-B10 alloantisera and by an adsorbent prepared from normal B10.A serum. These AEF were then compared to unabsorbed AEF for biological activity on the *in vitro* response to SRBC of DBA/2 B lymphocytes. As shown in Figure 4.13, cultures of untreated control whole spleen cells developed primary IgG anti-SRBC responses of around 1200 PFC; anti-θ treatment diminished this response to around 150 PFC. The addition of unabsorbed AEF to such anti-θ serum-treated B cells reconstituted and enriched the response markedly and in a dose-related manner at all three concentrations of AEF employed. The AEF subjected to the adsorbent prepared from (B6A)F$_1$ anti-B10.D2 serum retained essentially normal biological activity at the highest concentration (1:5), but the lowest concentration subjected to absorption (1:20) was around 45% lower in activity than the normal serum control. The AEF subjected to the B10.A anti-B10 (anti-Ia) immunoadsorbent, on the other hand, exhibited markedly diminished (80% or more) activity at all three concentrations indicating substantial reactivity of this anti-serum with the biologically active component(s) of AEF[103].

The identification of a small molecular weight component that is present in AEF and apparently required for full expression of biological activity (Figure 4.12), prompted us to determine the relationship of this component to β_2-microglobulin. The discovery of the association of β_2-microglobulin with histo-

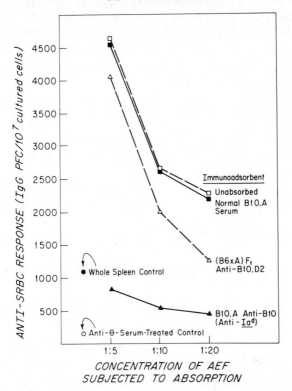

Figure 4.13   Removal of biological activity of AEF derived from DBA/2 (H-2^d) T cells by an anti-Ia^d immunoadsorbent. Three different concentrations of AEF were subjected to immunoadsorbents prepared from either normal B10.A serum or from (B6A)F$_1$ anti-B10.D2 or B10.A anti-B10 (anti-Ia^d) ascites. These AEF were then tested and compared to unabsorbed AEF for activity on the *in vitro* response to SRBC of anti-θ serum-treated DBA/2 spleen cells. Control responses of whole spleen cells and anti-θ-treated cells in the absence of AEF are shown to the left. The IgG antibody responses are presented and paralleled the IgM response pattern of these same cultures (not shown). (Taken from reference 103.)

compatibility molecules in several species and the demonstration of remarkable homology of its amino acid sequence with the constant homology regions of immunoglobulins have raised intriguing questions concerning the significance and function of this small protein (for review, see references 118 and 119). In preliminary experiments performed in collaboration with Dr. Howard Grey, we have tested the capacity of antisera directed against a murine β_2-microglobulin-like component to specifically adsorb the biologically active component of AEF. The results of these experiments indicate, indeed, that the activity of AEF can be removed on such immunoadsorbents[120]. We are reserving conclusions on these data, however, until evidence is obtained that will establish that the murine cell surface product with which these antisera have been prepared is in fact the homologue of β_2-microglobulin. If such is the case, then our results would indicate that a component in AEF is (or is highly cross-reactive with) β_2-microglobulin. Whether the specificities removed by these latter antisera are present on the heavy or light molecular weight components of AEF (or both) is presently being determined.

4.8.3 Conclusions

The studies presented above have demonstrated the existence of a class of molecules, produced by antigen-activated T cells, which exert biological activity in the regulation of immune responses. These molecules are in some cases antigen-specific and in other cases non-specific, but nevertheless share remarkable similarity in terms of molecular size, the presence on them of determinants coded for by genes in the major histocompatibility complex and their lack of identifiable immunoglobulin determinants. The existence of antigen-specific molecules that are non-immunoglobulin in nature clearly points to a new distinct class of molecules capable of performing receptor functions, most likely on T cells. The functional effects of these molecules are either suppressive or enhancing depending on the manner in which they are induced, and they are capable of acting on T lymphocytes and on B lymphocytes in various circumstances. What is not yet known is whether there are distinct molecules for each type of target cell and for different biological functions.

A final point that we must consider about such factors is whether or not their capacity to function is genetically restricted to the same extent as has been shown for cooperative T–B cell interactions (Section 4.6). The evidence thus far indicates that such restrictions may not exist, at least to the same extent, for the biological activity of the T cell factors as is the case for cooperative T–B cell interactions. Thus, as discussed above, Taussig et al.[33] have shown that the (T,G)-A- -L-specific factor obtained from T cells from donors of the H-2^k haplotype is capable of enhancing responses of bone marrow cells from donors of the *H-2^b* haplotype. Moreover, although the initial studies of Armerding and Katz[38] indicated some degree of strain preference in the action of AEF, more recent and extensive genetic analysis on this point has failed to reveal a clear pattern of genetic restrictions for the activity of this factor[105]. Whereas these findings appear to be contradictory to the observations on genetic restrictions of T–B cell interactions, there are two crucial points to emphasize here. First, it must be recognized that all of the experiments that have demonstrated the activity of T cell factors have been carried out *in vitro* where the factor(s) have been exposed to the target cell populations under conditions where the opportunity for interactions have been maximized. Second, and perhaps more germane, is the fact that the physiologic interactions between T and B cells under normal circumstances may well involve actual membrane-membrane contact to a great extent in addition to release of soluble T cell products. Thus, it must be considered that the conformational structure of a biologically active molecule within a cell membrane may be sufficiently different after being released from the cell to account for a difference in the degree of genetic restrictions observed.

4.9 FUNCTIONS OF PRODUCTS OF H-LINKED *Ir* GENES AND OTHER *I* REGION GENE PRODUCTS: RELATIONSHIP OF THESE PRODUCTS TO ACTIVATION OF IMMUNOCOMPETENT CELLS

The identification of specific H-linked *Ir* genes posed a considerable challenge to the unitarian concepts of classical immunology, as the recognition of immunogenicity controlled by different genes for different antigens was demonstrated to be distinct from, and independent of, the specificity system represented by the immunoglobulin receptor molecules on B cells. The hypothesis was therefore entertained that such genes were coding for the antigen receptor on T cells, a molecule whose nature has been controversial. This earlier interpretation was based largely upon the following circumstantial evidence:

(1) All responses controlled by H-linked *Ir* genes have been to thymus-dependent antigens; in no case have H-linked *Ir* genes been identified controlling responses to thymus-independent antigens although the latter responses have been shown, in some instances, to be controlled by allotype linked (Section 4.2) and sex chromosome-linked *Ir* genes[121,122].

(2) *Ir* gene functional expression in T lymphocytes has been amply demonstrated in many laboratories, particularly in responses involving cell-mediated immunity and the regulation of humoral immunity (discussed in Section 4.7).

These two lines of evidence indicated therefore a definite association of *Ir* genes with the activity of T cells themselves in immune responses and/or with the manner in which this activity is exercised on other cells. The approach to this question was subsequently directed to the identification of the cell types in which *Ir* gene defects can be detected in non-responders and to the analysis of the processes controlled by these genes. Evidence was presented that depending upon the strains and the antigens studied such defects could be detected in T cells alone, T and B cells, or even only in B cells of non-responder animals (Section 4.7). However, in the cases where the defect was detected in B cells, it appeared to be concerned with the ability of these cells to be effectively regulated by activated T cells and their products; it is pertinent to emphasize that the T cells concerned in the latter circumstance are those activated by the antigen under *Ir* gene control. These observations led to the conclusion that the function of *Ir* genes is intimately related to the mechanisms by which T cell regulation of immune responses is effected.

The studies directed to delineation of the mechanisms of T and B cell cooperative interactions led initially to the hypothesis that the primary role of T cells in such responses was that of antigen-focusing, either directly or indirectly via macrophages (discussed in reference 54). The weight of evidence, however, has subsequently demonstrated that T cell regulation of immune responses is mediated via factors which are active on both T cells and B cells. These factors have properties of either enhancing or suppressing responses and may be either specific or non-specific (Section 4.8).

The studies in recent years on the genetic control of the cooperative interactions between T cells and B cells and between macrophages and T cells demonstrated that genes in the major histocompatibility complex, which map in precisely the region where the majority of *Ir* genes have been identified, are responsible for this vital phenomenon (discussed in Section 4.6). Such findings motivated us to propose the existence of a distinct class of molecules on surface membranes of T cells, B cells and macrophages concerned with their effective interactions and the differentiation in immunocompetent cells that are regulated by such interactions. These cell interaction or CI molecules were also postulated by us to be coded for by genes in the *I* region of the *H-2* complex, and to possess antigenic specificities determined by genes in this region. We further speculated that the products of *Ir* genes and CI molecules would be intimately related both phenotypically and functionally[31,32]. Indeed, the hypothesis was formulated that such gene products i.e. *Ir* and *CI*, would, if not identical, be expressed together in the same molecular complex(es)[31].

This hypothesis has been supported by the recent demonstrations in our own laboratories as well as those of others of a newly recognized class of biologically active molecules obtained from activated T cells with distinctive properties (discussed in Section 4.8). These molecules are in the size range of 40 000–50 000 daltons, bear determinants of gene products of the *I* region, are endowed with either helper or suppressor activity depending on the experimental conditions and operate on both cell-mediated and humoral immune responses. These molecules do not react with anti-immunoglobulin reagents. Although studies on the antigen specificity of these molecules have been thus far limited, evidence has been presented demonstrating that certain of these can be specifically adsorbed by antigen-immunoadsorbent columns and appear to be most effective in regulating responses to the antigen used to stimulate their production.

It is clear that our understanding of the relationship between *Ir* and *CI* gene products is evolving very rapidly based upon the increasing availability of new data concerning these entities. Nevertheless, we feel that certain definitive conclusions can be drawn from what has been discussed in this chapter. (1) There is a class of molecules distinct from immunoglobulins that is capable of interacting specifically with antigen and which is composed, at least in part, of gene products of the major histocompatibility complex. (2) These molecules are produced by activated T cells; and (3) Their functions are to interact with appropriate CI molecules on other T cells, B cells and macrophages to control the differentiation of immunocompetent cells in immune responses. (4) The antigen specificities of such molecules may be relevant to the process of selective concentration onto other cells which have bound antigen, but the biological activity of such molecules need not depend upon their antigen specificity.

There are certain major problems to be resolved which primarily concern the structure of this molecule and the relationships of the *Ir* and CI gene products within this structure. The molecule can be considered to consist of two distinct functional entities, namely the portion concerned with the interactions between cells and the regulation of responses (i.e. *CI* entity) and the portion of the molecule with antigen-binding properties. The Ir gene product might be considered to be coding for the latter, except for the fact that even though the recognition controlled by *Ir* genes is highly specific, the number of identified *Ir* genes is considerably more limited than would be expected if this were the case. Moreover, the specificities of cellular immune responses controlled by H-linked *Ir* genes has been shown to be more extensive than the number of genes that control these responses. The possibility must be considered, therefore, that the *Ir* gene product in this molecule does not code for the combining site but rather introduces restrictions in the system by limiting the number of variable regions that CI molecules can possess. This can be done by either coding for CI molecules themselves or, alternatively, by coding for a constant portion of the variable region concerned with antigen recognition in a manner analogous to that which occurs in immunoglobulins. An example of this second model is the manner in which the allotype sequences controlled by the α locus in the rabbit place restrictions in the affinity of antibodies produced bearing these allotypic specificities[123].

Finally, the very recent demonstration that two genes located within the *H-2* complex are required for responses to GLϕ in mice (Section 4.3) raises intriguing possibilities concerning both the function of H-linked *Ir* genes and the nature of the T cell receptor. The need for two genes may simply reflect the required expression of cooperative genes in different classes or subclasses of lymphocytes for immune responses to develop or, alternatively, if these distinct genes are coding for the variable regions of T cell receptors, then the generation of receptor specificity may conceivably evolve from the cooperative interactions between such gene products on the cell surface as earlier suggested by Simonsen[124].

Acknowledgments

We are extremely grateful to our colleagues and collaborators who participated in the studies cited herein performed in our laboratories. We are particular indebted to Drs. Dieter Armerding and Martin Dorf for their invaluable contributions in the performance of many of the recent studies presented here and for help in preparing Figures 4.1, 4.2, 4.3 and 4.4. We thank Miss Deborah Maher for excellent secretarial assistance. The work performed in our laboratories was supported by Grants AI-10630 and AI-09920 from The National Institutes of Health.

References

1. McDevitt, H. O. and Benacerraf, B. (1969). *Advan. Immunol.*, **11**, 31
2. Benacerraf, B. and McDevitt, H. O. (1972). *Science*, **175**, 273
3. Benacerraf, B. (1974). *Ann. Immunol. (Inst. Pasteur)*, **125C**, 143
4. McDevitt, H. O. and Tyan, M. L. (1968). *J. Exp. Med.*, **128**, 1
5. Ellman, L., Green, I., Martin, W. J. and Benacerraf, B. (1970). *Proc. Nat. Acad. Sci. (USA)*, **66**, 322
6. Armerding, D. and Rajewsky, K. (1970). In H. Peeters (ed.). *Protides of the Biological Fluids, Proceedings of the 17th Colloqium, Bruges, 1969*, p. 185. (Oxford and New York: Pergamon Press)
7. Günther, R., Rüde, E. and Stark, O. (1972). *Eur. J. Immunol.*, **2**, 151
8. Armerding, D., Katz, D. H. and Benacerraf, B. (1974). *Immunogenetics*, **1**, 329
9. Dorf, M. E., Balner, H., de Groot, L. and Benacerraf, B. (1974). *Transpl. Proc.*, **6**, 119
10. Balner, H., Dorf, M. E., de Groot, M. L. and Benacerraf, B. (1973). *Transpl. Proc.*, **5**, 1555
11. Levine, B. B., Ojeda, A. and Benacerraf, B. (1963). *J. Exp. Med.*, **118**, 953
12. Benacerraf, B., Bluestein, H. G., Green, I. and Ellman, L. (1971). *Progr. Immunol.*, **1**, 485
13. Shevach, E. M. (1975). (Personal communication).
14. Green, I., Paul, W. E. and Benacerraf, B. (1969). *Proc. Soc. Nat. Acad. Sci. (USA)*, **64**, 1095
15. Shearer, G. M. (1975). (Personal communication).
16. McDevitt, H. O. and Sela, M. (1965). *J. Exp. Med.*, **122**, 517
17. McDevitt, H. O., Deak, B. D., Shreffler, D. C., Klein, J., Stimpfling, J. H. and Snell, G. D. (1972). *J. Exp. Med.*, **135**, 1259
18. Benacerraf, B. and Dorf, M. E. (1974). *Progr. Immunol. II*, **2**, 181
19. Klein, J. and Shreffler, D. C. (1971). *Transpl. Rev.*, **6**, 3
20. Dorf, M. E., Plate, J. M. D., Stimpfling, J. H. and Benacerraf, B. (1975). *J. Immunol.*, **114**, 602
21. Blomberg, B., Geckeler, W. R. and Weigert, M. (1972). *Science*, **177**, 178
22. Eichmann, E. (1972). *Eur. J. Immunol.*, **4**, 301
23. Pawlak, L. L. and Nisonoff, A. (1973). *J. Exp. Med.*, **137**, 855
24. Landucci Tosi, S., Mage, R. G. and Dubiski, S. (1970). *J. Immunol.*, **104**, 641
25. McDevitt, H. O. (Personal communication).
26. Hämmerling, G. J. and McDevitt, H. O. (1974). *J. Immunol.*, **112**, 1734
27. Kennedy, J., Dorf, M. E., Unanue, E. R. and Benacerraf, B. (1975). *J. Immunol.* (In Press).
28. Shevach, E. M., Paul, W. E. and Green, I. (1972). *J. Exp. Med.*, **137**, 1207
29. Shevach, E. M., Green, I. and Paul, W. E. (1974). *J. Exp. Med.*, **139**, 679
30. Bluestein, H. (1974). *J. Immunol.*, **113**, 1410
31. Katz, D. H. and Benacerraf, B. (1975). *Transpl. Rev.*, **22**, 175
32. Katz, D. H. and Benacerraf, B. (1974). In E. E. Sercarz, A. R. Williamson and C. Fred Fox (eds.). *The Immune System: Genes, Receptors, Signals*, p. 569. (New York: Academic Press)
33. Taussig, M. J., Mozes, E. and Isac, R. (1974). *J. Exp. Med.*, **140**, 301
34. Munro, A. J., Taussig, M. J., Campbell, R., Williams, H. and Lawson, Y. (1974). *J. Exp. Med.*, **140**, 1579

35. Mozes, E., Isac, R. and Taussig, M. J. (1975). *J. Exp. Med.,* **141,** 703
36. Tada, T. (1974). In D. H. Katz and B. Benacerraf (eds.). *Immunological Tolerance: Mechanisms and Potential Therapeutic Applications,* p. 471. (New York: Academic Press)
37. Tada, T. (1975). In A. S. Rosenthal (ed.). *Immune Recognition. Proceedings of the Ninth Leukocyte Culture Conference.* p. 771 (New York: Academic Press)
38. Armerding, D. and Katz, D. H. (1974). *J. Exp. Med.,* **140,** 19
39. Katz, D. H. and Armerding, D. (1975). In A. S. Rosenthal (ed.). *Immune Recognition. Proceedings of the Ninth Leukocyte Culture Conference.* p. 727 (New York: Academic Press)
40. McDevitt, H. O. and Chinitz, A. (1969). *Science,* **163,** 1207
41. Shreffler, D. C. and David, C. S. (1975). *Advan. Immunol.,* **20,** 125
42. Lieberman, R., Paul, W. E., Humphrey, W., Jr. and Stimpfling, J. H. (1972). *J. Exp. Med.,* **136,** 1231
43. Dorf, M. E., Lilly, F. and Benacerraf, B. (1974). *J. Exp. Med.,* **140,** 859
44. Zaleski, M., Fuji, J. and Milgrom, F. (1973). *Transpl. Proc.,* **5,** 201
45. Rüde, E. and Günther, E. (1975). *Progr. Immunol.,* **II. 2,** 223
46. Stimpfling, J. H. and Durham, T. (1972). *J. Immunol.,* **108,** 947
47. Dorf, M. E., Stimpfling, J. H. and Benacerraf, B. (1975). *J. Exp. Med.,* **141,** 1459
48. Yunis, E. J. and Amos, D. B. (1971). *Proc. Nat. Acad. Sci. (USA),* **68,** 3031
49. Bach, F. H., Widmer, M. B., Bach, M. L. and Klein, J. (1972). *J. Exp. Med.,* **136,** 1430
50. Seaver, S. S., Brown, A., Hämmerling, G. and McDevitt, H. O. (1975). (In preparation)
51. Mozes, E., Schwartz, M. and Sela, M. (1974). *J. Exp. Med.,* **140,** 349
52. Hill, S. and Sercarz, E. E. (1975). *Eur. J. Immunol.* (In press)
53. Keck, K. (1975). *Nature,* **254,** 78
54. Katz, D. H. and Benacerraf, B. (1972). *Advan. Immunol.,* **15,** 1
55. Gershon, R. K. (1974). *Contemp. Topics in Immunobiol.,* **3,** 1
56. Basten, A. (1974). In D. H. Katz and B. Benacerraf (eds.). *Immunological Tolerance: Mechanisms and Potential Therapeutic Applications,* p. 107. (New York: Academic Press)
57. Claman, H. M., Phanuphak, P. and Moorehead, J. W. (1974). In D. H. Katz and B. Benacerraf (eds.). *Immunological Tolerance: Mechanisms and Potential Therapeutic Applications,* p. 123. (New York: Academic Press)
58. Gershon, R. K., Maurer, P. H. and Merryman, C. F. (1973). *Proc. Nat. Acad. Sci.* (USA), **70,** 250
59. Kapp, J. A., Pierce, C. W. and Benacerraf, B. (1974). *J. Exp. Med.,* **140,** 172
60. Kapp, J. A., Pierce, C. W., Schlossman, S. and Benacerraf, B. (1974). *J. Exp. Med.,* **140,** 648
61. Kapp, J., Pierce, C. W. and Benacerraf, B. (1975). *J. Exp. Med.,* (In press)
62. Kindred, B. and Shreffler, D. C. (1972). *J. Immunol.,* **109,** 940
63. Katz, D. H., Hamaoka, T. and Benacerraf, B. (1973). *J. Exp. Med.,* **137,** 1405
64. Katz, D. H., Hamaoka, T., Dorf, M. E. and Benacerraf, B. (1973). *Proc. Nat. Acad. Sci. (USA),* **70,** 2624
65. Rosenthal, A. S. and Shevach, E. M. (1973). *J. Exp. Med.,* **138,** 1194
66. Toivanen, P., Toivanen, A. and Vainio, O. (1974). *J. Exp. Med.,* **139,** 1344
67. Katz, D. H., Hamaoka, T., Dorf, M. E., Maurer, P. H. and Benacerraf, B. (1973). *J. Exp. Med.,* **138,** 734
68. Katz, D. H., Hamaoka, T., Dorf, M. E. and Benacerraf, B. (1974). *J. Immunol.,* **112,** 855
69. Katz, D. H., Dorf, M. E. and Benacerraf, B. (1974). *J. Exp. Med.,* **140,** 290
70. Dorf, M. E., Katz, D. H., Graves, M., DiMuzio, H. and Benacerraf, B. (1975). *J. Immunol.,* **114,** 1717
71. Katz, D. H., Graves, M., Dorf, M. E., DiMuzio, H. and Benacerraf, B. (1975). *J. Exp. Med.,* **141,** 263
72. Benacerraf, B. and Katz, D. H. (1975). *Advan. Cancer Res.,* **21,** (In press)
73. Rosenthal, A. S. and Shevach, E. M. (1973). *J. Exp. Med.,* **138,** 1194

74. Shevach, E. M. and Rosenthal, A. S. (1973). *J. Exp. Med.*, **138**, 1213
75. Erb, P. and Feldmann, M. (1975). *Nature* (In press)
76. Katz, D. H. and Unanue, E. R. (1973). *J. Exp. Med.*, **137**, 967
77. Kapp, J. A., Pierce, C. W. and Benacerraf, B. (1973). *J. Exp. Med.*, **138**, 1121
78. Lonai, P. and McDevitt, H. O. (1974). *J. Exp. Med.*, **140**, 977
79. Pierce, C. W., Kapp, J. A., Solliday, S. M., Dorf, M. E. and Benacerraf, B. (1974). *J. Exp. Med.*, **140**, 921
80. Bechtol, K. B., Freed, J. H., Herzenberg, L. A. and McDevitt, H. O. (1974). *J. Exp. Med.*, **140**, 1660
81. Ellman, L., Green, I. and Benacerraf, B. (1970). *Cell. Immunol.*, **1**, 445
82. Kapp, J. A., Pierce, C. W. and Benacerraf, B. (1973). *J. Exp. Med.*, **138**, 1107
83. Levine, B. B. and Benacerraf, B. (1965). *Science*, **147**, 517
84. Green, I. and Benacerraf, B. (1971). *J. Immunol.*, **107**, 374
85. Green, I., Paul, W. E. and Benacerraf, B. (1969). *Proc. Nat. Acad. Sci. (USA)*, **64**, 1095
86. Dunham, E. K., Unanue, E. R. and Benacerraf, B. (1972). *J. Exp. Med.*, **136**, 403
87. Mitchell, G. F., Grumet, F. C. and McDevitt, H. O. (1972). *J. Exp. Med.*, **135**, 126
88. Ordal, J. C. and Grumet, F. C. (1972). *J. Exp. Med.*, **136**, 1195
89. Shearer, G. M., Mozes, E. and Sela, M. (1972). *J. Exp. Med.*, **135**, 1109
90. Dutton, R. W., Falkoff, R., Hirst, J. A., Hoffmann, M., Kappler, J. W., Kettman, J. R., Lesley, J. F. and Vann, D. (1971). *Prog. Immunol.*, **1**, 355
91. Tada, T., Okumura, K. and Taniguchi, M. (1973). *J. Immunol.*, **111**, 952
92. Okumura, K. and Tada, T. (1974). *J. Immunol.*, **112**, 783
93. Taniguchi, M. and Tada, T. (1974). *J. Immunol.*, **113**, 1757
94. Feldmann, M. (1972). *J. Exp. Med.*, **136**, 737
95. Feldmann, M., Cone, R. E. and Marchalonis, J. J. (1973). *Cell Immunol.*, **9**, 1
96. Tada, T. and Takemori, T. (1974). *J. Exp. Med.*, **140**, 239
97. Takemori, T. and Tada, T. (1974). *J. Exp. Med.*, **140**, 253
98. Tada, T. (1975). (Personal communication)
99. Zembala, M., Asherson, G. L., Mayhew, B. and Krejci, J. (1975). *Nature*, **253**, 72
100. Taussig, M. J. and Munro, A. (1975). In A. S. Rosenthal (ed.). *Immune Recognition. Proceedings of the Ninth Leukocyte Culture Conference*, p. 791. (New York: Academic Press)
101. Schimpl, A. and Wecker, E. (1972). *Nature (London) New Biol.*, **237**, 15
102. Schimpl, A. and Wecker, E. (1972). *J. Exp. Med.*, **137**, 547
103. Armerding, D., Sachs, D. H. and Katz, D. H. (1974). *J. Exp. Med.*, **140**, 1717
104. Katz, D. H., Dorf, M. E., Armerding, D. and Benacerraf, B. (1974). In E. E. Smith and D. W. Ribbons (eds.). *Molecular Approaches to Immunology, Miami Winter Symposia, Vol. 9.* (New York: Academic Press)
105. Armerding, D. and Katz, D. H. (In preparation)
106. Armerding, D., Dorf, M. E. and Katz, D. H. (In preparation)
107. Katz, D. H. (1972). *Transpl. Rev.*, **12**, 141
108. Katz, D. H. and Benacerraf, B. (1974). In D. H. Katz and B. Benacerraf (eds.). *Immunological Tolerance: Mechanisms and Potential Therapeutic Applications*, p. 189. (New York: Academic Press)
109. Katz, D. H. and Benacerraf, B. (1974). In D. H. Katz and B. Benacerraf (eds.). *Immunological Tolerance: Mechanisms and Potential Therapeutic Applications*, p. 249. (New York: Academic Press)
110. Katz, D. H., Davie, J. M., Paul, W. E. and Benacerraf, B. (1971). *J. Exp. Med.*, **134**, 201
111. Osborne, D. P., Jr. and Katz, D. H. (1973). *J. Exp. Med.*, **137**, 991
112. David, C. S., Shreffler, D. C. and Frelinger, J. A. (1973). *Proc. Nat. Acad. Sci. (USA)*, **70**, 2509
113. Hauptfield, V. D., Klein, D. and Klein, J. (1973). *Science*, **181**, 167
114. Sachs, D. H. and Cone, J. L. (1973). *J. Exp. Med.*, **138**, 1289

115. Hämmerling, G. J., Deak, B. D., Mauve, G., Hämmerling, U. and McDevitt, H. O. (1974). *Immunogenetics*, **1**, 68
116. Unanue, E. R., Dorf, M. E., David, C. S. and Benacerraf, B. (1974). *Proc. Nat. Acad. Sci.* (*USA*), **71**, 5014
117. Sachs, D. H., Fathman, C. G., Cone, J. L. and Dickler, H. B. (1975). *Transpl. Proc.* (In press)
118. Cunningham, B. A. and Berggard, I. (1974). *Transpl. Rev.*, **21**, 3
119. Strominger, J. L., Cresswell, P., Grey, H., Humphreys, R. H., Mann, D., McCune, J., Parham, P., Robb, R., Sanderson, A. R., Springer, T. A., Terhorst, C. and Turner, M. J. (1974). *Transpl. Rev.*, **21**, 126
120. Armerding, D., Grey, H. M. and Katz, D. H. (Unpublished observation)
121. Amsbaugh, D. F., Hanse, C. T., Prescott, B., Stashak, P. W., Barthold, D. R. and Baker, P. J. (1972). *J. Exp. Med.*, **136**, 931
122. Mozes, E. and Fuchs, S. (1974). *Nature* (*London*), **249**, 167
123. Werblin, T. P., Kim, Y. T., Mage, R., Benacerraf, B. and Siskind, G. W. (1973). *Immunology*, **25**, 17
124. Simonsen, M. (1974). *Allergology*, **146**. (Amsterdam: Excerpta Medica)

5
Selection of Lines of Mice with High and Low Antibody Responses to Complex Immunogens

G. BIOZZI, C. STIFFEL, D. MOUTON and Y. BOUTHILLIER

5.1   INTRODUCTION

The cellular basis of the immune response consists essentially in a phenomenon of multiplication and differentiation of T and B lymphocytes stimulated by the antigen processed in macrophages. The selection of the specific clone of lymphocytes is made by the stereospecific combination of antigen determinants with pre-existing receptors on the lymphocyte surface. In B lymphocytes, these receptors are immunoglobulins; the nature of the receptors in T lymphocytes is still controversial.

Intracellular and intercellular reactions are therefore integrated in the phenomenon of immune response. The efficiency and coordination of such a complex phenomenon are controlled and regulated at different levels by genetic factors.

The structural genes coding for the polypeptide chains forming the molecules of antigen receptors are thus involved in antigen recognition. Immune responsiveness to antigens of restricted specificity is regulated by specific immune response genes (*Ir* genes). Specific *Ir* genes linked to the major histocompatibility locus control the antigen recognition by T lymphocytes[1-6]. Other specific *Ir* genes linked to the immunoglobulin allotype regulate the fine structure of antibody molecules affecting specificity, homogeneity, affinity and idiotypic antigenicity[7-16]. Each of these genes regulates the specific responsiveness to a single or a few antigens.

The experimental results reviewed in this chapter demonstrate that a two-way selective breeding for quantitative antibody response to a complex multideterminant immunogen has produced lines of mice endowed with High or Low responsiveness to many other unrelated complex immunogens. The genetic selection has therefore modified the general immune responsiveness irrespectively of the specificity of the antibody synthesized. General immune responsiveness is a polygenic character determined by a group of about ten independent loci.

The immune response to a multideterminant immunogen is not the mere result of the additive effect of *Ir* genes specific for each antigenic determinant. Specific and general regulations of immune responsiveness thus operate at different levels. Nevertheless, recent results indicate that specific and general regulations have some common genetic mechanisms. We have demonstrated that among the group of genes regulating general antibody synthesis, one is linked with the *H-2* locus and another one with the immunoglobulin allotype. Provisional unpublished experiments, made in collaboration with P. H. Maurer, show that High and Low responder lines of mice, separated by selective breeding for general antibody synthesis are also separated for antibody response to polymers of restricted specificity such as GAT[10] and GLPhe. On the other hand, the control of antibody response to antigens of restricted specificity may also be a polygenic trait[17–21] including allotype-linked and *H-2* linked loci[16,21,22].

The rapid accumulation of experimental studies demonstrating the analogies between the genetic control of specific and general antibody synthesis preludes the formulation in the near future of a unified theory of the genetic regulation of immune responsiveness.

5.2 TWO-WAY SELECTION FOR AGGLUTININ PRODUCTION

The selective breeding for the character 'agglutinin production' was carried out on individual merit by mating at each generation the mice giving the highest titres (High line) or the lowest titres (Low line). The titre of serum agglutinins was measured 5–7 days and 14 days after i.v. immunization with an optimal dose of heterologous erythrocytes. The agglutinin titres were expressed either as the highest serum dilution giving a positive agglutination or as the $\log_2$ of this dilution starting from $1 = 1/10$ serum dilution. For each line and at each generation five pairs at least were formed. Though brother–sister mating was excluded, an increasing coefficient of consanguinity was produced by the closed colony breeding. Two types of selection were performed: Selection I and Selection II.

Selection I

The foundation population was composed of 62 random-bred albino mice of both sexes obtained from several commercial breeders. The mice were immunized intravenously with optimal doses of sheep erythrocytes (SE) ($10^8 - 5 \times 10^8$). Their offspring were weaned at 30 days of age. For the first 6 generations the immunization was made about 30 days after weaning. In these generations, the antibody response was biased by maternal-transmitted antibody, especially in High line. Nevertheless, responsiveness of the two lines was different in F_6. It was then noticed that the two lines also differed for their responsiveness to non-cross-reacting pigeon erythrocytes (PE). In order to speed up the selective breeding without interference of maternal-transmitted antibody, from the 6th generation onwards SE and PE (10^8) were alternated at each generation and mice were immunized 35–45 days after birth[23-24].

Selection II

The foundation population was constituted of 50 random-bred albino mice of both sexes (from Charles River, Elbeuf, France). The selective breeding was carried out for agglutinin response to SE. The animals were weaned when 30 days old and immunized 60–70 days after weaning in order to obtain the elimination, by natural decay, of the maternal-transmitted antibody[25,26].

At present, Selection I has been carried out for 30 successive generations and Selection II for 16 successive generations. In both cases, selective breeding proved to be a very efficient method for separating High and Low responder lines of mice. No significant difference in agglutinin titres was observed between males and females; therefore, the character was established by the combined means of males and females.

Selective breeding produces a strong modification in the kinetics of agglutinin synthesis, both the peak titre and the duration of agglutinin production are affected (Figure 5.1). In Low responders, the peak is reached 5 days

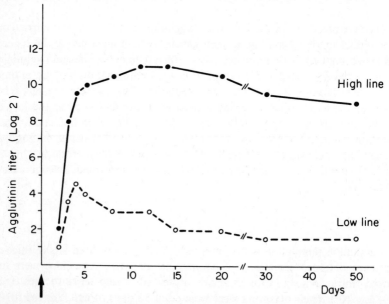

Figure 5.1 Kinetics of anti SE-agglutinin production in F_{18} High and Low responders of Selection I. From Biozzi *et al.* (1971). In *Progress in Immunology*, p. 529, by courtesy of Academic Press, New York.

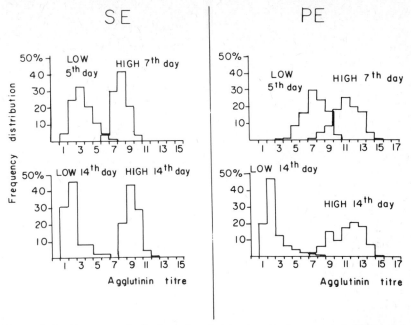

Figure 5.2 Frequency distribution of agglutinin titres in 'homozygous' High and Low responders of Selection I. $F_{20-22-26-28-30}$ mice were immunized with SE (204 High responders–230 Low responders). $F_{21-23-25-27-29}$ mice were immunized with PE (197 High responders–217 Low responders). From Feingold *et al. Eur. J. Immunol.* (submitted for publication).

post-immunization. Afterwards, the agglutinin titre drops rapidly to almost the pre-immunization level on the 20th day. In High responders, the agglutinin titre rises until the 14th day and persists at a very high level for months.

In Figure 5.2 is represented the frequency distribution of SE and PE agglutinin titres 5–7 days and 14 days post-immunization in homozygous F_{20}–F_{30} of Selection I. An important quantitative difference in immune responsiveness to both SE and PE is evident. The maximal inter-line difference is found in the agglutinin titres measured 14 days post-immunization since, by that time, both the level and the duration of antibody synthesis are taken into account. In consequence, the 14th day agglutinin titres are considered as the best measure of the phenotypic character and used in the following genetic analysis of immune responsiveness.

5.2.1 Inter-line separation produced by selective breeding

Selection I

The divergence between High and Low responder lines produced by 30 generations of selection is represented in Figure 5.3. The data of the first 6

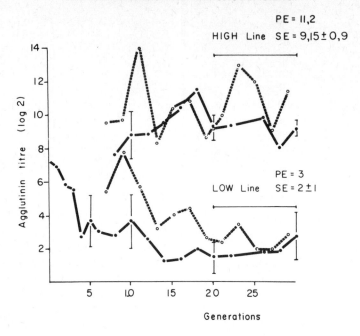

Figure 5.3 Mean SE or PE agglutinin titres 14 days post-immunization in successive generations of High and Low responders of Selection I. Vertical bars indicate standard deviation. Dotted line = PE, solid line = Se. From Feingold *et al. Eur. J. Immunol.* (submitted for publication).

generations of High line are not represented since immune responsiveness was affected by maternal antibody[23]. From the 6th generation onwards, SE and PE were alternated and the corresponding data are reported on Figure 5.3. In spite of the erratic fluctuations due to environmental factors it is evident that the inter-line separation occurs progressively during the selective breeding and becomes maximal after about 20 generations. This demonstrates that the character investigated is submitted to polygenic regulation. All the genes favourable to responsiveness have been progressively accumulated in the High line F_{20} while all the unfavourable ones have been segregated in the Low line F_{20}. The continuation of selective breeding for ten generations (F_{20}–F_{30}) did not significantly increase the inter-line difference. Thus, the F_{20}–F_{30} generations may be considered as homozygous for the character investigated. The data established in F_{20}–F_{30} are consequently cumulated and considered as the best measure of the final effect of the selective breeding. It is evident that this effect is asymmetrical since immune responsiveness is decreased in Low line to a larger extent than it is increased in High line. The mean titre of SE agglutinins is 7.3 (1/900) in the foundation population, 9.15 (1/3,200) in homozygous High responders and 2.0 (1/20) in homozygous Low responders.

Selection II

A more exact appreciation of inter-line separation produced by selective breeding is obtained in Selection II where the data of all generations are available for both lines. The inter-line separation is represented in Figure 5.4. Unfortunately, Selection II is less advanced and at present it only includes 16 generations. Nevertheless, the inter-line separation of F_{16} is about the same as in homozygous mice of Selection I. It may therefore be supposed that F_{16} mice of Selection II are close to homozygosity for the character investigated; this assumption will be verified by continuing the selective breeding.

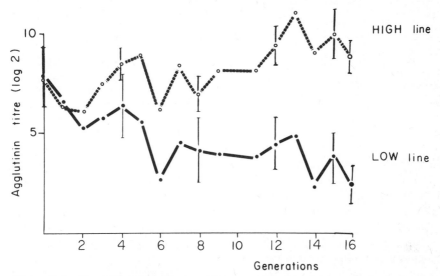

Figure 5.4   Mean SE agglutination titres 14 days post-immunization in successive generations of High and Low lines of Selection II. Vertical bars indicate standard deviation. From Feingold *et al. Eur. J. Immunol.* (submitted for publication).

The results of Selection II are very similar to those of Selection I. The mean value and individual variability of the two foundation populations are very close. Likewise, in Selection II, the effect is asymmetrical; starting from the value of 7.8 (1/1,000) in the foundation population, the titre of agglutinin is reduced to 2.4 (1/30) in F_{16} Low responders and is increased to 8.6 (1/1,920) in F_{16} High responders.

It is remarkable that Selections I and II give results so similar despite the different origin of their foundation populations. This similarity suggests that the frequency of the genes involved in antibody synthesis is comparable in the two foundation populations of outbred albino mice.

To verify whether homozygous High and Low responders of Selection I had a similar or a different genetic constitution to their homologues of Selection II, the following experiment was performed[25]: High responders of Selection I were mated with High responders of Selection II and Low responders of both Selections were also mated. The first progeny was not tested. The production of anti-SE agglutinins was determined on their second descent. The results are reported on Table 5.1 in comparison with those obtained in High and Low

Table 5.1 Mean SE agglutinin titres in High and Low responder mice of Selections I and II and in mice born from homologous crosses between the two selections

	Agglutinin titre High line	14 Days Low line
Selection I mean F_{20}–F_{30}	9.15 ±0.9 (204*)	2 ±1 (230)
Selection II mean F_{13}–F_{15}	9.9 ±0.8 (181)	3.6 ±1.5 (196)
High I × High II Low I × Low II	9.7 ±0.7 (57)	4.9 ±1.8 (64)

* Figures in brackets indicate the number of mice
From Feingold *et al. Eur. J Immunol.* (submitted for publication)

mice of both Selections. It is evident that immune responsiveness is not substantially modified by crossing High responders or Low responders of the two Selections. These results suggest that the genes responsible for High or Low antibody synthesis are the same in both selections since no additive effect could be obtained in two generations of inter-selection homologous crosses. The similarity of the results of Selections I and II and the demonstration of the equivalence of the genes segregated in each line in both selections strongly support our belief that the genes regulating antibody synthesis are represented in relatively small populations of 50–60 random-bred albino mice of various origins. Therefore, it would seem that these genes are evenly distributed in the mouse.

5.2.2 Measure of heritability and estimation of the number of loci controlling agglutinin synthesis

The progressive inter-line separation produced by selective breeding in both Selections I and II clearly indicates that the character investigated is submitted to polygenic control. The realized heritability (h_2) of this character is measured according to the formula proposed by Falconer[27], $h_2 = R/S$ where S is the selection differential expressing the deviation of the parents from the mean value of their generations and R is the response to selection of their progeny. The number of independent loci involved is directly proportional to the max-

186

imal response to selection R and inversely proportional to the h_2. An approximate evaluation of the number of loci may be done according to the formula

$$n = \frac{1}{8} \times \frac{R^2}{VP \times h_2}$$

where VP is the phenotypic variance of the foundation population. For details of calculation and for a correct interpretation of the results within the limitations inherent in the method, see Falconer[27].

Selection I

An accurate analysis is made difficult by the lack of unbiased data concerning the first 6 generations of High line. Another difficulty arises from the alternation of two immunogens SE and PE from the 6th generation onwards. For a correct calculation of cumulated values of S in successive generations two methods are used, referred to as M1 and M2 in Table 5.2. According to M1, the titres of PE agglutinins are converted into SE agglutinin equivalents using a regression coefficient (0.5) established in F_7 mice which were immunized successively with SE and PE. According to M2, the cumulated values of S are calculated by considering the S values of the generations immunized with PE as the mean values of S in the two adjacent generations immunized with SE (for details of calculation, see reference 26). The alternate use of the two immunogens does not interfere with the calculation of the response to selection, R, since this may be correctly done with every other generation immunized with the same immunogen.

The data of S calculated according to M1 and M2 are reported on Table 5.2. The cumulated response to selection is the difference between the mean responsiveness of homozygous High and Low mice of the 22nd generation. The mean realized heritability (h_2) is the average of the regression between R and S. This analysis has been applied to the first 22 generations of selective breeding (at that stage mice of each line can be considered as homozygous since the maximal inter-line separation is attained). The two methods used, M1 and M2, give concordant results; the value of h_2 for the High line is 0.26 and 0.24 according to M1 and M2 respectively. It is somewhat higher in the Low line, 0.30 and 0.36 respectively from M1 and M2. The estimation of the number of independent loci determining the character depends on the value of h_2. Taking the extreme values of h_2, 0.36 and 0.24, the resulting number of loci is comprised between seven and ten.

Selection II

The value of h_2 may be more accurately measured in Selection II since all generations were immunized with SE. Directly comparable data are therefore

Table 5.2   Calculation of heritability from 14 days mean agglutinin titres in High and Low lines of Selection I

	Generation number	Generation† mean	Weighted mean § of selected parents	S: Selection differential cumulated	
				M1*	M2**
HIGH LINE	8	7.60	8.31	0	0
	9‡	9.43	11.20	0.71	0.71
	10	8.78	9.96	1.60	1.66
	11	13.93	15.03	2.78	2.84
	12	8.80	9.50	3.33	3.78
	13	8.22	9.24	4.03	4.48
	14	9.55	9.52	4.54	4.82
	15	10.36	11.21	4.51	4.79
	16	10.70	10.55	4.94	4.70
	17	10.80	11.57	4.79	4.55
	18	11.65	12.82	5.18	5.06
	19	8.54	9.63	6.35	6.23
	20	9.19	9.54	6.90	6.99
	21	10.17	11.09	7.25	7.34
	22	9.34	9.83	7.71	7.76
			Calculated heritability	0.26 ±0.16	0.24 ±0.17
LOW LINE	0	7.36	6.05	0	0
	1	7.17	5.80	1.31	1.31
	2	5.69	4.47	2.68	2.68
	3	5.58	3.70	3.90	3.90
	4	2.53	2.37	5.78	5.78
	5	3.72	2.50	5.94	5.94
	6	3.19	1.30	7.16	7.16
	7‡	5.58	3.05	9.05	9.05
	8	2.87	2.70	10.32	10.08
	9	7.84	5.34	10.49	10.25
	10	3.79	2.67	11.74	10.90
	11	5.67	4.96	12.86	12.02
	12	2.82	2.75	13.22	12.62
	13	3.17	1.98	13.29	12.69
	14	1.18	0.66	13.89	12.99
	15	4.01	2.11	14.41	13.51
	16	1.53	1.57	15.36	13.75
	17	3.83	2.00	15.32	13.71
	18	2.02	1.55	16.24	13.93
	19	2.60	1.50	16.70	14.40
	20	1.51	1.58	17.26	14.60
	21	2.36	1.61	17.19	14.53
	22	1.58	1.13	17.57	14.72
			Calculated heritability	0.30 ±0.04	0.36 ±0.05

Values of S in PE immunized generations are:
* M1: converted into SE equivalent agglutinins using the regression coefficient of 0.5
** M2: supposed to be the mean value of the two adjacent generations immunized with SE
† R is the difference between successive generations
‡ From the 7th generation onwards, even generations are immunized with PE and odd generations with SE
§ The deviation of selected parents has been weighted according to litter size
  From Feingold *et al. Eur. J. Immunol.* (submitted for publication)

available for the whole course of selective breeding. The h_2 values calculated separately for each line from the regression R/S are 0.22 ± 0.07 in High line and 0.18 ± 0.04 in Low line[25]. The h_2 may also be calculated from the inter-line divergence by plotting the cumulated values of R against the cumulated values of S established in both lines as represented in Figure 5.5.

Since it eliminates the erratic fluctuations due to environmental factors, the calculation used in Figure 5.5 is more precise and gives a h_2 value of

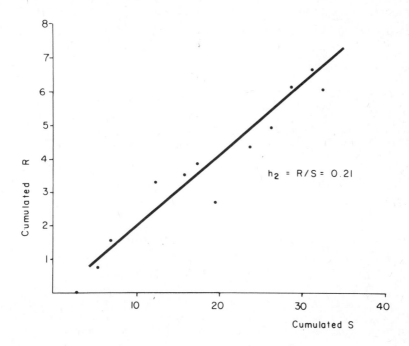

Figure 5.5 Calculation of heritability (h_2). Plot of cumulated R against cumulated S from inter-line divergence between High and Low lines of Selection II. From Feingold *et al. Eur. J. Immunol.* (submitted for publication).

0.21 ± 0.015. The precision of this measure is reflected by the small standard deviation. The number of loci is 11 when calculated from the h_2 value in High line, 13 from the h_2 value in Low line and 12 when h_2 is estimated from inter-line divergence.

The results of the genetic analysis, applied to Selection I and Selection II, are concordant. Taking the extreme values obtained in both selections, we may estimate that the heritability of the character antibody synthesis in the mouse is comprised between 0.36 and 0.18. The number of independent loci involved in the genetic regulation of this quantitative trait is comprised between seven and 13. It will be referred to as a group of about ten loci.

5.2.3 Estimation of global dominance in inter-line crosses with mice of Selection I

The two-way selective breeding was carried out according to the level of agglutinin titre. Nevertheless, it produced important changes in several different parameters of immune responsiveness. The modification of two of these parameters, sensitivity to antigen stimulation and duration of antibody synthesis, are evident in the experiment represented in Figure 5.6. Groups of F_{16} mice of both lines were immunized i.v. with increasing doses of SE from

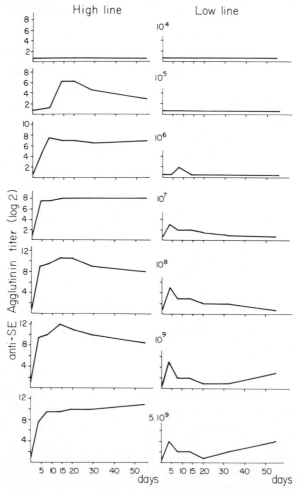

Figure 5.6 Dynamics of agglutinin production after intravenous immunization with increasing doses of SE in F_{16} High and Low responders of Selection I. From Biozzi *et al.* (1972). *J. Exp. Med.*, **135**, 1071.

the subimmunogenic one (10^4) up to the maximal tolerated one (5×10^9). Considering the mean agglutinin responses induced, it is obvious that the High line is more sensitive to antigen stimulation. The dose of 10^5 SE induces a strong antibody synthesis in most of the High responders while it is subimmunogenic in Low responders in which a 10^6 SE dose hardly induces a detectable response. A more detailed study indicates that there is an inter-line difference of about 50-fold in the threshold immunogenic dose of SE.

The dominance in inter-line crosses was therefore studied, using the optimal dose of antigen 5×10^8 SE and the threshold dose of antigen 10^6 SE. The results summarized in Figure 5.7 demonstrate that the dominance effect depends on the dose of antigen administered. The agglutinin titre was measured in F_1 hybrids, F_2 hybrids and $(F_1 \times$ High$)$Bc, $(F_1 \times$ Low$)$Bc and compared with responsiveness of homozygous High and Low lines $(F_{20}-F_{30})$.

For the optimal dose of antigen, the responsiveness of F_1 hybrids is intermediate between the parental lines but is higher than the mid-parental value.

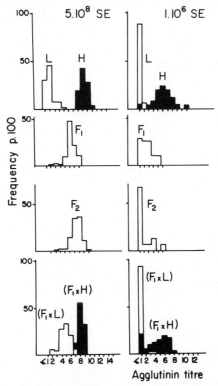

Figure 5.7 Frequency distribution of SE agglutinin titres in mice of High line, Low line and inter-line crosses (F_1, F_2 and backcrosses) in response to intravenous injection of either an optimal dose of SE (5×10^8) or a threshold dose of SE (1×10^6). From Stiffel *et al.* (1974). *Progress in Immunology, Vol II — Proceedings of 2nd International Congress of Immunology,* p. 205 (by courtesy of ASP Biological and Medical Press, Amsterdam).

This indicates that global high responsiveness is incompletely dominant. Owing to this dominance effect $(F_1 \times High)$ Bc respond almost as well as High responders whereas responsiveness of $(F_1 \times Low)$ Bc is intermediate. The degree of global dominance of high responsiveness calculated using High, Low and F_1 mean values as follows:

$$\frac{1}{2} \left(\frac{High + Low - 2F_1}{(High - Low)} \right)^2 \qquad \text{(see ref. 26)}$$

is 0.23. The maximal value of this ratio in case of complete dominance is 0.5. The responsiveness of F_2 hybrids is similar to that of F_1 hybrids but surprisingly the variance is not as great as it should be expected in F_2 hybrids. This may be due to the relatively small number of F_2 tested in relation with the large number (about ten) of independent loci involved.

As previously mentioned, another parameter of immune responsiveness that has been modified by the selective breeding is the duration of antibody response. In that respect the High line is characterized by a 'Long kinetics' and the Low line by a 'Short kinetics' of agglutinin production (see Figure 5.1).

The study of the distribution in hybrids of the 'Long' or 'Short' kinetics of the response indicates that in F_1 hybrids the 'Long kinetics' is also dominant and that very few segregating hybrids show the 'Short kinetics' characteristic of the Low line.

The dominance effect is completely different when the mice are immunized with the threshold dose of antigen (Figure 5.7). In this case, low responsiveness is dominant in F_1 hybrids. Using this immunizing dose 96% of Low responders are negative (agglutinin titre $\leqslant 2$) while all the High responders produce a high titre of agglutinin (6.25 ± 1.8). Fifty-five per cent of F_1 hybrids are negative, the remainders giving only a very low response (mean 3.5 ± 0.85). The distribution of responsiveness in F_2 hybrids and backcrosses is compatible with a two-loci model. If these two loci are a and b in High line and A and B in Low line, then due to the dominance effect of low responsiveness the following phenotypes may be postulated: A,A–Bb and A,a–BB are equal to Low responders, a,a–B,b and A,a–b,b are intermediate between F_1 hybrids and High responders and A,A–b,b and a,a–BB are intermediate between F_1 hybrids and Low responders. A two-loci model gives the best correlation between the percentages of the observed/theoretical distribution of non-responders that are respectively 73/53 in F_2 hybrids, 26/29 in $(F_1 \times High)$ Bc and 93/76 in $(F_1 \times Low)$ Bc. A single-locus model and a three-loci model give a greater divergence between the theoretical and experimental data[26]. The results are thus compatible with the hypothesis that, at threshold antigen stimulation, the antibody response is controlled by the action of only two loci. This finding opens the way to a more detailed analysis of the genetic regulation of the different parameters of immune responsiveness enabling to individualize the particular effect of sub-groups of loci. At present, it seems possible to advance that two out of the group of about ten loci that have been separated in each line by the selective breeding, are particularly involved in the genetic regulation of the sensitivity to immunogenic stimulation.

5.2.4 Calculation of the degree of consanguinity induced by selective breeding in High and Low lines

The inbreeding coefficient is computed in successive generations of both lines by applying the classical formula to every genetically efficient individual giving at least one descent in the last generation. The remote consanguinity of the foundation population is considered as equal to zero. Though brother–sister mating was excluded, an increasing degree of consanguinity is produced in each line because of closed colony breeding. The calculation of the inbreeding coefficient is applied to the first 21 generations of selection. The results are reported on Table 5.3 as well as the size of each generation and the number of genetically efficient pairs.

Table 5.3 Size of each generation — number of efficient parents and mean coefficient of inbreeding in High and Low lines of Selection I

Generation number	High line			Low line		
	Size	Number of pairs	Mean coef. of inbreeding	Size	Number of pairs	Mean coef. of inbreeding
0	62	—	0	62	—	0
1	63	3	0	36	2	0
2	22	3	0.208	18	2	0.250
3	31	3	0.015	20	3	0.313
4	42	4	0.195	16	3	0.406
5	58	4	0.240	43	3	0.359
6	34	3	0.267	32	4	0.406
7	42	4	0.299	34	5	0.457
8	34	5	0.353	48	4	0.480
9	56	5	0.379	41	4	0.497
10	56	6	0.385	26	4	0.533
11	46	5	0.446	35	4	0.550
12	58	6	0.441	17	2	0.579
13	82	7	0.459	58	6	0.640
14	43	7	0.471	48	5	0.649
15	73	9	0.498	43	5	0.656
16	53	9	0.519	46	5	0.663
17	62	9	0.526	53	8	0.682
18	71	7	0.531	66	6	0.691
19	81	11	0.544	58	7	0.696
20	57	8	0.549	35	5	0.709
21	53	7	0.551	32	4	0.714
22	37	6		53	8	

From Feingold et al. Eur. J. Immunol. (submitted for publication)

The inbreeding coefficient increases progressively in both lines during the course of the selection. It is higher in Low line because of the smaller number of efficient pairs. Consequently, 50% of the genetic homogeneity is reached at the 9th generation in Low line and at the 15th generation in High line. At the 20th generation, when the selection for agglutinin production is completed, the inbreeding coefficient is 0.55 in High line and 0.71 in Low line.

The high level of consanguinity produced by the closed colony breeding implies a corresponding level of homogeneity in many genetic traits inside each line. The majority of these traits are not involved in the regulation of immune responsiveness; nevertheless, the association of two genetic characters with immune responsiveness has been demonstrated in inter-line segregating hybrids, as described in the following paragraph.

5.3 ASSOCIATION OF SE AGGLUTININ SYNTHESIS WITH THE *Ig* ALLOTYPE AND WITH THE LOCUS OF THE MAJOR HISTOCOMPATIBILITY ANTIGEN (*H-2*)

The genetic analysis, previously described, demonstrates that the quantitative synthesis of SE agglutinins is regulated by a group of about ten independent loci; thus, the linkage of one of them with another genetic trait can only account for a part of the inter-line difference in immune responsiveness (1/10 in the theoretical case of ten equivalent loci). Two positive associations of SE agglutinin production in segregating inter-line hybrids have been demonstrated; one with the allotype marker of Ig heavy chain accounting for about 10% of the inter-line difference and another one with the *H-2* locus that is quantitatively more important since it accounts for about 20% of the inter-line difference in agglutinin synthesis. Since the *H-2* locus and the locus of the structural genes of Ig heavy chains are independent from each other, we are dealing with two out of the group of about ten loci regulating antibody synthesis.

The first allotype analysis made by Lieberman *et al.* in F_{18} mice demonstrated that the Low responders were homozygous for the heavy chain linkage group ($G^{3,5,7,8}H^9$, $^{11}A-F^f$) rarely found in Swiss mice but observed as a recombinant type among wild mice. High responders presented two phenotypes: the linkage group of Balb/c: ($G^{1,6,7,8}H^9$, $^{11}A^{12,13,14}F^f$) for 8% and the linkage group of C57B1 ($^2G-H^9$, $^{16}A^{15}F^s$) for 43%, the remainders were hybrids of these two phenotypes[24].

The correlation between *Ig* allotype and responsiveness to SE was demonstrated in F_2 hybrids, ($F_1 \times$ High)Bc and ($F_1 \times$ Low)Bc derived from F_{18} as shown in Table 5.4.

In recent experiments, still unpublished, made in collaboration with R. Lieberman, this correlation was confirmed in inter-line crosses obtained from $F_{27}-F_{29}$. In these generations, High responders have become homozygous for

Table 5.4 Correlation between *Ig* allotypes and SE agglutinin titres in F_2 hybrids and backcrosses between High and Low responder lines in Selection 1

Inter-line cross	Sex	Number of mice	Allotype*	Titre of SE agglutinin 5 days post-immunization	
F₂ hybrids	Female	33	H/H	7.45	
		66	H/L	6.60	$p < 0.01$
		17	L/L	6.40	
	Male	37	H/H	7.65	
		52	H/L	7.30	$p < 0.001$
		20	L/L	6.70	
(F₁ × High)Bc	Female	10	H/H	8.00	$p < 0.05$
		12	H/L	7.1	
	Male	11	H/H	7.55	not sig-
		10	H/L	7.7	nificant
(F₁ × Low)Bc	Female	12	L/L	4.5	$p < 0.1$
		9	H/L	5.3	
	Male	21	L/L	4.6	$p < 0.01$
		18	H/L	5.25	

* H = allotype of High responders   L = allotype of Low responders
From Lieberman *et al.* (1972). *J. Exp. Med.*, **136**, 790

the allotype marker. The quantitative difference in responsiveness associated with the allotype is small.

The analysis shows that about 10% of the inter-line divergence is determined by either the structural genes of Ig heavy chains or by a closely-linked locus. The determination of allotypic markers in mice of Selection II is in progress, it will discriminate between these two hypotheses. The importance of allotype-linked specific immune response genes has recently been confirmed by several authors (see review in reference 28). Dorf *et al.*[16] have recently studied the immune responsiveness to the terpolymer GAT in various inbred strains of mice. The recognition of this antigen is determined by a *H-2*-linked *Ir* gene. The fundamental finding of this study is that among the responder strains, the quantitative regulation of antibody synthesis is a polygenic character independent from the *H-2* locus but correlated with the heavy chain allotype markers of Ig.

A considerable amount of data have been published on the *H-2*-linked specific immune response genes (reviewed in references 15, 28, 29). We have, therefore, investigated a possible association between immune responsiveness to SE and the *H-2* locus in inter-line segregating hybrids. Preceding unpublished preliminary experiments, made in collaboration with J. G. Howard and D. A. L. Davies, suggested homozygosity (or large homogeneity) for the

H-2 locus inside High and Low mice, each line presenting a different antigenic *H-2* profile. The analysis of SE agglutinin titres in inter-line F_2 hybrids suggested a positive association between *H-2* locus and immune responsiveness.

Recently, in our laboratory, the positive association between SE immune responsiveness and the major histocompatibility antigen was clearly demonstrated[25]. A specific immune serum against histocompatibility antigens of Low line was prepared in High responders hyperimmunized with pooled spleen cells from Low responders. An efficient anti-High line histocompatibility antigen immune serum could not be prepared in Low responders because of their very poor humoral responsiveness to histocompatibility antigens (see Section 6). Therefore, anti-High line immune serum was prepared in C_3H mice hyperimmunized with pooled spleen cells from High line mice. This immune serum was absorbed with Low line spleen cells. Using a cytotoxicity test on lymph node cells in presence of guinea pig C', these immune sera were specific: they were highly cytotoxic for all the mice of the corresponding line and without effect for all the mice of the other line. The cytotoxicity test used detects essentially the major histocompatibility antigens of the *H-2* locus. Thus, these immune sera could be used to identify the distribution of the *H-2* phenotypes in inter-line hybrids. Seventy-three F_2 hybrids, 63 (High $\times$ F_1)Bc and 59 (Low $\times$ F_1)Bc were immunized with 5×10^8 SE i.v. The SE agglutinin titres were measured individually at different times after immunization. Then, the *H-2* type of each animal was determined by studying the cytotoxicity of the two specific immune sera on isolated lymph node cells. The results of this experiment represented in Table 5.5 show a distribution of the *H-2* phenotypes

Table 5.5 Correlation between SE agglutinin titres and *H-2* phenotypes in inter-High and Low line crosses (F_2 and backcross) of Selection 1

Cross	H-2 *Phenotype*	Mean SE agglutinin titre (20th day)		Weighted difference**	
F_2	†H.H (13)* ††L.L (22)	8.54 7.00	$p < 10^{-3}$	1.38	$p < 10^{-7}$
	H.H (13) H.L (38)	8.54 7.83	$p > 0.05$	0.66	$p < 10^{-3}$
	L.L (22) H.L (38)	7.00 7.83	$p = 10^{-3}$	0.77	$p < 10^{-4}$
($F_1 \times$ H)	H.H (40) H.L (23)	9.71 9.11	$p < 10^{-3}$	0.57	$p < 10^{-5}$
($F_1 \times$ L)	L.L (25) H.L (34)	5.50 6.44	$p = 10^{-2}$	1.01	$p < 10^{-6}$

* Figures in brackets represent the number of mice in each group
** Differences weighted by the agglutinin titres measured at different times after immunization and by the number of mice
† H phenotype of High responders
†† L phenotype of Low responders
From Stiffel *et al.* (1974). *Progr. Immunol., Vol. II — Proceedings of 2nd International Congress of Immunology*, p. 205 (ASP Amsterdam: Biological and Medical Press)

among the inter-line hybrids approaching the Mendelian ratios. A definite correlation is evident between *H-2* locus and agglutinin titres established 20 days post-immunization. A more impressive statistical signification of this correlation is obtained by weighting the inter-hybrid differences according to the agglutinin titres measured at different times post-immunization and to the number of mice in each group. A highly significant statistical difference for all the combinations may then be demonstrated. From these results, it appears that one of the group of about ten loci regulating the antibody synthesis is either the *H-2* locus itself or a closely-linked locus. It is different from the previously demonstrated one linked with Ig allotype marker and its effect on antibody synthesis is more important since it accounts for about 20% of the inter-line divergence.

A positive correlation between immune responsiveness to SE and the *H-2* locus was also demonstrated in congenic lines of mice by Sabolovich *et al.*[30]

5.4 PHENOTYPIC EXPRESSION OF GENES REGULATING THE SYNTHESIS OF SE AGGLUTININS

The effect of the genes, segregated in each line during the selective breeding, is at least partially expressed in the populations of isolated lymphoid cells. In fact, the *in vitro* immune response to SE is stronger with lymph node or spleen cells isolated from High than from Low responders[31]. It should, however, be stressed that the inter-line difference of responsiveness is considerably smaller *in vitro* than *in vivo*.

In vivo experiments have demonstrated that the functions of both lymphocytes and macrophages were deeply affected by the genetic selection.

5.4.1 Phenotypic expression at lymphocyte level

The result of an adoptive immunization experiment obtained by transferring an equivalent number of spleen cells from immunized High line donors into normal Low line recipients and vice versa is shown in Figure 5.8. The transmitted cells go on producing antibody in the host until they are destroyed by homograft reaction. The results of Figure 5.8 demonstrate that the amount of antibody produced is determined by the phenotype of the population of transferred cells even if they survive in a host of the opposite phenotype. Control experiments proved that High and Low line recipients have the same ability to destroy allogeneic isolated spleen cells (from random-bred albino mice) as measured by adoptive immunization assay.

Cell transfer experiments indicate that lymphoid cells from the two lines have diverse potentialities.

Figure 5.9 illustrates results obtained in a typical experiment of this kind.

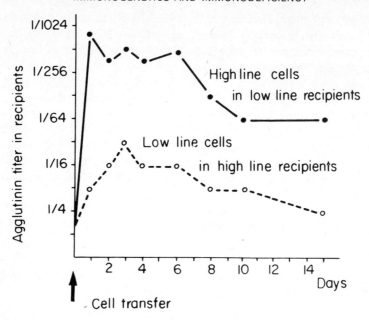

Figure 5.8 Adoptive immunization experiment: production of SE agglutinins after transfer of pre-immunized spleen cells of High or Low responder into normal recipients of the opposite line. Donor immunization: 5×10^8 SE intravenously 14 and 4 days before transfer. Transfer: one spleen equivalent per recipient intraperitoneally. From Biozzi *et al.* (1971). In *Progress in Immunology*, p. 529, by courtesy of Academic Press, New York.

Random-bred albino mice were immunologically suppressed either by X-ray irradiation or by cyclophosphamide treatment. Then, equivalent numbers (4×10^7) of spleen cells from High or Low donors were injected intravenously together with an immunizing dose of SE. Figure 5.9 shows the titres of SE agglutinins in the sera of the recipient mice. It is evident that a better immune restoration is obtained when High line cells are injected. In the heterologous populations of cells transmitted, macrophages and lymphocytes only may be considered as involved in the immune response. However, macrophages have little chance to play a role and in fact identical results are obtained if spleen or lymph node cells are deprived of macrophages by filtration through a glass beads column before transfer. Thus, it should be concluded that genes regulating responsiveness to SE are at least partially expressed in lymphocytes. Nevertheless, the experiments reported on Figure 5.9 may be criticized since SE agglutinins are synthesized in recipients during the period of GVH reaction. This reaction is more severe in the recipients of Low line cells as shown by the cumulative mortality curves also reported on Figure 5.9. It is difficult to evaluate the interference of the GVH reaction on responsiveness to SE.

Several attempts were undertaken in order to delay or reduce the rate of

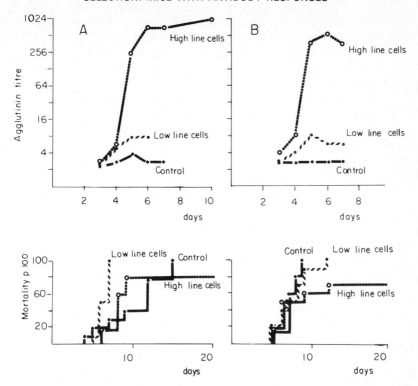

Figure 5.9 Cell-transfer experiment: transfer of spleen cells from normal High or Low responders into outbred immuno-suppressed recipients. 3×10^8 SE are injected intravenously together with spleen cells. A: X rays: 950 rad 24 hours before transfer; B: Cyclophosphamide treatment: 6 mg per mouse intraperitoneally 6 hours before transfer.

mortality in recipients, especially by varying the recipient strains, the number or the origin of transmitted cells (bone marrow–thymus mixtures instead of spleen cells). Unfortunately, in all cases the mortality occurred in the phase of agglutinin production and it occurred earlier in the Low line cells recipients.

5.4.2 Phenotypic expression at macrophage level

Different modifications of macrophage functions have been induced by the selection for SE agglutinin production. This underlines the important participation of macrophages in the mechanism of the immune response.

High and Low line macrophages differ essentially in antigen processing and/or antigen presentation rather than in antigen phagocytosis.

The phagocytic function of liver and spleen macrophages measured *in vivo* by the kinetics of blood clearance of colloidal carbon[32] is similar in both lines (phagocytic index $K = 0.015 \pm 0.005$ and 0.020 ± 0.006 in High and Low line respectively). The rate of phagocytosis of radiolabelled SE is also identical in High and Low responders (0.063 and 0.058 respectively). After complete blood clearance a similar distribution of SE in liver and spleen is observed in both lines: 90% and 91% of SE in liver macrophages and 7.4% and 6% in spleen macrophages respectively in High and Low responders. No important modifications have therefore been demonstrated in the phagocytosis of the antigen used for the genetic selection. Nevertheless, other antigens such as pneumococcus polysaccharide (SIII)[33], keyhole limpet haemocyanin and levan[34] are phagocytized faster by Low line macrophages. In contrast with the minor changes in antigen phagocytosis, the intracellular metabolism of the phagocytized antigens is very different in the two lines.

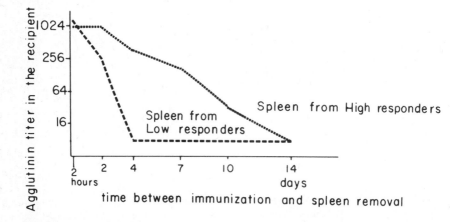

Figure 5.10 Persistence of SE immunogenicity in the spleen of High and Low responders: SE agglutinin production in primed outbred albino mice after injection of irradiated spleen (1/4 spleen equivalent per recipient) from High or Low responders immunized at different times before spleen removal (for details: see text).

The results reported on Figure 5.10 show that the persistence of the immunogenicity of SE in the spleen macrophages is much longer in High than in Low responders.

Groups of High and Low responders were immunized intravenously with the same dose of SE (2×10^8). Subgroups of animals were sacrificed at different times after immunization comprised between 2 hours and 14 days. The spleens were removed and irradiated with 10 000 rad, then, homogenized and injected (as 1/4 spleen equivalent) to groups of outbred albino mice pre-immunized with a subimmunogenic dose of SE (10^5). The persistence of immunogenicity of SE in the spleen of the donors results in the induction of secondary agglutinin production in the recipients. As shown on Figure 5.10, the immunogenicity of SE lasts only 4 days in Low line while it persists for 10 days in High line.

It is known that intravenously injected SE are rapidly phagocytized by spleen macrophages and that their antigens persist in these cells since no significant amounts of antigen could be demonstrated in antibody synthesizing cells[35].

Recent experiments carried out *in vitro* by Wiener and Bandieri[34] using another antigen, keyhole limpet haemocyanin (^{125}I-KLH) have confirmed and extended the preceding results. This antigen is phagocytized at a higher rate by peritoneal macrophages of Low responders. After uptake, the overall degradation of ^{125}I-KLH also occurred considerably faster in Low line macrophages, in which after 5 hours all the ^{125}I-KLH is broken down into TCA-soluble derivatives while at the same time about 20% of the antigen is still in a macromolecular form in the High line macrophages.

The importance for the immunogenicity of the portion of the undegraded antigen attached to the outer membrane of macrophages was definitely demonstrated by Unanue and Cerrottini[36]. Consequently, this phenomenon was studied by Wiener and Bandieri in peritoneal macrophages from High and Low responders. The ^{125}I-KLH bound to the outer macrophage membrane was determined by trypsin treatment of the intact cells following antigen uptake. The results of this experiment are reported on Figure 5.11.

About the same percentage (approximately 30%) of ^{125}I-KLH phagocytized is fixed to the surface of macrophages of both lines. However,

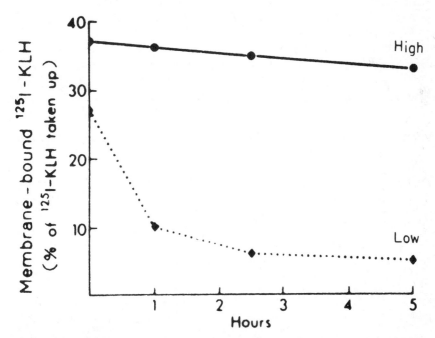

Figure 5.11   Retention of membrane-bound ^{125}I-KLH after its uptake by macrophages from High and Low responders. From Wiener *et al.* (1974). *Eur. J. Immunol.*, **4**, 457, by courtesy of Verlag Chemiè, Weinheim.

the amount of antigen bound to the membrane of Low line macrophages decreases rapidly while it persists for a longer period in the membrane of High line macrophages. This difference in antigen degradation and presentation is probably a major factor in the regulation of the antibody synthesis in the two lines.

The same authors have also noticed important morphological differences in cultured peritoneal macrophages from High and Low responders, the latter, in addition, showed higher lysosomal enzyme activities.

Other modifications of macrophage activity in these lines of mice have been reported. Howard *et al.* showed that living T_4 bacteriophage is killed much more rapidly inside the Low line than High line macrophages (mentioned in reference 33). Likewise, R. Fauve observed that living *Listeria* monocytogenes multiply faster in the spleen and liver macrophages of High than in those of Low responders[37]. In fact, in spite of a similar initial distribution of injected *Listeria* in High and Low macrophages the number of living micro-organisms 48 h after inoculation is 54×10^6 in the liver and 15×10^6 in the spleen of High responders, whereas in Low responders the figures are respectively: 2.4×10^6 and 2.8×10^6.

The modifications of macrophage activity resulting from the selective breeding may also be demonstrated by another experimental approach as shown in Figure 5.12. This is based on the facts that macrophage phagocytic activity[38] and macrophage antigen processing[39] are radioresistant phenomena.

Mice of High and Low lines were irradiated in order to suppress their immune responsiveness. This suppression is only due to the lymphocytes' destruction since it is reversed by the transfer of pure populations of small lymphocytes[40]. Irradiated mice of each line received i.v. 4×10^7 spleen cells from (High × Low)F_1 hybrids together with an immunizing dose of 3×10^8 SE.

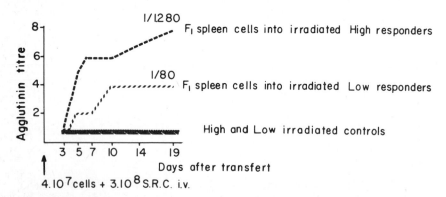

Figure 5.12 Cell-transfer experiment: production of SE agglutinin in irradiated High and Low responders after transfer of (High × Low)F_1 spleen cells (4×10^7 per recipient). 3×10^8 SE are injected intravenously together with spleen cells. X rays: 950 rad 24 hours before transfer. From Biozzi *et al.* (1974). In *La Génétique des Immunoglobulines et de la Réponse Immunitaire. Ann. Immunol.* (Inst. Pasteur) **125C**, 107, by courtesy of Masson et Cie, Paris.

(The responsiveness of F_1 hybrids to this dose of SE is intermediate between that of High and Low lines.) The agglutinin response is markedly stronger in High than in Low recipients. The transmitted cells are responsible for antibody synthesis since the two irradiated control groups do not respond at all. Thus, in this experiment, the difference in the intensity of the immune response is related to macrophage functions in the recipients.

All the above-reported findings demonstrate that some macrophage functions, namely those concerning the metabolism and presentation of the antigen, have been profoundly modified by selective breeding for antibody production. Some of the loci characterizing High and Low responders are therefore probably expressed phenotypically at macrophage level. On the other hand, the experiments of lymphocytes transfer suggest that lymphocytes potentialities as well have been altered by selective breeding. Moreover, different intrinsic characteristics of B lymphocytes have been found out in non-immunized mice of High and Low lines[41]. Our present opinion is that some of the genes separated by selective breeding are expressed in lymphocytes and others in macrophages. On the basis of the role played by the *H-2*-linked and *Ig*-allotype-linked specific *Ir* genes, it is possible to hypothesize that in our lines of mice the two loci associated with the *H-2* locus and *Ig* allotype are expressed in lymphocytes. They participate in the regulation of specific immune response to the antigens used for the selection. Other genes expressed in macrophages regulate the efficiency of antigen processing and consequently play the main role in the control of general responsiveness to many unrelated immunogens that will be described in Section 6.

5.5   CYTODYNAMICS OF IMMUNE RESPONSE

The sharp difference in SE agglutinin synthesis between High and Low responders might be due to a difference either in the number of antibody-producing immunocytes or in the amount of antibody produced by each immunocyte. A combination of the two mechanisms is also possible.

The study of the immune response at cellular level was therefore undertaken by two methods: the haemolysin plaque forming cells (PFC) assay using the modified Jerne technique[42,43] and the rosette forming cells (RFC) test using the method described previously[44,45]. The PFC are the antibody secreting cells (mature or immature plasmocytes) derived from antigen-induced differentiation of B lymphocytes.

The rosettes are formed by a larger and more heterogeneous population of antibody-synthesizing cells including secreting and non-secreting immunocytes derived from both T and B lymphocytes[46-48]. Our experimental conditions reduce to a negligible percentage ($\leqslant 3\%$) the number of rosettes formed by cells passively coated with antibody. The RFC found in non-immunized animals (natural RFC) are essentially small lymphocytes ($\leqslant 10\,\mu$). Among

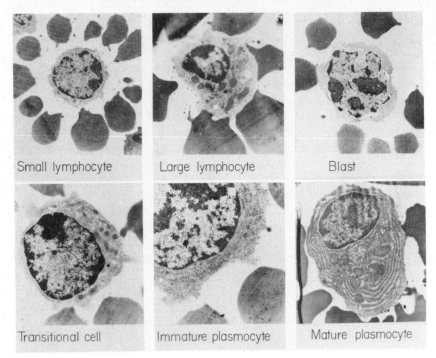

Figure 5.13 Ultrastructural morphology of the different types of RFC. From Biozzi *et al.* [*1972*]. *Transpl. Proc.*, **4**, 339, by courtesy of Grune and Stratton Inc., New York.

these are the receptor-bearing antigen sensitive cells (target cells) initiating the immune response to SE[49–51]. After immunogenic stimulation, rosettes are formed by immunocytes at all the stages of differentiation starting from small lymphocytes and ending in mature plasmocytes. In Figure 5.13 are shown the principal ultrastructural aspects of RFC throughout the whole process of cell differentiation during the immune response. In stained preparations with an optical microscope, it is easy to classify the RFC as small, medium and large lymphocytes, blasts and plasmocytes[52,53].

The initial exponential phase of the immune response to intravenously injected SE occurs exclusively in the spleen. The rate of multiplication and differentiation of immunocytes induced by the immunogenic stimulation can be measured, during this phase, by the quantitative study of the number and morphology of RFC[43,49,54]. The comparison of the number of RFC and PFC in the spleen with the titre of serum antibody at the end of the exponential phase gives information on the relationships between cellular and humoral aspects of the immune response.

In Table 5.6, the immune response of High and Low lines to SE is expressed at humoral and cellular levels by the mean titre of serum haemolysins and agglutinins and by the mean number of PFC and RFC in the spleen at the end

Table 5.6 Comparison of the number of PFC and RFC in High and Low responder mice before immunization and 4 days post-immunization

		High line	Low line	High line / Low line
Non-immunized mice	Natural PFC/spleen	$\leqslant 70$	$\leqslant 70$	—
	Natural RFC/spleen	23 000	30 000	—
	Natural serum haemolysins	$\leqslant 1/10$	$\leqslant 1/10$	—
	Natural serum agglutinins	1/10	1/5	—
4th day post-immunization 5×10^8 SE i.v.	PFC/spleen	130 000	6500	20
	RFC/spleen	3 000 000	270 000	11
	Serum haemolysins	1/8000	1/200	40
	Serum agglutinins	1/3600	1/120	30

From Biozzi *et al.* (1972). *J. Exp. Med.* **135**, 1071

of the exponential phase (4th day post-immunization). The corresponding values found in non-immunized mice are also reported. No difference is observed between non-immunized High and Low responders in both serum antibody titres (natural agglutinins and haemolysins) and in the number of active immunocytes (natural RFC and PFC). At the end of the exponential phase, the number of immunocytes detected by both methods and the serum antibody titres are markedly higher in High than in Low responders. This finding demonstrates that in High responders the expansion of the population of specific immunocytes occurs at a higher rate than in Low responders.

The inter-line difference is about two-fold larger in terms of serum haemolysin than in terms of haemolysin secreting cells (PFC). This point will be discussed later. The inter-line difference is still larger (about 3-fold) between the humoral agglutinin level and the number of RFC. This discrepancy is probably due to the equivalent T cell mediated immune responsiveness of the two lines (see Section 8). In consequence, the presence of the same number of T cells in the expanding population of T and B lymphocytes lowers the inter-line difference measured in terms of rosettes which are formed by both B and T lymphocytes.

The essential conclusion drawn from the data of Table 5.6 concerns the difference in the rate of immune response between High and Low lines at both cellular and humoral levels. Using the rosette method, we have previously proposed a model of cytodynamic analysis allowing the measure of the principal parameters governing the kinetics of the immune response to SE in the mouse, namely: the doubling time of RFC, the duration of the exponential phase and the number of antigen sensitive cells initially stimulated by the antigen (target cells)[49]. The results obtained by applying this cytodynamic analysis to the response of High and Low lines are represented in Figure 5.14.

The only parameter modified by the genetic selection is the doubling time of RFC which is markedly shorter in High than in Low responders. The other

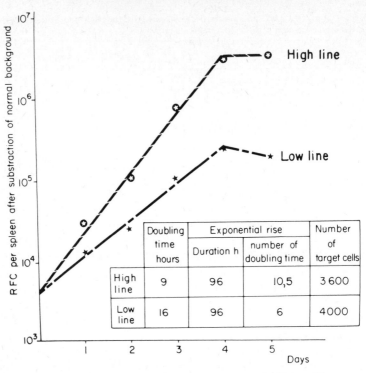

Figure 5.14 Cytodynamic parameters of the immune response in High and Low responders immunized with an optimal dose of SE (5 × 10⁸). From Biozzi *et al.* (1972). *J. Exp. Med.*, **135**, 1071, by courtesy of The Rockefeller University Press, New York.

parameters, i.e. the duration of the exponential phase and the number of target cells are the same in both lines. The doubling time of RFC measured in this way corresponds to the mean multiplication time of RFC populations[43,49]. Thus, the physiological effect of the group of genes regulating antibody synthesis concerns the rate of immunocyte multiplication during the exponential phase of the immune response.

Another important physiological modification induced by the genetic difference between High and Low responders is related to the rate of immunocyte differentiation which also occurs faster in High than in Low responders as shown in Figure 5.15.

High and Low responders have an equivalent number of natural rosettes formed exclusively by small lymphocytes. At the end of the exponential phase, 650 000 RF plasmocytes have differentiated in High line and only 15 400 in Low line. The inter-line difference in the number of RF plasmocytes is 40-fold, which does correspond with the inter-line difference in humoral antibody titre (see Table 5.6). These results indicate that the sharp inter-line difference in antibody synthesis is due to the number of antibody producing cells rather than

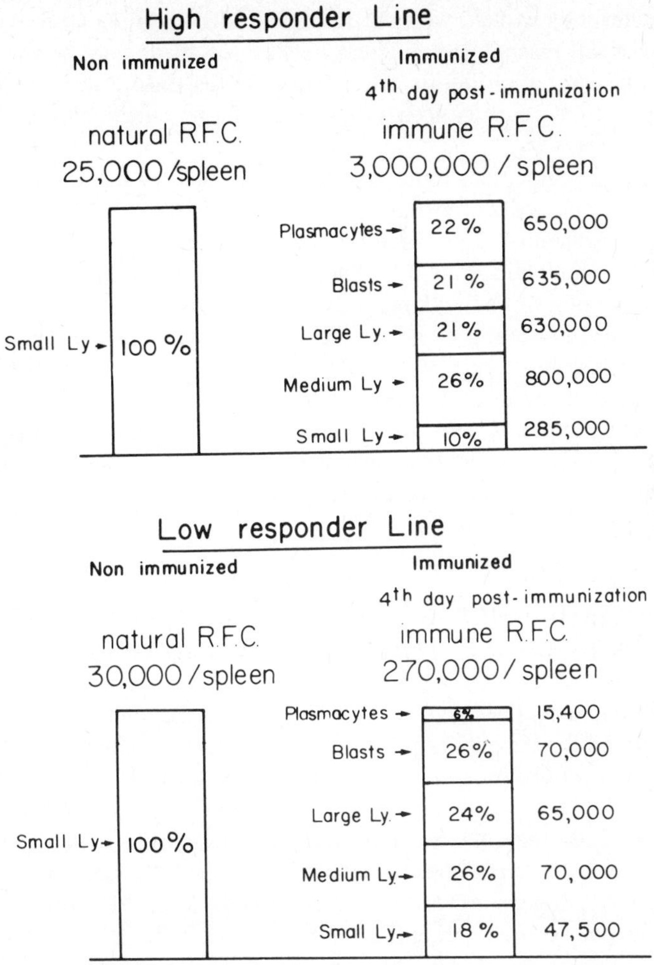

High responder Line

Non immunized   Immunized

4th day post-immunization

natural R.F.C.   immune R.F.C.

25,000 /spleen   3,000,000 / spleen

Plasmacytes →	22 %	650,000
Blasts →	21 %	635,000
Large Ly. →	21%	630,000
Medium Ly →	26%	800,000
Small Ly →	10%	285,000

Small Ly → 100 %

Low responder Line

Non immunized   Immunized

4th day post-immunization

natural R.F.C.   immune R.F.C.

30,000 /spleen   270,000/ spleen

Plasmacytes →	6%	15,400
Blasts →	26%	70,000
Large Ly. →	24%	65,000
Medium Ly →	26%	70,000
Small Ly →	18 %	47,500

Small Ly → 100%

Figure 5.15 Distribution of the different types of RFC before immunization and 4 days post-immunization in the spleen of High and Low responders. From Biozzi *et al.* (1972). *Transpl. Proc.,* **4,** 339, by courtesy of Grune and Stratton, New York.

to the amount of antibody synthesized by each cell. The humoral antibodies are secreted by the population of RF plasmocytes that have differentiated from the antigen sensitive small lymphocytes. In both lines, the number of RF plasmocytes is higher than that of PFC reported on Table 5.6. This discrepancy probably comes from the low sensitivity of the plaque assay; in fact, more sensitive methods of PFC detection have been described.

The rosettes formed by the cell in the intermediate steps of differentiation are about ten-fold more numerous in High than in Low responders. Both the process of plasmocyte maturation itself and the contribution of T derived lymphocytes may explain why this ratio is smaller than the 40-fold difference observed in RF plasmocyte numbers. A more detailed study on the dynamics of RFC differentiation during the exponential response clearly indicates that the inter-line difference concerns essentially the transformation of blast cells into plasmocytes[54].

The experimental data summarized in this section demonstrate that the genetic difference between High and Low responders affects essentially the rate of multiplication and differentiation of immunocytes induced by immunogenic stimulation. This difference may be due to intrinsic modifications of the potentialities of either lymphocytes or macrophages, or both. A more efficient antigen processing by macrophages may result in an acceleration of the rate of lymphocytes response. In both cases, it can be predicted that the High and Low responders to SE will also be High and Low responders to other non-cross-reacting immunogens since the process of immunocyte multiplication and differentiation is also a general phenomenon independent from immune specificity. This prediction is confirmed by the experiments reported in the next section.

5.6 ANTIBODY RESPONSE OF HIGH AND LOW LINES TO OTHER NON-CROSS-REACTING IMMUNOGENS

The High and Low lines genetically separated for SE agglutinin synthesis are also separated for the antibody response to all the other non-cross-reacting immunogens tested so far, apart from the two exceptions which will be mentioned later.

A clear inter-line difference in antibody response to the following immunogens was observed: pigeon, rat and human erythrocytes, somatic (O) and flagellar (H) antigens of *Salmonella*, antigens extracted from *Trichinella spiralis*, bovine serum albumin (BSA), bovine γ-globulin (BGG), haemocyanin, hen egg albumin (HEA), T_4 bacteriophage, pneumococcus polysaccharide (SIII), histocompatibility antigens, amino acid polymers such as GAT and GLPhe, dinitrophenyl hapten (DNP) and picryl chloride (administered by skin painting). A few examples will be described in this paragraph.

Haemocyanin

In Figure 5.16 is reported the antibody response to *Limulus polyphemus* haemocyanin measured by passive haemagglutination. The superiority of the High line in both primary and secondary responses is evident.

The response to keyhole limpet haemocyanin was also measured quantitatively by a Farr method; 7 days after secondary challenge the percentage of KLH bound by a 1/2 serum dilution was 29.6 and 0.6 respectively in High and Low responders[41].

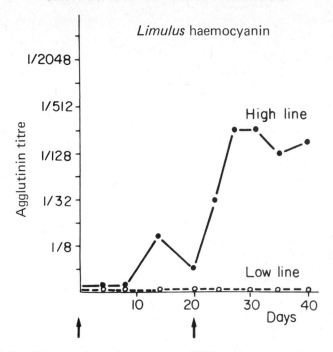

Figure 5.16 Primary and secondary responses of High and Low responders immunized with *Limulus* haemocyanin (0.2 mg/mouse intravenously) measured by passive haemagglutination using KLH coated SE. From Biozzi *et al.* (1971). In *Progress in Immunology*, p. 529, by courtesy of Academic Press, New York.

Bovine serum albumin

A detailed study of the primary response to BSA is reported in Figure 5.17. Increasing doses of alum precipitated BSA are injected intraperitoneally in groups of mice of both lines.

For the whole antigen range, High responders produce more antibody than Low responders. In Low line mice only the two highest antigen doses induce a significant antibody synthesis while a wider range of antigen doses is efficient in High line. Thus, as for the response to sheep erythrocytes, the threshold antigen dose is much lower in High line (10^{-5} mg) than in Low line (10^{-3} mg).

Hen egg albumin

A study of primary IgE antibody production is performed by immunizing the mice with alum precipitated HEA. Two doses of antigen are used: 1 μg and 100 μg. The titre of IgE antibody is evaluated by heterologous passive cutaneous anaphylaxis in rat skin[55,56]. High responders injected with the high

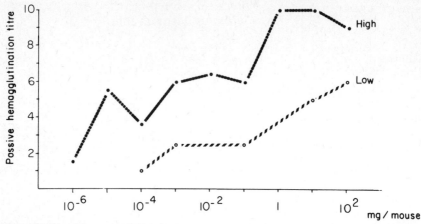

Figure 5.17 Responses of High and Low responders to intraperitoneal injection of increasing doses of alum precipitated BSA. Passive haemagglutination titres (using BSA coated SE) 7 days post-immunization, in High line and 21 days post-immunization in Low line. (No detectable antibody is produced in Low line on the 7th day.) From Heumann, A. M. (unpublished results).

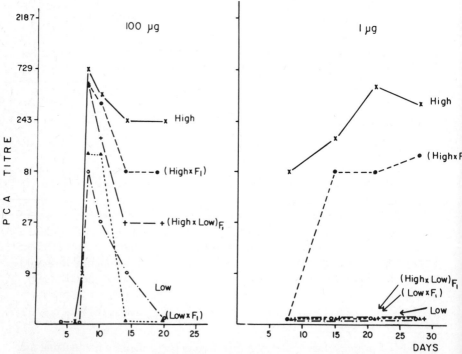

Figure 5.18 Synthesis of IgE antibody in High line, Low line and inter-line crosses after immunization with 100 μg or 1 μg of alum precipitated HEA. From Prouvost-Danon *et al. Proceedings of the 9th European Congress of Allergology and Clinical Immunology — London September 1974*, in press.

dose of antigen produce a greater amount of antibody than Low responders (Figure 5.18.). With this antigen dose, the response of F_1 hybrids, at the peak level, is close to that of the High line. Therefore, there is an incomplete dominance of the response. This dominance effect of high response is confirmed in F_1 backcrossed with the parental lines.

The low dose of antigen induces a strong and persistent IgE response in High line while in Low line no antibody, or a very small amount only, is produced (Figure 5.18). The study of the response in inter-line crosses shows that low responsiveness is completely dominant since neither the F_1 hybrids, nor the ($F_1 \times$ Low) backcrosses respond. The heritability of responsiveness to 1 μg of HEA is therefore similar to that observed for the threshold dose of SE (10^6, see Figure 5.7).

Dinitrophenyl hapten

In Table 5.7 are summarized some data on responsiveness to DNP hapten in High and Low lines[57]. The superiority of High line in anti-DNP precipitin synthesis appears especially in the secondary response where an extremely high

Table 5.7 Primary and secondary responses to DNP–BGG: serum concentration and characteristics of antibody produced

	7 days primary*			14 days secondary†		
	anti-DNP (mg/ml)‡	K_0	a	anti-DNP (mg/ml)‡	K_0	a
High line	0.04–0.21	$(0.86)10^7$	1.00	12.5–13.9	$(1.4–3.6)10^7$	0.68–0.70
Low line	0	—	—	0.57–3.00	$(1.3–2.6)10^7$	0.78–0.96

K_0 = Association constant (litre/mol)
a = Heterogeneity index
* Primary immunization: 1 mg DNP–BGG in complete Freund's adjuvant intraperitoneally
† Secondary immunization: same dose 75 days after priming
‡ Quantitative precipitation technique with DNP–BSA
From Del Guercio et al. (1972). Immunochemistry, 9, 769

concentration of serum antibody is produced. In spite of this quantitative difference the affinity and the heterogeneity of the antibodies synthesized are similar in the two lines.

T_4 bacteriophage

The production of antibody to T_4 bacteriophage has been measured by Howard et al. in terms of phage inactivation constant (K). Twenty-three days after intravenous immunization with 5×10^8 T_4 phage particles, the mean K titre was 5.59 in High responders and 0.033 in Low responders[58].

Histocompatibility antigens

In Figure 5.19 is represented the production of cytotoxic antibody against histocompatibility antigens in mice of both lines after primary immunization

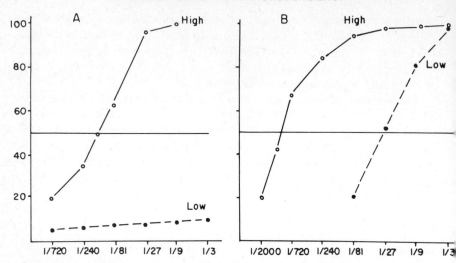

Figure 5.19 Titration of cytotoxic antibodies in the serum of High and Low responders. A. 10 days after injection of 5×10^7 spleen cells from the opposite line. B. 9 days after 5 injections of 5×10^7 spleen cells from outbred albino mice. From Liacopoulos-Briot *et al.* (1972). *Transpl.* **14**, by courtesy of Williams and Wilkins Co., Baltimore.

(Figure 5.19A) and after hyperimmunization (Figure 5.19B) with allogeneic lymphoid cells.

After the primary immunization, only High responders synthesize cytotoxic antibody. In hyperimmunized mice, the superiority of High responders is evident since the 50% cytotoxic titre of the serum is 40-fold higher than that of Low responders[59].

Pneumococcus polysaccharide (SIII)

The antibody response to all the aforesaid antigens is T cell dependent. However, the two lines of mice are also markedly separated in their antibody

Table 5.8 Responses to various doses of i.v. administered pneumococcus polysaccharide SIII in High and Low responder mice

	Number of PFC per spleen ($\times 10^3$)								
	SIII doses (µg)								
	—	0.1	0.5	2	5	20	50	250	1,000
High line	4.2 (3–9)	14.5	35.2	144	167	850	940	1,502	13.6
Low line	12 (5–20)	12	6.2	12.5	13	63	35	1	—

Responses are expressed as the number of PFC per spleen, using SE coated with SIII
From Howard *et al.* (1972). *Eur. J. Immunol.*, **2**, 269

response to T independent antigens such as pneumococcus polysaccharide SIII[33]. This antigen induces the synthesis of only IgM antibody in mice.

The results in Table 5.8 show the responses to various doses of SIII from the subimmunogenic up to the tolerogenic ones. At the optimal antigen dose (20 μg), the number of PFC per spleen in High responders is 13-fold higher than in Low responders. It is also of interest to remark that the threshold dose of SIII is about 40-fold lower in High than in Low responders, 0.5 μg and 20 μg respectively. A similar phenomenon was observed for the responsiveness to SE (Figure 5.6) and to BSA (Figure 5.17). The dose of SIII required to induce immunological paralysis is greater in High than in Low responders.

Levan and dextran

Howard *et al.* studied the antibody response of High and Low lines to native levan (mol. wt. 2×10^7) and native dextran (mol. wt. 8×10^7). The specificities of these antigens are respectively determined by β 2–6-linked fructose and α1–3-linked glucose. As SIII, levan and dextran are T independent antigens eliciting the synthesis of only IgM antibody in the mouse but unlike SIII, levan and dextran produce equivalent antibody response in High and Low lines (Figure 5.20).

The antibody responsiveness to these two antigens is measured 4–5 days post-immunization by counting the number of PFC per spleen using SE coated with the corresponding antigen. No significant inter-line difference appears on Figure 5.20A in the PFC response for the doses of 1–3 μg of levan. The

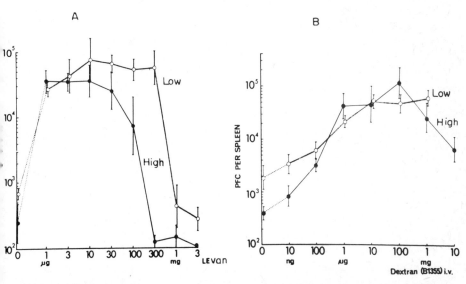

Figure 5.20 PFC per spleen in High and Low responders immunized: A. with increasing doses of levan 4 days before; B. with increasing doses of dextran 5 days before. From Howard *et al.* 1974. *Eur. J. Immunol.*, **4**, 453, by courtesy of Verlag Chemie, Weinheim.

response to higher doses shows that High line is more susceptible to tolerance induction than Low line, so while High responders are fully tolerized by 300 μg, this dose optimally immunizes Low responders. The equivalent response of the two lines was confirmed by using decreasing doses of levan from 1 μg to 100 ng (results not shown in Figure 5.20). The results of Figure 5.20B illustrate the equivalent PFC response of High and Low lines to dextran over the dose range 100 ng–1 mg. Partial tolerance is induced by 10 mg in High line mice, the effect in Low line is unknown since these mice do not tolerate such a high dose.

The anti-levan response is also similar in both lines immunized with *Pseudomonas levanicum* vaccine, a micro-organism which contains levan. Levan and dextran are the first antigens so far tested eliciting equivalent responses in High and Low lines. Moreover, no significant difference between the two lines is observed in the synthesis of anti-DNP antibody after immunization with DNP-levan conjugate whereas the usual superiority of High responders is confirmed in anti-DNP antibody production after immunization with DNP conjugated with polymerized flagellin or BGG. The inter-line difference in the production of anti-DNP antibody depends, in consequence, on the responsiveness to the carrier[58].

On the basis of their results with levan and dextran, Howard *et al.*[58] have proposed that the marked inter-line difference in the rate of multiplication and differentiation of immunocytes (see Section 5) is not due to intrinsic genetic differences at the level of lymphocytes themselves but results from genetic modifications of antigen handling by macrophages. This hypothesis would account for the inter-line difference in general immune responsiveness to many unrelated antigens. The identical response to levan and dextran (which is an exception) might be explained by one of the two following hypotheses.

(1) Levan and dextran are macrophage-independent antigens *in vivo*. Owing to their high degree of molecular branching they have a multi-point binding with B lymphocytes that become directly stimulated.
(2) Levan and dextran are independent of the genetic differences in antigen handling by macrophages. This hypothesis has received direct support from the experiments of Wiener and Bandieri[34] showing that KLH and SIII, which induce different responses in High and Low mice, are processed in different ways by peritoneal macrophages *in vitro* while levan has a similar fate in the macrophage of both lines.

The study of Howard *et al.* is of interest since it indicates that the two lines of mice do not differ in general immune-responsiveness to all the antigens. However, experiments presently in progress in our laboratory in F_{30} mice seem to indicate some difference between High and Low line in humoral responsiveness to dextran and levan. This discrepancy, if confirmed, could result from genetic divergence between the lines maintained in our laboratory and the colonies established in Howard's laboratory deriving from our F_{17} generation.

In the interpretation of these findings, other factors should be considered besides the exclusive role of macrophages: dextran and levan are antigens of restricted specificity and therefore they may be submitted to the control of specific *Ir* genes which might interact with the polygenic regulation of antibody response, as recently demonstrated[16].

5.7 REGULATION OF THE CLASS OF ANTIBODY SYNTHESIZED AND OF THE CONCENTRATION OF SERUM IMMUNOGLOBULINS

Whatever may be the phenotypic expression of the genes controlling the antibody synthesis, their major physiological effect is the regulation of the immune response rate in terms of immunocyte multiplication and differentiation. The cells synthesizing the various classes or sub-classes of antibody are all controlled by the same genetic regulation since the inter-line difference in antibody production between High and Low responders has been demonstrated for the classes of IgM, IgG and IgE antibody and also for the sub-classes IgG1, IgG2[32,55,56]. The study of IgA synthesis is in progress. An example of the genetic control of the synthesis of both IgM and IgG classes of antibody is represented in Figure 5.21.

Total serum agglutinins and mercaptoethanol-resistant agglutinins to SE are measured during the primary and secondary responses in High and Low lines. During the primary response only IgM antibody is produced by Low responders while both IgM and IgG are synthesized by High responders. After the secondary immunization, the High line synthesizes only IgG antibody while the Low line produces the two classes of antibody.

These experiments demonstrate that the group of genes governing antibody synthesis regulates the production of antibody molecules belonging to the two main classes of Ig. The study of the antibody response to other protein antigens: hen egg albumin, BSA and DNP–BGG have confirmed the preceding conclusion and extended these results to the other classes and sub-classes of antibody previously mentioned.

The quantitative study of the immune response to SE at cellular level has demonstrated that the increase in the number of cells synthesizing anti SE antibody (RFC) represents only 2–3% of the total enlargement of the spleen cell population produced by the intravenous injection of this immunogen[43,49,60]. This phenomenon implies modifications of the serum concentration of immunoglobulins in the two lines, particularly after immunization. In fact, these differences have been found, as demonstrated in the data of Table 5.9 where the serum levels of the various classes and sub-classes of Ig in High and Low responders are indicated[61].

The titres of Ig have been measured by radial diffusion using immune sera monospecific of each Ig class.

In non-immunized mice, the serum concentration of the different Ig is

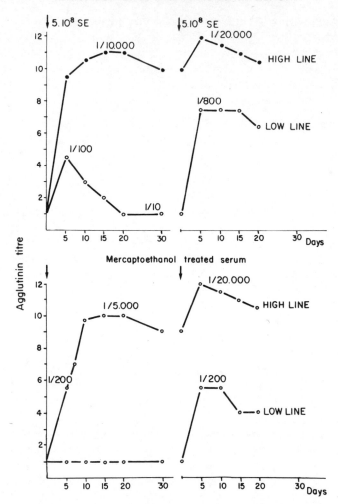

Figure 5.21 Kinetics of total mercaptoethanol resistant agglutinin synthesis, during primary and secondary responses to SE in High and Low responders. From Biozzi *et al.* (1974). In *La Génétique des Immunoglobulines et de la Réponse Immunitaire. Ann. Immunol.* (Inst. Pasteur) **125C**, 107, by courtesy of Masson et Cie, Paris.

slightly higher in High line except for IgM. This leads to a two-fold difference in the total concentration. The inter-line difference augments markedly 14 days after immunization when the total serum level of Ig is not significantly modified in Low responders while it is considerably increased in High responders. The difference is then of about 7-fold for the total Ig concentration and reaches 15-fold for the IgG1.

These findings have been confirmed in various conditions of immunization with several antigens. Two weeks after the secondary intraperitoneal immunization with 1 mg DNP–BGG in complete Freund's adjuvant the total

Table 5.9 Levels of classes and sub-classes of Ig in High and Low F_{14} responder mice (before immunization or 14 days after injection of 5×10^8SE)

| | Serum immunoglobulins (mg/ml) | | | |
| | Before immunization | | After immunization | |
	High line	Low line	High line	Low line
IgM	0.17	0.14	0.40	0.14
IgG1	0.78	0.31	3.60	0.24
IgG2	1.45	0.61	6.00	0.75
IgGA	0.54	0.34	0.90	0.46
Total	2.94	1.40	10.90	1.59

From Biozzi et al. (1970). J. Exp. Med., 132, 752

level of Ig was 14.6 mg/ml in High responders and 2.82 mg/ml in Low responders[57].

Since the catabolism of Ig is similar in both lines[32], th difference of Ig serum levels is due to an impairment of the general Ig synthesis in Low responders. The inter-line difference in serum concentrations of Ig corresponds to a parallel modification in both weight and cell content of the spleen. In non-immunized mice, the spleen weight is somewhat smaller in the Low line. The antigen stimulation produces an important augmentation of the spleen weight in High responders in which the spleen cell content doubles in three days. Such an effect is much more reduced in Low responders since the spleen size only increases by about 40%[43].

In order to gain some information on the inheritance of the regulation of Ig synthesis, Ig levels were measured in F_1 hybrids, F_2 hybrids, ($F_1 \times$ High)Bc and ($F_1 \times$ Low)Bc 10 days post-immunization with SE. The results are presented in Table 5.10. The data of Table 5.10 have been obtained in F_{18} and those of Table 5.9 in F_{14} which explains the difference in the serum levels of Ig. As shown in Table 5.10, the serum concentrations of Ig in F_1 hybrids are closer to those of Low responders, thus, the character 'low level' is dominant.

Table 5.10 Levels of classes and sub-classes of Ig in F_1, F_2 and backcrosses between F_{18} High and Low responder lines (10 days post-immunization with 5×10^8SE)

| | Serum immunoglobulins (mg/ml) | | | | | |
	High line	Low line	$(High \times Low)F_1$	F_2	$(High \times F_1)$	$(Low \times F_1)$
IgM	0.60	0.25	0.30	0.35	0.60	0.25
IgG1	6.00	0.70	0.95	1.00	3.20	1.30
IgG2	7.00	1.30	2.50	2.70	6.00	2.40
IgA	1.20	0.90	0.90	0.95	1.40	0.70
Total	14.80	3.15	4.65	5.00	11.20	4.65

From Lieberman et al. (1972). J. Exp. Med., 136, 790

In the backcrosses, the Ig levels tend to approach those of the parental lines. Thence, the serum level of all the Ig after immunogenic stimulation is submitted to genetic regulation. However, the inheritance pattern is probably different for each class or sub-class of Ig.

The defect in the synthesis of Ig in Low responders after immunogenic stimulation reflects the general inter-line difference in specific antibody response of the two lines to many unrelated immunogens. If this defect is partially or entirely produced by genetic modifications expressed phenotypically in macrophages, the role of these cells in the Ig synthesis and eventually in the pathogenesis of hypogammaglobulinaemia should have to be considered.

5.8 DISSOCIATION BETWEEN ANTIBODY SYNTHESIS AND CELL MEDIATED IMMUNITY IN HIGH AND LOW RESPONDER LINES

Several aspects of T cell mediated immunity have been studied in the two lines.

5.8.1 Skin graft rejection

As previously shown, High and Low lines differ in their histocompatibility antigens. The serum antibody response against the histocompatibility antigens of the other line is markedly stronger in High than in Low responders (see Figure 5.19A). Despite this fact, Low responders reject grafted skin quite efficiently. The mean rejection time of skin grafts exchanged between the two lines is 10.4 days in Low responder recipients and 12.6 days in High responder recipients. This difference is significant at $p = 0.01$. Low responders are therefore significantly better at mounting this immune response usually considered as mediated by T lymphocytes. When the skin graft rejection is achieved, the superiority of High responders in the humoral antibody synthesis is confirmed: their serum is cytotoxic for Low line lymphocytes up to a 1/50 dilution, while the serum of Low responder recipients even undiluted, is devoid of detectable cytotoxic effect for High line lymphocytes. The shorter time of skin graft rejection in Low responder recipients may be caused either by the lack of synthesis of facilitating antibody or by the possible participation of host macrophages[59].

5.8.2 Graft-versus-host (GVH) reaction

Another reaction of transplantation immunity mediated by T lymphocytes is the GVH reaction which may be evaluated quantitatively by the spleen weight increase (Spleen Index) produced by the injection of allogeneic lymphocytes in neonatal recipients. Byfield and Howard measured the spleen index in (High $\times$ DBA)F_1 and (Low $\times$ DBA)F_1 injected with an equivalent number of spleen cells from High or Low donors. The spleen index was 1.34 (range 1.1–2.2) and 1.71 (range 1.3–2.0) in recipients receiving High or Low cells respectively[62]. No significant difference was therefore demonstrated in the capacity of T lymphocytes of the two lines for the induction of GVH reaction in F_1 hybrids. These results have been confirmed in our laboratory when GVH reaction was induced by High or Low line lymphocytes transferred in allogeneic adult recipients previously immunosuppressed. In this case, the reaction induced by Low responder lymphocytes was markedly stronger than that induced by an equivalent number of High responder lymphocytes (see Figure 5.8).

5.8.3 Delayed hypersensitivity

A pure delayed hypersensitivity without simultaneous production of humoral antibody is not easily induced in mice. The experimental model chosen was that described by Asherson and Ptak[63] where the delayed hypersensitivity reaction is measured by the increase in ear thickness 24 hours after a local application of picryl chloride in mice pre-sensitized 6–7 days previously by skin painting with this antigen.

The increase in the ear thickness was slightly larger in High responders than in Low responders, 36×10^{-3} cm and 25×10^{-3} cm respectively. At the time of challenge, a small amount of antibody was detected in the serum, 29 μg protein/ml and 4 μg protein/ml in High and Low responders respectively. In consequence, the reaction measured was not one of pure delayed hypersensitivity. In contrast with the 7-fold difference in antibody level only a slight inter-line difference was observed in the ear thickness. This might be imputed to the participation of either B lymphocytes or humoral antibody in the complex mechanism of the local reaction. An important change at the level of T lymphocyte responsiveness was thus excluded[64].

5.8.4 Responsiveness to phytohaemagglutinin (PHA)

Another way of investigating the potentialities of T lymphocytes is the study of their responsiveness to PHA *in vitro*. This reaction was measured by the incorporation of tritiated thymidine in populations of spleen and lymph node cells from High and Low responder mice. The cells were incubated during 48 hours in the presence of various doses of PHA in tissue culture medium without any protein addition. No significant difference in responsiveness was detected in the two lines under these experimental conditions[65]. Consequently, the genetic difference between High and Low lines does not affect their responsiveness to PHA *in vitro*.

5.8.5 Thymic hormone

A new parameter of thymus function *in vivo* is the determination of the serum level of the hormone secreted by thymus epithelial cells[66], by its property to inhibit the rosette formation[67]. Identical levels of this thymic hormone have been found in the serum of High and Low responders, similar to the hormone concentration of conventional outbred albino mice[68].

The results of the various experiments reported in this paragraph are concordant. They demonstrate that in High and Low responder mice, the potentialities of T cells are similar, in contrast with the striking difference observed in the antibody response to both T dependent and T independent antigens. On these grounds, we had proposed the hypothesis that the responsiveness of B lymphocytes was affected by the group of genes regulating antibody synthesis[69]. It should be stressed, however, that the reactions of the T cell mediated immunity studied do not necessarily investigate the potentiality of T cells as helpers or suppressors of B cell activity. The study of the regulatory function of T lymphocytes on the activity of B lymphocytes may be of primary importance to understand the mechanism of genetic regulation of antibody synthesis in the two lines of mice. This study is in progress but made difficult by the strong histoincompatibility existing between the two lines.

The results presented in this section demonstrate a complete dissociation between the genetic regulation of humoral and cell mediated immunity. This implies that the two responses have fundamentally diverse immunobiological significances. If the inter-line difference in antibody synthesis is exclusively due to genetic modifications of antigen processing in macrophages, as suggested by Howard *et al.*[58] then we must admit that the metabolic pathway of the antigen-inducing antibody synthesis is different from that inducing cell-mediated immunity.

5.9 RESISTANCE OF HIGH AND LOW RESPONDER LINES TO EXPERIMENTAL TUMOURS AND INFECTIONS

Up to now only incomplete and provisional data have been obtained on the modification of host resistance against tumours and infections. Nevertheless, we shall report some examples illustrating the usefulness of the two lines of mice for the study of the mechanisms of host resistance[70,71]. The dissociation of humoral and cell mediated immunity characterizing the two lines would permit evaluation of the relative importance of each type of response in the resistance against experimentally induced diseases.

5.9.1 Allogeneic tumours

The rate of growth and the mortality observed in High and Low responders implanted subcutaneously with Sarcoma 180 is represented in Figure 5.22.

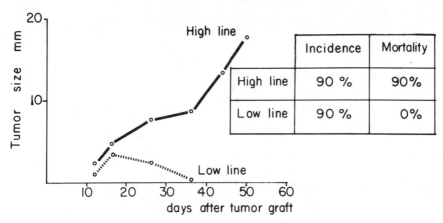

Figure 5.22 Growth of Sarcoma 180 grafted subcutaneously in High and Low responders. From Biozzi *et al.* (1972). *Ann. Inst. Pasteur,* **122,** 685, by courtesy of Masson et Cie, Paris.

The tumours grow at the same rate in both lines for about two weeks. Afterwards, growth continues in High responders inducing high mortality. On the contrary, in Low responders all the tumours regress and eventually disappear. The regression of the tumour in Low responders may be caused by the lack of synthesis of facilitating antibody since the Sarcoma 180 is particularly sensitive to enhancement. Cell-mediated immunity may therefore play its full role and destroy the tumour. This interpretation is substantiated by the study of resistance to Erlich ascitic tumour in High and Low responder lines. This tumour which is resistant to the enhancing effect of facilitating antibody grows at the same rate and induces a similar mortality in both lines[71].

5.9.2   Syngeneic tumours

The allogeneic immune reactivity inhibits the growth of tumours originated in inbred strains of mice when transplanted in both High or Low responders. As we know that F_1 hybrids between the two lines and an inbred strain retain a substantial difference in antibody response, characteristic of High or Low line (see Table 5.11), we used such hybrids to study host resistance against leukaemia of AKR and DBA/2 mice.

First generation hybrids between High or Low responders and AKR or DBA/2 mice were inoculated with an equivalent number of leukaemic cells from AKR or DBA/2 donors respectively. One hundred per cent mortality was attained in both hybrids without any modification of the survival time. Thus, in spite of their different humoral responsiveness the susceptibility of these hybrids to invasion by leukaemic cells is not modified[71].

We demonstrated several years ago that pretreatment with *Mycobacterium tuberculosis* BCG strain or with *Corynebacterium parvum* (*C. parvum*) protects mice against different types of tumours (reviewed in reference 72) in-

Table 5.11   Maximal titre of SE agglutinin in F_1 hybrids between High and Low responders and AKR and DBA/2 mice

	Maximal titre of SE* agglutinin
High line	1/10 000
Low line	1/100
(High × AKR)F_1	1/2000
(Low × AKR)F_1	1/100
(High × DBA/2)F_1	1/3840
(Low × DBA/2)F_1	1/480

* Immunization with 5×10^8 SE i.v.
From Biozzi et al. (1972). Ann. Inst. Pasteur, 122, 685

cluding AKR leukaemia transmitted in AKR or (AKR × CBA)F_1 mice[73,74]. In an attempt to analyse the possible role of immune responsiveness in this type of protection, we studied the effect of C. parvum treatment on AKR leukaemia transmitted in (AKR × High)F_1 and (AKR × Low)F_1.

The results of this experiment reported on Table 5.12 show that the protective effect of C. parvum pretreatment is evident in both F_1 hybrids. Furthermore, the Low responder hybrids are somewhat more resistant in terms of survival than High responder hybrids. It has previously been demonstrated that C. parvum had an adjuvant effect on both humoral antibody synthesis and cell-mediated immunity[75]. In High and Low lines, the pretreatment with C. parvum markedly amplifies the inter-line difference in antibody production. This adjuvant effect is very small in Low responders while it is extremely strong in High responders[43]. Thus, it may be supposed that the antibody response against tumour antigens is also very different in C. parvum pretreated High and Low responder F_1 hybrids. The strong protection of C. parvum treated F_1 hybrids is therefore caused by cell-mediated immunity rather than by humoral anti-tumour antibody response. The probable cooperation of macrophages in the anti-tumour immunity induced by C. parvum may account for the higher resistance of (AKR × Low)F_1 since Low responders have more active macrophages (see Section 4).

Table 5.12   Resistance of normal and C. parvum treated (AKR × High)F_1 and (AKR × Low)F_1 mice to leukaemia induced by i.p. injection of 100 leukaemic cells

	C. parvum*	Mortality (%)	Mean harmonic time to death (days)
(High × AKR)F_1	−	100	29
	+	31	—
(Low × AKR)F_1	−	100	27
	+	16	—

* C. parvum: 500 μg intraperitoneally 6 days before intraperitoneal injection of leukaemic cells
From Biozzi et al. (1972). Ann. Inst. Pasteur, 122, 685

5.9.3 Carcinogen-induced tumours

Intramuscular injection of 200 μg of oil solution of 3,4-benzpyrene in High and Low lines induced a tumour incidence of 16% in High responders and of 52% in Low responders. The resulting mortality 9 months after the benzpyrene injection was 13% and 52% in High and Low lines respectively. High responders are therefore more resistant to this type of tumour. In order to establish whether this resistance is correlated with the immune responsiveness, the carcinogen was injected in groups of F_1 hybrids, F_2 hybrids, $(F_1 \times High)Bc$ and $(F_1 \times Low)Bc$. F_1 hybrids, which have an intermediate antibody response to optimal dose of SE (see Figure 5.7) are as susceptible as Low responders. Moreover, no correlation was found between tumour incidence and immune responsiveness in the two backcrosses and in F_2 hybrids. It was concluded that the two characters 'antibody response to SE' and 'tumour resistance' are dissociated[71]. This conclusion must be revised on the basis of the data obtained since then on the importance of the antigen dose on the inheritance of immune responsiveness (see Figure 5.7 and Figure 5.18). For the threshold dose of antigen, Low responsiveness is dominant as well as high tumour incidence.Then, the resistance to tumour induction would be related to the two loci regulating immune responsiveness at weak antigenic stimulation. Therefore, it is difficult to recognize the nature of the inter-line difference in the resistance to benzpyrene induced tumours, namely if it is connected with the genes involved in the regulation of antibody synthesis at weak antigenic stimulation or if it is related to any other genetic trait resulting from the high consanguinity characterizing each line of mice (see Table 5.3).

5.9.4 Bacterial infections

The experiments reported on Table 5.13 summarize the study of the resistance of High and Low responders to *Salmonella typhimurium* infection. *S. typhimurium* is a natural pathogen in mice. Defence against this infection is probably due either to cell mediated immunity or to macrophage activity or to an association of both mechanisms[76,77]. As shown in Table 5.13, the natural resistance against this infection is greater in Low than in High responders. Because of the extreme severity of intraperitoneal challenge, this difference is only manifest in terms of mean survival time. When the severity of the infection is reduced as in intradermal challenge a greater resistance of Low responders is evident in terms of definitive survival.

Quite surprisingly, the higher resistance of Low responders is amplified by the specific vaccination made either with non-virulent strain of *S. typhimurium* or with an active fraction prepared by Dodin in the Pasteur Institute. The vaccination is scarcely effective in High responders, in which the survival time is

Table 5.13 Resistance of normal or vaccinated High and Low responder mice to
S. typhimurium **infection**

No. of micro-organisms injected	Route of infection	Vaccination	High line		Low line	
			Mortality (%)	Mean time to death days	Mortality (%)	Mean time to death days
5000	i.d.	—	100	10.4	50	16.2
200	i.p.	—	100	5.4	100	9
1000	i.p.	—	100	5.4	100	8.7
1000	i.p.	+*	100	8.7	10	—
1000	i.p.	+‡	100	8	10	—

* Vaccination with living non-virulent strain of *S. typhimurium*
‡ Vaccination with an active fraction of *S. typhimurium*
From Dodin *et al.* (1972). *Ann. Inst. Pasteur*, **123**, 137 and Biozzi, JG. (1972), in H. O. McDevitt and M. Landy (eds.).
Genetic Control of Immune Responsiveness, p. 317. (New York and London: Academic Press)

slightly prolonged, whereas it is extremely efficient in Low responders since 90% of definitive protection is obtained[78].

Similar results were observed in High and Low responders infected with a virulent strain of *Yersinia pestis* (*Y. pestis*) (Table 5.14).

The inoculation of *Y. pestis* causes 100% mortality in both lines, again the natural resistance being weaker in High than in Low responders as indicated by the mean survival time. Specific vaccination with an immunogenic fraction of *Y. pestis* prepared by Dodin produces complete protection of Low responders while it is ineffective in High responders.

If cell mediated immunity alone is responsible for resistance to these infections, no significant inter-line difference could reasonably be expected unless a larger synthesis of facilitating antibody in High responders would protect the micro-organisms against cell mediated immunity. This hypothesis is not very likely since no clear-cut effect of passively-administered antibody has been demonstrated in these types of infections.

The higher resistance of Low responders seems therefore to result from the participation of the macrophages in both natural or vaccination induced host

Table 5.14 Resistance of normal or vaccinated High and Low responders to *Y. pestis* infection
(1000 microorganisms injected intraperitoneally)

	High line		Low line	
	Mortality	Mean time to death days	Mortality	Mean time to death days
Controls	100%	4.6	100%	7.7
Vaccinated 500 μg fraction from *Y. pestis*	100%	5	0	—

From Biozzi, G. (1972). In H. O. McDevitt and M. Landy (eds.). *Genetic Control of Immune Responsiveness*, p. 317. (New York and London: Academic Press)

resistance. The higher activity of Low line macrophages was described in Section 4. In connection with antibacterial immunity, it is relevant to underline the quicker destruction of living T_4 bacteriophages and the slower rate of growth of *Listeria monocytogenes* in Low responder macrophages. The overall results so far obtained rule out the intervention of antibody in the protection against these infections. They emphasize the importance of cell-mediated immunity and the role of macrophages in the mechanism of host resistance.

Acknowledgment

The excellent secretarial assistance of Mrs J. Albert in the preparation of the manuscript is greatly appreciated.

References

1. McDevitt, H. O. and Benacerraf, B. (1969). *Advan. Immunol.,* **11**, 31
2. Lieberman, R. and Humphrey, W., Jr. (1971). *Proc. Nat. Acad. Sci. (USA),* **68**, 2510
3. Sela, M. (1972). *Harvey Lectures,* (New York: Academic Press)
4. Benacerraf, B. (1973). *Harvey Lectures,* (New York: Academic Press)
5. Melchers, I., Rajewsky, K. and Shreffler, D. C. (1973). *Eur. J. Immunol.,* **3**, 754
6. Benacerraf, B. (1974). *Ann. Immunol. (Institut Pasteur),* **125C**, 143
7. Mozes, E., McDevitt, H. O., Jaton, J. C. and Sela, M. (1969). *J. Exp. Med.,* **130**, 493
8. Eichmann, K., Braun, D. C. and Krause, R. M. (1971). *J. Exp. Med.,* **134**, 48
9. Blomberg, B., Geckeler, W. R. and Weigert, M. (1972). *Science,* **177**, 178
10. Eichmann, K. (1972). *Eur. J. Immunol.,* **4**, 301
11. Sher, A. and Cohn, M. (1972). *Eur. J. Immunol.,* **2**, 319
12. Pawlak, L. L. and Nisonoff, A. (1973). *J. Exp. Med.,* **137**, 855
13. Lieberman, R., Potter, M., Mushinski, E. E., Humphrey, Jr., W. and Rudikoff, S. (1974). *J. Exp. Med.,* **139**, 983
14. Rihova-Skarova, B. and Riha, I. (1974). *Ann. Immunol. (Institut Pasteur),* **125C**, 195
15. Gasser, D. L. and Silvers, W. K. (1974). *Advan. Immunology.,* **18**, 1
16. Dorf, M. E., Dunham, E. K., Jonson, J. P. and Benacerraf, B. (1974). *J. Immunol.,* **112**, 1329
17. Gill, T. J., Kunz, H. W., Stechschulte, D. J. and Austen, K. F. (1970). *J. Immunol.,* **105**, 14
18. Gill, T. J. and Kunz, H. W. (1971). *J. Immunol.,* **106**, 980
19. Sloan, B. P. and Gill, T. J. (1972). *Immunochemistry,* **9**, 677
20. Stimpfling, J. H. and Durham, T. (1972). *J. Immunol.,* **108**, 947
21. Fuji, H., Zaleski, M. and Milgrom, F. (1972). *J. Immunol.,* **108**, 223
22. Mozes, E., Shaltiel, S. and Sela, M. (1974). *Eur. J. Immunol.,* **4**, 463
23. Biozzi, G., Stiffel, C., Mouton, D., Bouthillier, Y. and Decreusefond, C. (1970). In H. Peeters (ed.), *Protides of the Biological Fluids,* p. 161. (Oxford & New York: Pergamon Press)
24. Lieberman, R., Stiffel, C., Asofsky, R., Mouton, D., Biozzi, G. and Benacerraf, B. (1972). *J. Exp. Med.,* **136**, 790
25. Stiffel, C., Mouton, D., Bouthillier, Y., Heumann, A. M., Decreusefond, C., Mevel, J. C. and Biozzi, G. (1974). *Progress in Immunology,* Vol. II — *Proceedings of 2nd International Congress of Immunology,* p. 205 (Amsterdam: ASP Biological and Medical Press)

26. Feingold, N., Feingold, J., Mouton, D., Bouthillier, Y., Stiffel, C. and Biozzi, G. (1975). *Eur. J. Immunol.* (submitted for publication)
27. Falconer, D. S. (1960). *Introduction to Quantitative Genetics,* Ch. 11 (New York: The Ronald Press)
28. H. O. McDevitt and M. Landy (eds.). *Genetic Control of Immune Responsiveness* (1972). (New York and London: Academic Press)
29. Benacerraf, B. and Katz, D. H. (1974). *Advan. Cancer Res.*
30. Sabolovic, D., Oth, D. and Burg, C. (1971). *Immunology,* **20,** 341
31. Bandieri, A. Personal communication.
32. Biozzi, G., Stiffel, C., Mouton, D., Bouthillier, Y. and Decreusefond, C. (1974). *Ann. Immunol., (Institut Pasteur),* **125C,** 107
33. Howard, J. G., Christie, G. H., Courtenay, B. M. and Biozzi, G. (1972). *Eur. J. Immunol.,* **2,** 269
34. Wiener, E. and Bandieri, A. (1974). *Eur. J. Immunol.,* **4,** 457
35. Nossal, G. J. V., Williams, G. M. and Austin, C. M. (1967). *Aust. J. Exp. Biol. Med. Sci.,* **45,** 581
36. Unanue, E. R. and Cerottini, J. C. (1970). *J. Exp. Med.,* **131,** 711
37. Fauve, R. Personal communication
38. Stiffel, C., Halpern, B., Mouton, D., Biozzi, G. and Mathé, G. (1959). *Rev. Franç. Etudes Clin. Biol.,* **4,** 164
39. Schmidtke, J. R. and Dixon, F. J. (1973). *J. Immunol.,* **110,** 848
40. Gowans, J. L. and McGregor, D. D. (1965). *Progr. Allergy,* **9,** 1
41. Unanue, E. R., Biozzi, G. and Benacerraf, B. (1974). *Proc. Soc. Exp. Biol. Med.,* **145,** 1243
42. Jerne, N. J., Nordin, A. A. and Henry, C. (1963). In Amos and H. Koprowski, (eds.), *Cell-Bound Antibodies,* p. 109 (Philadelphia: The Wistar Institute Press)
43. Biozzi, G., Stiffel, C., Mouton, D., Bouthillier, Y. and Decreusefond, C. (1972). *J. Exp. Med.,* **135,** 1071
44. Biozzi, G., Stiffel, C., Mouton, D., Liacopoulos-Briot, M., Decreusefond, C. and Bouthillier, Y. (1966). *Ann. Inst. Pasteur,* **110,** 7
45. Biozzi, G., Stiffel, C. and Mouton, D. (1967). In R. Mihich (ed.), *Immunity, Cancer and Chemotherapy,* p. 103 (New York: Academic Press)
46. Capalbo, E. E. and Makinodan, T. (1964). *J. Immunol.,* **92,** 234
47. Greaves, M. F. and Möller, E. (1970). *Cell. Immunol.,* **1,** 372
48. Bach, J. F. (1971). *Cell-mediated Immunity,* p. 51 (Basel: S. Karger A.G.)
49. Biozzi, G., Stiffel, C., Mouton, D., Bouthillier, Y. and Decreusefond, C. (1968). *Immunology,* **14,** 7
50. Ada, G. L. and Byrt, P. (1969). *Nature (London),* **222,** 1291
51. Bach, J. F., Muller, J. Y. and Dardenne, M. (1970). *Nature (London),* **227,** 1251
52. Pavlovsky, S., Binet, J. L., Decreusefond, C., Stiffel, C., Mouton, D., Bouthillier, Y. and Biozzi, G. (1970). *Ann. Inst. Pasteur,* **119,** 63
53. Decreusefond, C., Mouton, D., Binet, J. L., Pavlovsky, S., Stiffel, C., Bouthillier, Y. and Biozzi, G. (1970). *Ann. Inst. Pasteur,* **119,** 76
54. Biozzi, G., Stiffel, C., Mouton, D., Bouthillier, Y. and Decreusefond, C. (1972). *Transpl. Proc.,* **4,** 339
55. Prouvost-Danon, A., Stiffel, C., Mouton, D. and Biozzi, G. (1971). *Immunology,* **20,** 25
56. Prouvost-Danon, A. and Biozzi, G. (1974). *Proceedings of the 9th European Congress of Allergology and Clinical Immunology — London September 1974* (in press)
57. Del Guercio, P. and Zola, H. (1972). *Immunochemistry,* **9,** 769
58. Howard, G. J., Courtenay, B. M. and Desaymard, C. (1974). *Eur. J. Immunol.,* **4,** 453
59. Liacopoulos-Briot, M., Bouthillier, Y., Mouton, D., Lambert, F., Decreusefond, C., Stiffel, C. and Biozzi, G. (1972). *Transplantation,* **14,** 590
60. Dresser, D. W. and Wortis, H. H. (1965). *Nature (London),* **208,** 859

61. Biozzi, G., Asofsky, R., Lieberman, R., Stiffel, C., Mouton, D. and Benacerraf, B. (1970). *J. Exp. Med.*, **132**, 752
62. Byfield, P. E. and Howard, J. G. (1972). *Transplantation,* **14**, 133
63. Asherson, G. L. and Ptak, W. (1968). *Immunology,* **15**, 405
64. Mouton, D., Bouthillier, Y., Oriol, R., Decreusefond, C., Stiffel, C. and Biozzi, G. (1974). *Ann. Immunol. (Inst. Pasteur),* **125C**, 581
65. Liacopoulos-Briot, M., Mouton, D., Stiffel, C., Lambert, F., Decreusefond, C., Bouthillier, Y. and Biozzi, G. (1974). *Ann. Immunol. (Inst. Pasteur)* **125C**, 26
66. Bach, J. F. and Dardenne, M. (1973). *Immunology,* **25**, 353
67. Bach, J. F. and Dardenne, M. (1972). *Transpl. Proc.,* **4**, 345
68. Dardenne, M., Monier, J. C., Biozzi, G. and Bach, J. F. (1974). *Clin. Exp. Immunol.,* **17**, 339
69. Biozzi, G., Stiffel, C., Mouton, D., Bouthillier, Y. and Decreusefond, C. (1971). *Progress in Immunology,* p. 529 (New York: Academic Press)
70. Biozzi, G. (1972). In H. O. McDevitt and M. Landy (eds.). *Genetic Control of Immune Responsiveness,* p. 317 (New York and London: Academic Press)
71. Biozzi, G., Stiffel, C., Mouton, D., Bouthillier, Y. and Decreusefond, C. (1972). *Ann. Inst. Pasteur,* **122**, 685
72. Stiffel, C., Mouton, D. and Biozzi, G. (1971). *Ann. Inst. Pasteur,* **120**, 412
73. Lamensans, A., Stiffel, C., Mollier, M. F., Laurent, M., Mouton, D. and Biozzi, G. (1968). *Rev. Franç. Etudes Clin. Biol.,* **13**, 773
74. Lamensans, A., Mollier, M. F. and Laurent, M. (1968). *Rev. Franç. Etudes Clin. Biol.,* **13**, 871
75. Neveu, T., Branellec, A. and Biozzi, G. (1964). *Ann. Inst. Pasteur,* **106**, 771
76. Biozzi, G., Stiffel, C., Halpern, B. N. and Mouton, D. (1960). *Rev. Franç. Etudes Clin Biol.,* **5**, 876
77. Mackaness, G. B. (1970). In R. Van Furth (ed.). *Mononuclear Phagocytes* (Oxford: Blackwell Scientific Publications)
78. Dodin, A., Wiart, J., Stiffel, C., Bouthillier, Y., Mouton, D., Decreusefond, C. and Biozzi, G. (1972). *Ann. Inst. Pasteur,* **123**, 137

6
Immunodeficiency

FRED S. ROSEN

Supported by grant AI 05877 from the U.S.P.H.S. and the John Simon Guggenheim Foundation.

6.1 INTRODUCTION

The discovery of X-linked agammaglobulinaemia in 1952 was only a prelude to the discovery of a large number of deficiency states in the immunological systems. At present, almost all the well-defined immunodeficiencies in man and animals have a genetic basis. Despite this fact, it is curious that very few examples of structural gene defects have come to light. Most of the immunodeficiency diseases appear to result from the failure of some regulatory process, and a disproportionate number of them are X linked.

This chapter is concerned only with the primary defects in the cellular or humoral immune response. Thus, all hypercatabolic states or those due to exogenous agents, such as irradiation or drugs, are excluded as are immunodeficient states secondary to malignant processes. The primary immunodeficiencies are categorized in the accompanying table[1].

The study of immunodeficiency has resulted in several major contributions to the advancement of immunology. The age-old questions regarding the constituents of normal resistance to infection have been largely answered by the exquisite susceptibility of patients with B cell defects to pyogenic organisms as opposed to the susceptibility to opportunistic organisms observed in the T cell deficient. The immunoglobulin concept arose in part from the demonstration by immunoelectrophoresis of the absence of discrete groups of globulins from agammaglobulinaemic serum. And, finally, the cellular basis for the dichotomy between cellular and humoral immunity was first revealed by the study of immunodeficiency disease. Hopefully, further study of these immunological curiosities will continue to be of heuristic value to the progress of immunology.

6.2 B CELL DEFECTS

6.2.1 X-linked agammaglobulinaemia

X-linked agammaglobulinaemia usually manifests itself in the second year of life, although the onset of the characteristically severe, recurrent infections may begin at any age from eight months to three years. The infections are those caused by the common pyogenic organisms — *Staphylococcus aureus*, pneumococci, meningococci, *Hemophilus influenzae*, and less often beta haemolytic streptococci or *Pseudomonas*. They differ from infections in normal children only in their frequency, severity, and the tendency for infection with the same organism to occur more than once. Pyoderma, purulent conjunctivitis, pharyngitis, otitis media, sinusitis, bronchitis, pneumonia, empyema, purulent arthritis, meningitis, and sepsis occur with surprising frequency and may be associated with unusually high fever and unexpected elevation or depression of the leukocyte count. A rather indolent rheumatoid-like arthritis with sterile effusion into one of the large joints develops in about one third of

Table 6.1

Type	Suggested cellular defect			Inheritance		
	B cells					
	Circulating Ig-bearing B lymphocytes (a)*	(b)**	T cells	X-linked	Autosomal recessive	Other†
X-linked agamma	X	(X)††		X		X
Thymic hypoplasia			X			X
Severe combined immunodeficiency	X	X	X	X	X	
with dysostosis	X	?	X		X	
with ADA deficiency	X		X		X	
with generalized haematopoietic hypoplasia	X		X			
Selective Ig deficiency						
IgA	?	X	(X)			
Others		?				
X-linked immunodeficiencies — increased IgM		X		X		
Immunodeficiency with ataxia telangiectasia		X	X		X	
Immunodeficiency with thrombocytopaenia and eczema (Wiskott–Aldrich syndrome)	X	X*	X	X		X
Immunodeficiency with thymoma		X	X			X
Immunodeficiency with normal or hypergammaglobulinaemia	X	X	(X)			X
Transient hypogammaglobulinaemia of infancy		X			(X)	
Variable immunodeficiencies (largely unclassified and very frequent)	X	X	(X)			X

* Absent or very low
** Easily detectable or increased
† Some cases with circulating B lymphocytes without detectable surface Ig have been found
†† Implies multifactorial or unknown genetic basis or no genetic basis

patients and may be the presenting complaint. The children usually, but not always, handle most viral infections normally[2].

Provided the diagnosis is made before repeated infections have produced serious anatomical damage, the immediate prognosis for these children is excellent and they gain weight and grow normally. However, in later childhood, adolescence, or early adult life, complications may develop in some of these patients. Slowly progressive neurological disease, suggesting a 'slow virus' infection, accompanies a dermatomyositis-like syndrome with brawny edema, perivascular mononuclear infiltrates, and, terminally, severe systemic symptoms and death. Prolonged shedding of ECHO virus has been demonstrated in these cases. These enteroviruses can be repeatedly cultured from the cerebrospinal fluid over a prolonged period of time prior to death; these children are incapable of terminating the enterovirus infection[3].

A careful family history may uncover instances of death from overwhelming infection or multiple severe infections in other male siblings, maternal un-

Table 6.2   Incidence of C5 deficiency in inbred strains of mice (Data from Cinader et al., 1964)

C5 normal		C5 deficient
B10D2 — New line	SEA/Gn-se	B10D2 — Old line
BALB/CJ	SEC/1Gn	A/J
BDP/J	SJL/J	A/HeJ
BRVR/Sr	SL/R1	AKR/J
BSVS/Sr	SM/J	AU
BUB/Bn	STOLI/Lw	BUA/Wi
BUB/Bn-C	T6	BUC/Wi
BUB/Wi	WH/Ht	BUE/Wi
CBA/J	129/J	CE/J
C3H$_f$/BiOci	2BC3H	DBA/2J
C3H/HeJ	2C3H	DDK
C3H/HeN		DM/Ms
CHI/St		FAKI
C56BL/HaOci		GFF
C57BL/10J		JF/Bcr
C57BR/cdJ		I/FnLn
C57L/J		JU/Fa
C58/J		KK
DBA/1J		MaS/A
F/St		NBL/N
FU		NC
HR/De		NS/Fr
MA/J		NXB/B1
MO/Ko		PHH
NZO/B1		RF/J
PE/R1		SMA/Ms
PHL		ST/J
P/J		SWR/J
PL/J		YBR/HeWiHa
PS		
RIII/AnJ		
RIII/WyJ		

cles, or male offspring of maternal aunts. The syndrome is transmitted as an X-linked phenomenon. However, no linkage with other markers on the X chromosome has been shown. The agammaglobulinaemia gene is at least 30 centimorgans from the Xg(a) gene, an X linked red cell antigen[4].

The tissue findings are diagnostic. Removal of a stimulated regional lymph node discloses absence of the expected germinal centres, secondary follicles, and plasma cells[5]. The thymus is normal, but lymph nodes and spleen lack the usual follicular architecture. Germinal centres are absent, and there are few if any plasma cells in the medullary cords or red pulp. Although the number of lymphocytes in the tissues appears diminished, they are present in the thymus-dependent areas of lymphoid tissue, and normal numbers are found in the blood. Plasma cells are absent from the bone marrow, intestinal tract, spleen, and lymph nodes. Study of the circulating lymphocytes has revealed normal numbers of T cells. T cell function as measured by response to PHA, MIF production, and lymphocytotoxicity or allograft rejection is normal[6,7]. On the other hand, B cells cannot be found in the blood and tissues of almost all cases[8-11]. However, blood of a few cases of proved X-linked agammaglobulinaemia does contain normal numbers of B lymphocytes[11,12]. These B cells are unresponsive to pokeweed mitogen or the T cell mitogen in the presence of antigen[11]. Females in such kindred who are obligate heterozygotes may have a mixed population of normal and abnormal B lymphocytes; it appears from preliminary findings that the Lyon hypothesis applies to B lymphocytes and that B cells are subject to X chromosome inactivation.

6.2.2 Common, variable, unclassified immunodeficiency ('acquired' hypogammaglobulinaemia)

This is the most common form of immunodeficiency with serious clinical consequences and probably includes a number of entities; it occurs in either sex at any age without any known causative factor, either genetic or acquired, although a predisposition may be inherited since its development has been reported in siblings or among relatives[13-15].

The picture is that of the antibody deficiency syndrome associated with immunoglobulin deficiency, which may be somewhat less severe than in the X-linked form of agammaglobulinaemia. Pathologically, there is necrobiotic change in the follicular architecture of the lymph nodes and spleen, or lymphadenopathy and splenomegaly due to reticulum cell hyperplasia or giant cortical follicles. The predominant infections are sinusitis and pneumonia, often leading to bronchiectasis. A sprue like malabsorption syndrome and pernicious anaemia are common among these patients[16]. Recent work has demonstrated that this malabsorption syndrome is often due to *Giardia lamblia* demonstrated either in aspirates of duodenal fluid or in biopsy specimens of duodenal mucosa[17].

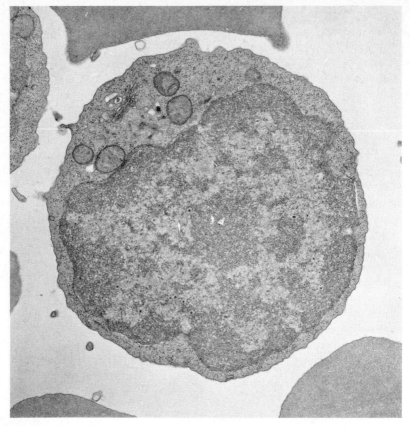

Figure 6.1a B lymphocyte from a patient with common variable hypogammaglobulinaemia following exposure to the T cell mitogenic factor. This B lymphocyte shows no response.

Patients with 'acquired' agammaglobulinaemia may have no B cells, but, more commonly, normal numbers of B cells or even increased numbers of B cells are found[18,19]. In some patients, the B cells do not respond to mitogenic stimuli and do not synthesize immunoglobulin; in others, mitotic responses and immunoglobulin synthesis is normal, but there is no secretion of the immunoglobulin formed[18,20] We have studied one patient whose B cells functioned normally *in vitro* when cultured in normal AB+ serum, but did not in the patient's serum[18]. His serum contains an inhibitor of his own, as well as normal B cells. Obviously a whole spectrum of B cell maturation failure is presented by these patients. In some patients, T cell function deteriorates progressively. This is particularly true of patients who have an associated thymoma. Other patients have been reported to have 'suppressor' T cells which inhibit normal B cell proliferation in culture[21]. The implication is that these patients have normal B cells, but evidence for this has not yet been presented.

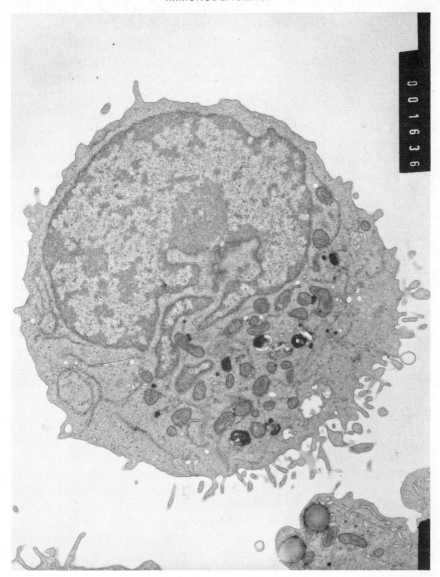

Figure 6.1b   B lymphocyte from a patient with common variable hypogammaglobulinaemia following exposure to the T cell mitogenic factor. The cell shows a response in new development of endoplasmic reticulum and enlargement of the nucleus but it has failed to secrete newly synthesized *γ*-globulin. Magnification × 10 200 (from Geha *et al., New Eng. J. Med.* **291,** by courtesy of the publishers).

6.2.3   X-linked immunodeficiency with increased IgM

In a few instances, patients have been observed with manifestations similar to those in X-linked agammaglobulinaemia, but with higher levels of immunoglobulins which, when analysed, turn out to reflect a marked deficiency of serum IgA and IgG but an elevation in the concentration of IgM. The congenital form of this disease seems to occur almost entirely in males and has an apparent X-linked pattern of inheritance. Except for a greater frequency of 'autoimmune' haematologic disorders (neutropenia, haemolytic anaemia, thrombocytopenia), the clinical course in these patients resembles that of X-linked agammaglobulinaemia[22]. Histologically, there is disorganization of the follicular architecture of the lymphoid tissues, but PAS positive plasmacytoid cells containing IgM are present, and even tonsillar hypertrophy due to infiltrates of these cells has been observed. Only B cells with IgM surface fluorescence are found. B cell lymphomas of the intestinal tract are a frequent cause of death in boys with this immunodeficiency. A similar syndrome of X-linked immunodeficiency with increased IgM has been found in mice.

6.2.4   Selective immunoglobulin deficiencies (Dysgammaglobulinaemia)

This term is used to describe cases in which there are consistent deficiencies of one or more of the recognizable plasma immunoglobulins. Although often associated with the clinical manifestations of the antibody deficiency syndrome, some instances of selective immunoglobulin deficiency may be chance laboratory findings in otherwise apparently normal individuals[23].

6.2.4.1   Selective deficiency of IgG subclasses

Selective deficiency of IgG subclasses may occur, in which the patient is unable to synthesize one or more of the IgG subclasses and thus fails to produce antibodies in one or more of the four presently identified IgG subclasses. This results in failure to respond to particular types of antigens, in increased susceptibility to a limited spectrum of bacterial infections, and in a reduction in total serum IgG concentration proportional to the percentage of the total IgG pool accounted for by the deficient IgG subclass. Of course, a deficiency in IgG1 is most severe, since this subclass constitutes over 70% of the IgG[24,25].

A further discussion of failure of allelic expression of some of the IgG subclasses and allelic control of IgG levels is given in the chapter by Kunkel and Kindt.

6.2.4.2   Selective IgA deficiency

Selective IgA deficiency is observed with considerable frequency (3–7 per 1,000 population). In a few patients, this may portend the development of ataxia telangiectasia, but an appreciable number of such individuals remain healthy throughout life. However, a high incidence of rheumatoid arthritis, systemic lupus erythematosus, and malabsorption syndrome has been observed among this group of patients[26-28]. A significant number of IgA deficient individuals have circulating antibodies to IgA and have anaphylactic reactions upon receiving whole blood or plasma[29]. IgA deficiency is not linked to the Am structural gene marker of IgA2[30].

6.2.5 Transient hypogammaglobulinaemia of infancy

The level of IgG globulin, which is passively acquired by transplacental passage, falls rapidly during the first month of life, levels off during the second month, and thereafter begins to rise. Rarely, there is delay in the maturation of B cells; the level of IgG globulins received by passive transfer from the mother continues to fall and is not adequately raised by immunoglobulins synthesized by the infant, so that within a few months the total γ-globulin level is much lower than usual for that age. The infants have overt infections, unexplained episodes of fever, and often bronchitis with wheezing. Normal numbers of B cells are present in the circulation of affected infants.

For unexplained reasons, there occurs an escape from the block in B cell maturation sometime between 18 and 30 months of age, and immunoglobulin levels rise rapidly to normal. This phenomenon resembles allotypic suppression in rabbits. A search for discordance in Gm alleles amongst the parents of affected infants or for the presence of Gm agglutinators in the mothers of affected infants revealed no significant differences from what would be expected by random events.

6.2.6 Transcobalamin II deficiency and agammaglobulinaemia

Hitzig *et al.* have described one kindred in which transcobalamin II deficiency is inherited as an autosomal recessive trait. In addition to megaloblastic anaemia, the propositus had profound agammaglobulinaemia. Enumeration of B and T cells yielded normal results, but plasma cells were absent and the patient formed no antibodies. Vitamin B12 corrected both the anaemia and agammaglobulinaemia. During the rise in immunoglobulin levels, the patient made antibodies to antigens used for sensitization prior to vitamin B12 therapy[31-33].

6.3 GENETICALLY DETERMINED DEFECTS IN THE COMPLEMENT SYSTEM

The complement system is one of the principal effector systems of antigen–antibody interactions. The sequential interaction of the nine complement components has been extensively reviewed elsewhere. All of these components have now been isolated and characterized. This has led to useful investigation of genetic variations and deficiencies of individual complement components. Although these deficiency states cannot properly be classified with the primary immunodeficiency diseases, the end result of defects in C3 synthesis or deficiency of the C3b inactivator much resembles defects in B lymphocytes; i.e. extraordinary susceptibility to pyogenic bacterial infection and a breakdown of the heat-labile opsonic system of the blood. Furthermore, there has been an extraordinary incidence of connective tissue disease in patients with other complement component deficiencies (C1r, C2, C4, C5, and C7), as is seen in selective IgA deficiency. However, more epidemiological data, such as has been obtained with selective IgA deficiency, are required to confirm these associations. Finally, important linkage information is just now coming to light. C3 levels in mice, allotypy of Factor B of the properdin system in man, and C2 deficiency are all intimately linked to the major histocompatibility complex.

6.3.1 Hereditary angioneurotic edema

Hereditary angioneurotic edema results from a genetically determined deficiency of the C1 inhibitor. The defect is transmitted as an autosomal dominant. The serum of affected patients contains anywhere from 5 to 30% of the normal concentration of C1 inhibitor (18 mg/100 ml).

Patients with this disease are prone to recurrent episodes of swelling. The edema fluid accumulates rapidly in the affected part, which becomes tense but not discoloured; no itching, no pain, and no redness are associated with the edema. Laryngeal edema may be fatal because of airway obstruction and consequent pulmonary edema. If the intestinal tract is involved, most often the jejunum, severe abdominal cramps and bilious vomiting ensue. Diarrhoea, which is clear and watery in character, occurs when the colon is affected. The attacks last 48–72 hours. Although they are often unheralded, they may occur subsequent to trauma, menses, excessive fatigue, and mental stress. Attacks of angioedema are infrequent in early childhood; the disease exacerbates at adolescence and tends to subside in the sixth decade of life. In children especially, a mottling of the skin reminiscent of erythema marginatum may be frequently noticed and not necessarily be associated with attacks of angioedema[34].

Attacks of angioedema are associated with the generation of activated C1 ($\overline{C1}$) in the plasma, an event which cannot be measured in normal plasma. The natural substrates of $\overline{C1}$, C4 and C2, are consumed so that their serum concentration falls precipitously as the attack progresses. The terminal components of the complement system remain unaffected[35]. Highly purified $\overline{C1}$ or $\overline{C1s}$, when injected intradermally into normal skin or into patients, induces angioedema[36]. This reaction does not occur in people genetically deficient in C2, or in guinea pigs genetically deficient in C4, thus suggesting that the interaction of $C\bar{1}$ with C4 and C2 generates one or more factors which enhance vascular permeability. The effect is on the postcapillary venule[37]. A polypeptide kinin-like substance which has vasopermeability inducing properties has also been generated in the plasma of the patients. Its origin from C2 appears likely but is not proved.

The autosomal dominant inheritance of hereditary angioneurotic edema presents an interesting puzzle. Obviously affected individuals are heterozygous for the abnormality. Despite this, their serum contains very little C1 inhibitor (average 17% of normal), and liver biopsies can be shown to contain a markedly reduced number of hepatic parenchymal cells engaged in C1 inhibitor synthesis[38,39].

The C1 inhibitor or α_2-neuraminoglycoprotein is the most highly glycosylated glycoprotein of serum. It contains over 40% carbohydrate, almost half of which is neuraminic acid. It has a molecular weight of 106 000 but behaves like a 7S protein on gel filtration. In addition to its capacity to inactivate $C\overline{1s}$, it also has an inhibitory effect on $C\overline{1r}$, plasmin, kallikrein, Factor XIa of the clotting system, and activated Hageman factor[40]. However, these other inhibitory activities can be replaced by α_2-macroglobulin or antithrombin III. It remains, nonetheless, the unique inhibitory substance in serum for C1. The inhibition of C1 may involve the formation of a covalent bond between $C\overline{1s}$ and the C1 inhibitor, analogous to the interaction between thrombin and antithrombin III. Both plasmin and trypsin cleave the C1 inhibitor and render it inactive. So does acidity; the protein loses its inhibitory activity when exposed to a pH below 7.0[41,42].

In 15% of affected kindred, sera of patients contain normal or elevated amounts of a cross-reacting, immunologically non-functional protein. The CRM+, non-functional C1 inhibitors differ among the different kindred with respect to their (1) electrophoretic mobilities, (2) their capacity to bind $C\overline{1s}$, and (3) their capacity to inhibit esterolysis by $C\overline{1s}$ of N acetyl tyrosine ethyl ester. However, all CRM+ C1 inhibitors fail to inhibit destruction of C4 by $C\bar{1}$[43,44]. The clinical course of the disease is the same in CRM+ and CRM− patients.

6.3.2 Hereditary C2 deficiency

Over 20 kindred have been discovered in which one or more members is homozygous for deficiency of the second component of complement, C2. The defect is transmitted as an autosomal recessive trait, but heterozygotes are easily detected by their having half the normal serum C2 concentration by functional or immunochemical measurements[45–48].

About half the affected kindred have been ascertained by the presence of connective tissue diseases, such as SLE, polymyositis, and Henoch Schonlein purpura in the propositi, suggesting that this genetic deficiency may predispose to these illnesses[49-51].

No genetically transmitted polymorphism of C2 has as yet been recognized. It has, therefore, been impossible to study the transmission of a 'null' gene in affected kindred. It is of considerable interest that a close linkage between HL-A haplotype and C2 deficiency has now been found in at least three affected kindred[52]. C2 is synthesized by fixed and wandering macrophages. Such phagocytic cells are normal in C2 deficient individuals, except for their inability to synthesize C2[53].

6.3.3   Hereditary C3 deficiency

A common, genetically determined polymorphism of C3 has been recognized in man and the Rhesus monkey, *Macaca mulatta*, by virtue of electrophoretic differences. The most common form of C3 migrates relatively slowly on prolonged electrophoresis in agarose and is designated C3S. It has a gene frequency of 0.77–0.80 in European or North American Caucasians and a much higher incidence in blacks (0.92–0.96) and Orientals (0.99)[54]. The other common or fast allele is C3F, and it has a gene frequency of 0.19–0.22 in Caucasian populations. A number of rare alleles have been identified and are designated by their mobilities relative to the S and F gene products; i.e. $C3F_{1.4}$, $F_{1.1}$, $F_{1.0}$, $F_{0.85}$, $F_{0.5}$, $S_{0.4}$, $S_{0.6}$, $S_{0.8}$, $S_{0.9}$ and $S_{0.10}$. The various allelic forms of C3 have normal C3 haemolytic activity[55]. Discrepancies between maternal and cord blood C3 types provide evidence for fetal synthesis of C3[56]. The recipient of an orthotopic liver transplant had a $C3FS_{0.6}$ genotype. The liver donor was C3SS. After 20 hours, the recipient's C3 typed SS, thereby providing convincing evidence of the hepatic origin of C3[57].

(+)

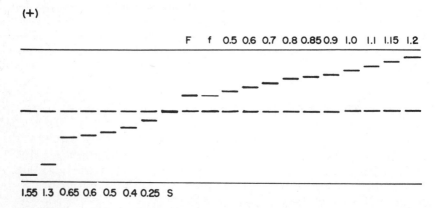

Figure 6.2   Relative electrophoretic positions of the known variants of C3 in man (from Alper and Parkman, *Hematology of Infancy and Childhood*, by courtesy of the publishers).

A kindred was reported to show segregation of a 'null' gene in six backcrosses, of which two were highly informative[58]. A hyposynthetic variant of C3F, designated C3f, was also found in three generations of one kindred where it was possible to show that the C3f was synthesized at one third the rate of C3S with ^{125}I labelled C3F and ^{131}I labelled C3S[59]. Individuals with the 'null' gene and the hyposynthetic variant are clinically normal.

C3 deficiency in the homozygous form has been found in three individuals recently[60]. Homozygotes contain no C3 in their serum by immunochemical measurement and less than 0.1% of normal by sensitive functional assay. Heterozygous individuals in these kindred are readily detected by their half normal levels of C3. About three dozen heterozygotes have been identified in one large kindred.

These deficient children are subject to recurrent pyogenic infections, and their clinical history has a striking resemblance to agammaglobulinaemia. C3 deficient serum is unable to sustain opsonization of bacterial particles. A defect in antibody formation has been reported to occur in cobra venom treated animals. This has been presumed to result from C3 depletion by cobra venom treatment[61]. However, C3 deficient children have normal antibody formation to both T dependent and T independent antigens. Furthermore, they have normal numbers of B lymphocytes with C3 receptors. The cobra venom experiments may require a more complex explanation for the phenomenon of depressed antibody synthesis.

Recently, Nussenzweig and his co-workers have reported that C3 levels in mice are linked to their H-2 type[62]. In man, however, there is no linkage

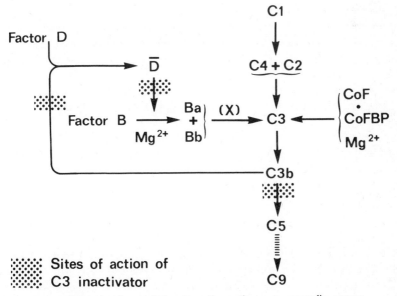

Figure 6.3 A scheme of the alternative pathway or properdin system.

between the HL-A locus and C3 genotype. It remains to be seen if this is also the case in mice so that the H-2 may be linked to some other factor controlling C3 synthesis rates.

The alternative pathway of C3 activation or the properdin system operates by a positive feedback in that the generation of small amounts of C3b accelerates the pathway and results in considerable conversion of C3 to C3b[63]. In the presence of C3b, an enzyme, designated Factor D, splits its substrate, Factor B, into γ (Bb) and α (Ba) conversion products[64]. The complex, $\overline{C3bBb}$, converts more C3 to C3b[65]. The feedback is controlled by the C3b inactivator, a β globulin of the blood, also designated KAF, which enzymatically destroys C3b in converting it to an inactive form, C3bi, and then to C3c[66,67]. Properdin may act to prevent decay of the $\overline{C3bBb}$ complex.

6.3.4 C3b inactivator deficiency

A patient homozygous for C3b inactivator deficiency has been found to have recurrent pyogenic infection due to the influenza bacillus, meningococci, and pneumococci, including mastoiditis, otitis, pneumonia, and septicaemia[68]. The consequence of his genetic deficiency is spontaneous activation of the alternative pathway at all times, so that his serum contains C3b and activated Factor D but no Factor B and very little C3. His catabolic rate of C3 is four times normal, as ascertained by injection of ^{125}I labelled C3. As a consequence of the accelerated C3 destruction, he releases increased amounts of the C3 anaphylatoxin or C3a, so that he has massive histaminuria and occasional showers of hives. The urticaria is particularly pronounced when he is exposed to hot or cold water[69]. Infusions of plasma or purified C3b inactivator halt the *in vivo* C3 hypercatabolism and cause the disappearance of C3b from his circulation[70]. Ordinarily, C3b produced in his circulation by the alternative pathway activation adheres to his erythrocytes so that they are Coombs' positive with an anti-C3 reagent[71]. This phenomenon disappears transiently following infusion of normal plasma. Despite C3b on his red cells, their survival is normal, and he has no haemolytic anaemia. The defect is inherited as an autosomal recessive characteristic. With antiserum to the C3b inactivator, several first degree relatives are known to be heterozygous for the deficiency by the presence of half normal serum levels of C3b inactivator[66].

6.3.5 Factor B polymorphism

A complex, genetically determined polymorphism has been found for Factor B[72]. The two common alleles are also designated S and F, as with C3, because of their relative electrophoretic mobilities. The gene is designated Bf with gene frequencies for Bf^S and Bf^F of 0.709 and 0.278 in the Caucasian population.

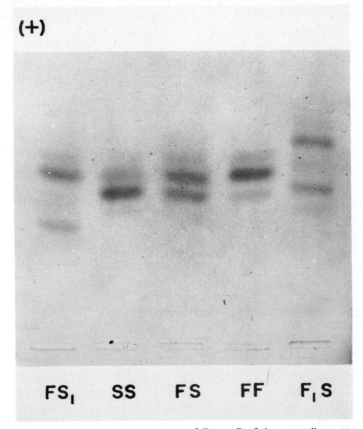

(+)

FS₁   SS   FS   FF   F₁S

Figure 6.4   The common genotypes of Factor B of the properdin system.

At least two rare alleles, F_1 and S_1, have been found. Significant differences between Bf types of maternal and cord blood suggest fetal synthesis of the protein. No deficiency of Factor B has as yet been found.

Factor B locus is closely linked to the HL-A locus[73]. In 30 families, no crossovers were noted between HL-A and Bf types. A similar close linkage is found in the Rhesus monkey[74].

6.3.6   Other genetic deficiencies of complement in man

Deficiencies of C1r, C4, C5, C6, and C7 have been found in various isolated kindred[75-79]. In all cases, heterozygous relatives of the propositi have been found. However, no genetic polymorphism is yet known for these human components so that it is not yet possible to demonstrate the inheritance of a 'null' gene. The propositi in kindred with C1r, C4, and C5 deficiency had a lupus-like syndrome. The proposita of the C6 deficiency kindred presented with gonococcal arthritis, and of the C7 deficiency kindred with Raynaud's phenomenon. A second kindred with C7 deficiency was discovered by chance in a normal child[80]. Certainly none of these deficiencies has been proved to result in undue susceptibility to infection.

6.3.7 C4 deficiency in guinea pigs

While screening guinea pig sera for possible allotypic antibody following immunization with normal guinea pig serum, a male NIH guinea pig was found to have antibody to guinea pig C4 and was subsequently shown to be C4 deficient[81]. Five other such guinea pigs were found among 250 animals in the NIH random bred colony. Several matings promptly revealed the defect to be transmitted as an autosomal recessive characteristic with easy detectability of the heterozygous state. Affected guinea pigs have no detectable haemolytic C4[82]. Affected guinea pigs had normal complement component titres, except for decreased C2 levels. Peritoneal macrophages have been shown to synthesize C4 normally. No C4 synthesis is detectable in macrophages of C4 deficient guinea pigs[83]. However, when C4 deficient macrophages are hybridized with HeLa cells, which do not normally synthesize C4, *human* C4 synthesis commences[84]. The molecular basis for this curious phenomenon is not yet known.

Because of the total obstruction in the activation of the classical complement pathway in their serum, C4 deficient guinea pig serum has played an important role in elucidating the function of the alternative or properdin pathway[85-87].

6.3.8 C5 deficiency in mice

Genetically determined complement deficiency was appreciated in mice before it was proved that the deficiency resided in the fifth component. Allotypic antisera revealed the absence of a β-globulin in several inbred strains, and the segregating locus was designated Hc' by one group of workers and MuB1 by another[88,89]. The gene product in both cases was determined to be C5 by Nilsson and Müller-Eberhard[90]. A large number of strains are known to be C5 deficient but the coisogenic B10·C2 'new' and 'old' lines have been extensively used in various investigations because the former have normal C5 and latter are C5 deficient. The strict coisogenicity of these two strains has been questioned. In any case, the C5 deficiency is transmitted as an autosomal recessive characteristic but antiserum to C5 readily distinguishes the heterozygotes.

Infusions of bone marrow cells from C5 sufficient strains (B10·D12 'new' or B6AF$_1$) into C5 deficient animals (B10·D2 'old' or A) results in prolonged appearance of C5 in serum of the formerly C5 deficient animals[91]. Apparently, the bone marrow cells which synthesize C5 lodge in the spleen. When 'old' line B10·D2 spleen cells are fused by Sendai virus with 'new' line kidney cells or chicken erythrocytes and the heterokaryotic cells are injected into 'old' line recipients, C5 is synthesized for about three weeks in the recipients[92]. These 'induction' effects are similar to the ones observed in the hybrid HeLa:guinea pig C4 deficient macrophages.

6.3.9 C6 deficiency in rabbits

Deficiency of C6 may be quite common in outbred rabbits[93,94]. Up to 5% of rabbits have the deficiency. The defect is inherited as an autosomal recessive but the heterozygotes can be easily detected[95]. C6 deficient rabbits produce antibody to homologous C6 so that the presence of CRM+ C6 in their serum is unlikely. Although C6 deficient rabbits appear healthy and have no gross immunological defect, they do have a clotting defect[96]. This appears to result from a peculiarity of the rabbit platelet which requires all complement components for the release of initiating factors. Blood from a C6 deficient human clots normally[97].

6.4 PRIMARY T CELL DEFICIENCIES

Patients with T cell deficiency have much more serious susceptibility to infection than patients with complete or partial B cell defects. In its most severe forms, T cell deficiency results in an inability to terminate opportunistic infections with organisms that are ordinarily innocuous. Consequently, varicella, vaccinia, and herpes and measles viruses can be fatal infections. The enterobacilli are commonly invasive in patients with T cell defects and infection with *Monilia* is almost universal. Malignancy of both the lymphoreticular organs and other viscera is also a common complication of the T cell disorders.

6.4.1 Severe combined immunodeficiency

Severe combined immunodeficiency (Swiss type agammaglobulinaemia, alymphocytosis, thymic alymphoplasia) is the most profound of the cellular defects. Affected patients usually have no T or B cells; the disease is invariably fatal. It is genetically determined, and there is clear evidence of autosomal recessive and X-linked recessive transmission of the disease. The clinical and laboratory findings may be quite variable from case to case, even among affected members of a single family. But, in man, the phenotypic expression of the disease is similar regardless of the inheritance pattern[2].

The onset of persistent infections of the lungs, monilial infection of the oropharynx, esophagus, and skin, chronic diarrhoea and wasting and runting begins in the early months of life and progresses with monotonous regularity to a fatal termination despite all attempts at routine therapy. Affected infants usually do not survive the first year or two of life. Examination usually reveals absence of tonsils, very small or absent lymph nodes despite chronic infection, chronic pneumonitis evidenced by a pertussis like cough, inspiratory retractions of the chest, rales, a somewhat distended abdomen with wasting and oral thrush[2].

Roentgenographic signs include pulmonary infiltration and absence of a thymic shadow. There is almost always an absolute decrease in the number of circulating lymphocytes, and occasionally neutropenia. In typical cases, the immunoglobulins are markedly decreased, but variants have been described in which circulating immunoglobulins are normal or there is selective immunoglobulin deficiency[98,99]. M components may be present in the circulation[100-102]. Plasma cells have been found in the tissues of such patients and some B lymphocytes may be detected in peripheral blood, but antibody formation is almost always impaired or absent. Tests of delayed hypersensitivity give negative results. Sensitization cannot be induced with dinitrochlorobenzene, cultured lymphocytes do not respond to phytohaemagglutinin, and skin allografts are not rejected. T cells are almost always absent from the circulation, and the few lymphocytes present in the blood usually have the characteristics of B cells.

B and T cell chimerism is readily established in affected infants with transplants of histoidentical sibling bone marrow[103-106]. As a matter of fact, maternal lymphocytes can be detected in affected male infants over a period of months[107]. Successful transplants from MLC-identical relatives have been accomplished despite HL-A non-identity between donor and recipient[108]. Administration of a suitable dose of bone marrow cells from the donor is accomplished with 50×10^6 nucleated cells per kg intravenously. More cells are optimal for intraperitoneal injection, perhaps 50×10^7. Evidence that the graft has become established and that immunological reconstitution has occurred usually requires 3–8 weeks.

These infants with severe combined immunodeficiency are exquisitely susceptible to graft-versus-host disease which has been observed in them following administration of peripheral blood, fetal liver cells, or histoincompatible bone marrow[109-111]. The course of the reaction much resembles the disease of mice and is rapidly fatal in 10–14 days. It is characterized by fever, a maculopapular rash involving the volar surfaces, diarrhoea with protein-losing enteropathy and edema, haemolytic anaemia and thrombocytopenia. Haemorrhage into the gut or lung is usually the terminal event. Donor cells are most abundantly evident in the spleen and liver and less so in skin and kidney. Splenic enlargement resembles also the observation in mice and correlates with the severity of the reaction.

At autopsy, the pathognomonic finding of severe combined immunodeficiency reveals itself in the thymus gland[112,113]. It usually fails to des-

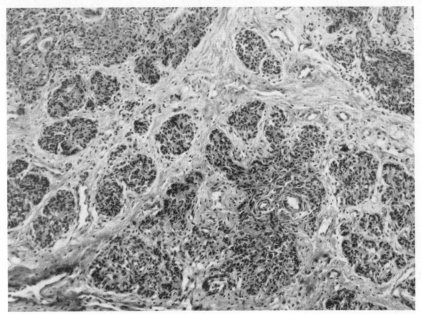

Figure 6.5   A section of the thymus gland from an infant with severe combined immuno-deficiency disease. Magnification × 400.

cend from the neck into the anterior mediastinum and remains just caudal to the thyroid isthmus. The organ is without lymphoid cells or Hassall's cor-puscles and the blood vessels are tiny, attesting to the fact that the thymus is fetal rather than involuted. Embryonal spindle cells are seen sometimes forming rosettes or nests in the connective tissue. The gland seems to be arrested at a stage where it resembles the thymus of a six- to eight-week fetus.

Recently, several but not all infants with the autosomal recessive form of the disease have been found to lack the enzyme adenosine deaminase (ADA) from their red cells and other tissues[114–116]. Heterozygosity was detectable in their parents by their half normal levels of ADA[117,118].

The enzyme in erythrocytes is genetically polymorphic and is known to occur in two different electrophoretic forms[119]. On the other hand, the tissue polymorphism is known to be due to post-transcriptional events[120]. It has been possible to trace the inheritance of a 'null' gene in at least two kindred with an affected child[117]. Despite the absence of ADA from the erythrocytes of affected infants, other tissues such as fibroblasts have a variant enzyme which may have abnormal stability[122]. Nonetheless, this finding has enabled the prenatal diagnosis in cultures of amnion cells[123]. Although thousands of Caucasians have been screened for ADA, no deficient individuals have been identified other than infants with severe combined immunodeficiency. Recently, a Kung boy in the Kalihari desert has been found to lack ADA from his erythrocytes[124]. However, he is immunologically normal[125]. It is quite

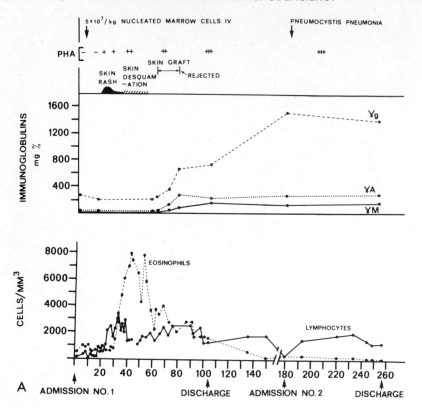

Figure 6.6 The course of immunological reconstitution in a child with severe combined immunodeficiency transplanted with histoidentical bone marrow cells (from Parkman *et al.* (1975). *New Eng. J. Med.*, **292**, 714, by courtesy of the publishers).

possible that he also has a variant enzyme in other tissues of greater stability than that found in infants with severe combined immunodeficiency.

The gene for ADA has been tentatively assigned to chromosome 20 so that there is no linkage with the major histocompatibility locus, assigned to chromosome 6 in man[126]. There is an independent assortment of HL-A haplotypes and ADA deficiency in families with infants affected with severe combined immunodeficiency[118]. Thus, it appears likely that the ADA deficiency has a causal relationship to severe combined immunodeficiency and that lymphoidal stem cells may be particularly vulnerable to the consequences of the absent or abnormal ADA.

ADA is involved in an important step in purine salvage by converting adenosine to inosine. ADA deficient erythrocytes accumulate adenosine triphosphate and convert inosine monophosphate to inosine triphosphate at an increased rate[127]. The accumulation of adenosine or another product in these infants may be lymphocytotoxic or interfere with pyrimidine biosynthesis by

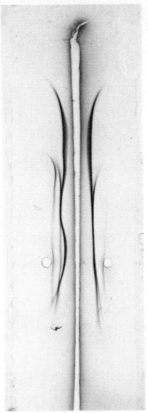

Figure 6.7   The appearance of multiple M components in the child whose course is depicted in Figure 6.6. The pattern was developed with goat anti-human immunoglobulins. Top: normal control. Anode to the right.

blocking conversion of orotic acid to orotidine[128]. Other interesting ideas stemming from this association of ADA deficiency and severe combined immunodeficiency remain to be explored, but the causative association between the ADA deficiency and the immunodeficiency is at present obscure.

Variant forms of severe combined immunodeficiency have been described. These include cases with dysostosis (short-limbed dwarfism) and rare cases with generalized haematopoietic hypoplasia[129-131]. The latter has been called reticular dysgenesia. Infants with this type of immunodeficiency also lack granulocytic precursors in the bone marrow and granulocytes from peripheral blood and survive for only a short time after birth. Nezelof syndrome, which is severe combined immunodeficiency with normal immunoglobulins is a specious diagnosis, and the term should be dropped. This variant is included in the term severe combined immunodeficiency.

Severe combined immunodeficiency has also been found in Arabian horses[132]. They have normal erythrocyte ADA levels. Horses normally lack

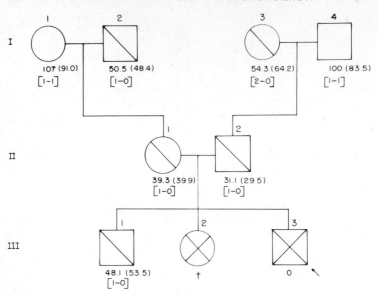

Figure 6.8 A family tree in which the proposita died of severe combined immunodeficiency. The arrow points to the infant in whom a prenatal diagnosis of adenosine deaminase deficiency was made. Under each symbol the ADA level is given by two different methods. The ADA genotype is given in brackets.

ADA from their serum. The syndrome is equally rapidly fatal in homozygous affected foals. As many as a third of Arabian horses may be heterozygotes for ADA deficiency.

6.4.2 Congenital thymic aplasia (DiGeorge syndrome)

Congenital thymic aplasia (DiGeorge syndrome) or (3rd and 4th pharyngeal pouch syndrome) results from a failure of the normal embryogenesis of the thymus and parathyroid glands, which are derived from the 3rd and 4th pharyngeal clefts. The syndrome is not genetically determined but appears rather to result from some intrauterine accident before the eighth week of gestation. Affected infants invariably have neonatal tetany. Anomalies of the great blood vessels are very frequently encountered, usually right sided aortic arch, or Tetralogy of Fallot[133]. These cardiac complications are the cause of late death in these children[134]. Mental subnormality also accompanies this syndrome.

The T cell defect in children with congenital thymic aplasia varies from the most profound to the barely discernible[135]. In any case, T cell function improves in these children with age, so that by five years of age no T cell deficit can be ascertained. It is not clear how this grossly retarded T cell maturation occurs in the absence of a thymus gland. Some children may have a small thymic remnant, but T cell maturation may occur at sites other than the thymus.

Transplants of fetal thymus into these infants result in the rapid acquisition of T cell function, even when implanted in a Millipore chamber[136-138].

6.4.3 Immunodeficiency with ataxia telangiectasia

This is an autosomal recessive disease in which abnormalities of the thymus have been found at post mortem examination. Gradually progressive cerebellar ataxia begins in early childhood. This is associated with increasing telangiectasia, which first becomes apparent as a rather inconspicuous dilatation of small blood vessels in the bulbar conjunctivae and ultimately is visible in the skin at about five years of age. Gonadal dysgenesis and failure of sexual maturation may be present in those who survive into the second decade. In late childhood, recurrent sinobronchial infections begin in many patients, often leading to bronchiectasis[139]. There is also a tendency to the development of malignant tumours, particularly of the lymphoid system. These reflect an immunological disturbance affecting T cell function, as shown by blunting of delayed hypersensitivity reactions, failure to reject allografts normally, and reduced response of the lymphocytes to phytohaemagglutinin. At post mortem examination late in the disease, the thymus is abnormally small and has a decreased number of thymocytes; there is a poor differentiation between cortex and medulla and decided diminution in the number of Hassall's corpuscles[140]. The most consistent B cell defect is a low level or absence of IgA globulin in the serum, which occurs in about 85% of affected patients and may precede clinical evidence of immunological deficiency by a number of years[141].

Chromosomal abnormalities of the D group are seen in karyotype analyses of these patients. The most frequently involved is chromosome 14, which is subject to frequent breaks and translocations in patients with ataxia telangiectasia[142]. All patients have elevated α-1-fetoprotein suggesting a generalized tissue maturation defect in this disease. In 20 patients with ataxia telangiectasia, the serum α-1-fetoprotein had a range of 44 to 2800 ng/ml (normal less than 30 ng/ml)[143].

6.4.4 Immunodeficiency with thrombocytopenia and eczema (Wiskott–Aldrich syndrome)

The Wiskott–Aldrich syndrome is an X-linked recessive disorder which usually is manifested by eczema, thrombocytopenia, and a wide variety of infections beginning late in the first year, although it may present rarely as thrombocytopenia alone. Death may occur from haemorrhage, infection, or the development of a malignant process similar to the Letterer–Siwe type of reticuloendotheliosis. The infections may be caused by a wide variety of micro-organisms, including viruses, bacteria, fungi and *Pneumocystis carinii*. Transient episodes of arthritis have been observed.

Results of studies of the pathogenesis of the Wiskott–Aldrich syndrome are confusing. The lymphoid tissues appear normal early in the course of the disease, but as the child grows there may be a loss of lymphocytes from the thymus and the paracortical areas of the lymph nodes. The peripheral lymphocyte count decreases, and there is a variable loss of cellular immunity, resulting in increased susceptibility to viral or fungal disease. Studies of immunoglobulin production in these patients suggest a normal response to a variety of antigens. IgA is usually elevated. IgM values are often low, and isohaemagglutinins and Forssman antibodies are usually lacking. The failure of these patients to respond to pneumococcal polysaccharides has led to the postulation that they have a general inability to respond to polysaccharide antigens, as opposed to normal responses to protein antigens. Whether this failure resides in the recognition system of the lymphocytes, in a deficit of the macrophages in processing such antigens, or in a qualitative deficiency of plasma cell function is not clear[144]. Since polysaccharides are widely distributed and important constituents of bacteria and fungi, it is reasonable that such a selective immunological deficiency might have a serious impact upon resistance. Transfer factor has been tried and found to induce cellular immunity and clinical improvement in some patients with this disease[145,146].

6.4.5 Nude mice

The clinical and immunological findings of thymic aplasia in human infants have an almost exact parallel in nude mice. However, nudity in the mouse is determined by an autosomal recessive gene in contrast to the absence of any apparent genetic basis for congenital thymic aplasia[147]. Nude mice, in addition to being hairless, lack a thymic epithelium[148]. They have no T cells but a normal complement of B lymphocytes and they respond well to thymus independent antigens but not at all to thymus dependent ones[149]. They accept xenografts[150]. They, like athymic infants, are readily restored to immunological health by implants of thymus. Theta-bearing T cells can be detected within hours of a nude mouse receiving a thymus graft and the T cells are of recipient origin[151].

Nude mice have provided some experimental evidence which calls into question the importance of immunological surveillance as a modality in resistance to oncogenesis. In both methylcholanthrene-induced skin carcinoma and Friend virus leukaemia, they have proved to be more resistant to the induction of tumours than controls. The results of methylcholanthrene carcinoma induction were quite striking; 7% in nudes versus 100% in controls[152].

6.4.6 Dwarf mice

Two strains of mice have a gene for dwarfism which is associated with a T cell defect. One strain, the Snell–Bagg mouse, is highly inbred since 1929 and is dwarfed when homozygous dw/dw. The other strain, the Ames mouse, is outbred and is also dwarfed when homozygous df/df. In both cases the affected mice are normal at birth. However, after weaning there is a progressive thymic atrophy and loss of T cell function[153,154]. The T cell deterioration can be prevented by injection of growth hormone which may have a thymotropic effect in mice, or by prolonged nursing or injections of mouse milk[155,156].

References

1. Cooper, M. D., Faulk, W. P., Fudenberg, H. H., Good, R. A., Hitzig, W., Kunkel, H. G., Roitt, I. M., Rosen, F. S., Seligmann, M. and Soothill, J. F. (1974). *Clin. Immunol. Immunopathol.,* **2**, 416
2. Rosen, F. S. and Janeway, C. A. (1966). *New Engl. J. Med.,* **275**, 709
3. Ziegler, J. B. and Penny, R. (1975). *Clin. Immunol. Immunopathol.,* **3**, 347
4. Rosen, F. S., Hutchison, G. and Allen, F. H. (1965). *Vox Sang.,* **10**, 729
5. Craig, J. M., Gitlin, D. and Jewett, T. (1954). *Amer. J. Dis. Child.,* **88**, 626
6. Rocklin, R. E., Rosen, F. S. and David, J. R. (1970). *New Engl. J. Med.,* **282**, 1340
7. Shannon, D. C., Johnson, G., Rosen, F. S. and Austen, K. F. (1966). *New Eng. J. Med.,* **275**, 690
8. Grey, H. M., Rabellino, E. and Pirofsky, B. (1971). *J. Clin. Invest.,* **50**, 2368
9. Froland, S. S. and Natvig, J. B. (1972). *Scand. J. Immunol.,* **1**, 1
10. Gayl-Peczalska, K. J., Park, B. H., Biggar, W. D. and Good, R. A. (1973). *J. Clin. Invest.,* **52**, 919
11. Geha, R. S., Rosen, F. S. and Merler, E. (1973). *J. Clin. Invest.,* **52**, 1725
12. Siegel, F. P., Pernis, B. and Kunkel, H. G. (1971), *Europ. J. Immunol.,* **1**, 482
13. Buehler, S. K., Fodor, G., Marshall, W. H., Firme, F., Fraser, G. R. and Vaze, P. (1975). *Lancet,* **i**, 195
14. Charache, P., Rosen, F. S., Janeway, C. A., Craig, J. M. and Rosenberg, H. A. (1965). *Lancet,* **i**, 234
15. Fudenberg, H. H., German, J. L. and Kunkel, H. G. (1962). *Arthritis Rheum.,* **5**, 656
16. Twomey, J. J., Jordan, P. H., Laughter, A. H., Meuwissen, H. J. and Good, R. A. (1970). *Ann. Int. Med.,* **72**, 499
17. Ochs, H. D., Ament, M. E. and Davis, S. D. (1972). *New Eng. J. Med.,* **287**, 341
18. Geha, R. S., Schneeberger, E., Merler, E. and Rosen, F. S. (1974). *New Eng. J. Med.,* **291**, 1
19. Preud'homme, J. L., Griscelli, C. and Seligmann, M. (1973). *Clin. Immunol. Immunopathol.,* **1**, 241
20. Cooper, M. D., Lawton, A. R. and Bockman, D. E. (1971). *Lancet,* **ii**, 791
21. Waldmann, T. A., Broder, S., Blaese, R. M., Durm, M., Blackman, M. and Strober, W. (1974). *Lancet,* **ii**, 609
22. Rosen, F. S., Kevy, S. V., Merler, E., Janeway, C. A. and Gitlin, D. (1961). *Pediatrics,* **28**, 182
23. Rockey, J. H., Hanson, L. A., Heremans, J. F. and Kunkel, H. G. (1964). *J. Lab. Clin. Med.,* **63**, 205

24. Schur, P., Borel, H., Gelfand, E. W., Alper, C. A. and Rosen, F. S. (1970). *New Engl. J. Med.,* **283,** 631

25. Yount, W. J., Hong, R., Seligmann, M., Good, R. A. and Kunkel, H. G. (1970). *J. Clin. Invest.,* **49,** 1957

26. Crabbe, P. A. and Heremans, J. F. (1967). *Amer. J. Med.,* **42,** 319

27. Ammann, A. J. and Hong, R. (1970). *Clin. Exp. Immunol.,* **7,** 833

28. Cassidy, J. T., Burtz, A., Petty, R. and Sullivan, D. (1968). *New. Eng. J. Med.,* **281,** 465

29. Vyas, G. N., Holmdahl, L., Perkins, H. A. and Fudenberg, H. H. (1969). *Blood,* **34,** 573

30. van Laghem, E. (1974). *Europ. J. Immunol.,* **4,** 57

31. Hitzig, W. H., Döhmann, U., Gimpert, E., Plüss, H. J. and Vischer, D. (1975). *J. Pediat.* (in press)

32. Gimpert, E., Jakob, M. and Hitzig, W. (1975). *Blood,* **45,** 71

33. Hitzig, W. H. and Kenny, A. B. (1975). (Submitted for publication)

34. Donaldson, V. H. and Rosen, F. S. (1966). *Pediatrics,* **37,** 1017

35. Donaldson, V. H. and Rosen, F. S. (1964). *J. Clin. Invest.,* **43,** 2204

36. Klemperer, M. R., Donaldson, V. H. and Rosen, F. S. (1968). *J. Clin. Invest.,* **47,** 604

37. Willms, K., Rosen, F. S. and Donaldson, V. (1975). *Clin. Immunol. Immunopathol.* (in press)

38. Rosen, F. S., Charache, P., Donaldson, V. and Pensky, J. (1965). *Science,* **148,** 957

39. Johnson, A. M., Alper, C. A., Rosen, F. S. and Craig, J. M. (1971). *Science,* **173,** 553

40. Ratnoff, O. D., Pensky, J., Ogston, D. and Naff, G. B. (1969). *J. Exp. Med.,* **129,** 315

41. Pensky, J., Levy, L. R. and Lepow, I. H. (1961). *J. Biol. Chem.,* **236,** 1674

42. Harpel, P. C. and Cooper, N. R. (1975). *J. Clin. Invest.,* **55,** 593

43. Rosen, F. S., Alper, C. A., Pensky, J., Klemperer, M. R. and Donaldson, V. H. (1971). *J. Clin. Invest.,* **50,** 2143

44. Harpel, P. C., Hugli, T. E. and Cooper, N. R. (1975). *J. Clin. Invest.,* **55,** 605

45. Klemperer, M. R., Woodworth, H. C., Rosen, F. S. and Austen, K. F. (1966). *J. Clin. Invest.,* **45,** 880

46. Klemperer, M. R., Austen, K. F. and Rosen, F. S. (1967). *J. Immunol.,* **98,** 72

47. Ruddy, S., Klemperer, M. R., Rosen, F. S., Austen, K. F. and Kumate, J. (1970). *Immunology,* **18,** 943

48. Cooper, N. R., ten Bensel, R. and Kohler, P. F. (1968). *J. Immunol.,* **101,** 1176

49. Leddy, J. P., Griggs, R. C., Klemperer, M. R. and Frank, M. M. (1975). *Amer. J. Med.,* **58,** 83

50. Agnello, V., de Bracco, M. and Kunkel, H. G. (1972). *J. Immunol.,* **108,** 837

51. Day, N. K., Geiger, H., McLean, R., Michael, A. and Good, R. A. (1973). *J. Clin. Invest.,* **52,** 1601

51a. Sussman, M., Jones, J. H., Almeida, J. O. and Lachmann, P. J. (1973). *Clin. Exp. Immunol.,* **14,** 531

52. Fu, S. M., Kunkel, H. G., Brusman, H. P., Allen, F. H. and Fotino, M. (1974). *J. Exp. Med.,* **140,** 1108

53. Einstein, L. P., Alper, C. A., Block, K. J., Herrin, J. T., Rosen, F. S., David, J. R. and Colten, H. R. (1975). *New Eng. J. Med.* (In press)

54. Alper, C. A. and Propp, R. (1968). *J. Clin. Invest.,* **47,** 2181

55. Colten, H. R. and Alper, C. A. (1972). *J. Immunol.,* **108,** 1184

56. Propp, R. and Alper, C. A. (1968). *Science,* **162,** 672

57. Alper, C. A., Johnson, A. M., Birtch, A. G. and Moore, F. D. (1969). *Science,* **163,** 286

58. Alper, C. A., Propp, R. P., Klemperer, M. R. and Rosen, F. S. (1969). *J. Clin. Invest.,* **48,** 553

59. Alper, C. A. and Rosen, F. S. (1971). *J. Clin. Invest.,* **50,** 324

60. Alper, C. A., Colten, H. R., Rosen, F. S., Rabson, A. R., Macnab, G. M. and Gear, J. S. S. (1972). *Lancet,* **ii,** 1179

61. Pepys, M. B. (1974). *J. Exp. Med.,* **140**, 126
62. Ferreira, A. and Nussenzweig, V. (1975). *J. Exp. Med.,* **141**, 513
63. Müller-Eberhard, H. J. and Götze, O. (1972). *J. Exp. Med.,* **135**, 1003
64. Alper, C. A., Goodkofsky, I. and Lepow, I. H. (1973). *J. Exp. Med.,* **137**, 424
65. Nicholson, A., Brade, V., Lee, G. D., Shin, H. S. and Mayer, M. M. (1974). *J. Immunol.,* **112**, 1115
66. Alper, C. A., Rosen, F. S. and Lachmann, P. J. (1972). *Proc. Nat. Acad. Sci. (USA),* **69**, 2910
67. Gitlin, J. D., Rosen, F. S. and Lachmann, P. J. (1975). *J. Exp. Med.* (in press)
68. Alper, C. A., Abramson, N., Johnston, R. B., Jr., Jandl, J. H. and Rosen, F. S. (1970). *New Engl. J. Med.,* **382**, 349
69. Alper, C. A., Abramson, N., Johnston, R. B., Jr., Jandl, J. H. and Rosen, F. S. (1970). *J. Clin. Invest.,* **49**, 1975
70. Ziegler, J. B., Alper, C. A., Rosen, F. S., Lachmann, P. J. and Sherington, L. (1975). *J. Clin. Invest.,* **55**, 668
71. Abramson, N., Alper, C. A., Lachmann, P. J., Rosen, F. S. and Jandl, J. H. (1971). *J. Immunol.,* **107**, 19
72. Alper, C. A., Boenisch, T. and Watson, L. (1972). *J. Exp. Med.,* **135**, 68
73. Allen, F. H. (1974). *Vox Sang.,* **27**, 382
74. Ziegler, J. B. and Alper, C. A. (1975). *Nature (London)* (in press)
75. Moncada, B., Day, N. K. B., Good, R. A. and Windhorst, D. B. (1972). *New Eng. J. Med.,* **286**, 689
76. Rosenfeld, S. I. and Leddy, J. P. (1974). *J. Clin. Invest.,* **53**, 67a
77. Hauptmann, G., Grosshans, E. and Reid, E. (1974). Personal communication
78. Leddy, J. P., Frank, M. M., Gaither, T., Baum, J. and Klemperer, M. R. (1974). *J. Clin. Invest.,* **53**, 544
79. Bayer, J. T., Gall, E. P., Norman, M. E., Nilsson, U. R. and Zimmerman, T. S. (1975). (Submitted for publication)
80. Wellek, B. and van Es, L. (1974). In Brent and Holborow (eds.). *Progress in Immunology II, Volume 1* (New York: American Elsevier)
81. Ellman, L., Green, I. and Frank, M. M. (1970). *Science,* **170**, 74
82. Frank, M. M., Mag, J., Gaither, T. and Ellman, L. (1971). *J. Exp. Med.,* **134**, 176
83. Colten, H. R. and Frank, M. M. (1972). *Immunology,* **22**, 991
84. Colten, H. R. (1972). *Proc. Nat. Acad. Sci. (USA),* **69**, 2233
85. Ellman, L., Green, I., Judge, F. and Frank, M. M. (1971). *J. Exp. Med.,* **134**, 162
86. Schreiber, A. D. and Frank, M. M. (1972). *J. Clin. Invest.,* **51**, 575
87. Diamond, R. D., May, J. E., Kane, M. A., Frank, M. M. and Bennett, J. E. (1974). *J. Immunol.,* **112**, 2260
88. Cinader, B. and Dubiski, S. (1963). *Nature (London),* **200**, 781
89. Erickson, R. P., Tachibana, D. K., Herzenberg, L. A. and Rosenberg, L. T. (1964). *J. Immunol.,* **92**, 611
90. Nilsson, U. and Müller-Eberhard, H. J. (1965). *Fed. Proc.,* **24**, 620
91. Phillips, M. E., Rother, U. A., Rother, K. O. and Thorbecke, G. J. (1969). *Immunology,* **17**, 315
92. Levy, N. L. and Ladda, R. L. (1971). *Nature (London) New Biology,* **229**, 51
93. Rother, K. O., Rother, U., Müller-Eberhard, H. J. and Nilsson, U. (1966). *J. Exp. Med.,* **124**, 773
94. Nelson, R. A. and Biro, C. E. (1968). *Immunology,* **14**, 527
95. Lachmann, P. J. (1969). *Protides Biol. Fluids,* **17**, 301
96. Zimmerman, T. S., Arroyave, C. M. and Müller-Eberhard, H. J. (1971). *J. Exp. Med.,* **134**, 1591
97. Heusinkveld, R. S., Leddy, J. P., Klemperer, M. R. and Breckenridge, R. T. (1974). *J. Clin. Invest.,* **53**, 554

98. Fireman, P., Johnson, H. A. and Gitlin, D. (1964). *Pediatrics*, **37**, 485
99. Nezelof, C., Jammet, M. L., Lortholary, P., Labrune, B. and Lamy, M. (1964). *Arch. Franc. Pediat.*, **21**, 897
100. Harboe, M., Pande, H., Brandtzaeg, P., Tveter, K. J. and Hjort, P. F. (1966). *Scand. J. Hemat.*, **3**, 351
101. Gelfand, E. W., Baumal, R., Huber, J., Crookston, M. C. and Shumak, D. (1973). *New Engl. J. Med.*, **289**, 1385
102. Geha, R. S., Schneeberger, E., Gatien, J., Rosen, F. S. and Merler, E. (1974). *New Engl. J. Med.*, **290**, 726
103. Gatti, R. A., Meuwissen, H. J., Allen, H. D., Hong, R. and Good, R. A. (1968). *Lancet*, **ii**, 1366
104. DeKoning, J., van Bekkum, D. W., Dicke, K. A., Dooren, L. J., van Rood, J. J. and Radl, J. (1969). *Lancet*, **i**, 1223
105. Stiehm, E. R., Lawlor, G. J., Kaplan, M. S., Greenwald, H. L., Neerhout, R. C., Sengar, D. P. S. and Terasaki, P. I. (1972). *New Engl. J. Med.*, **286**, 797
106. Levey, R. H., Gelfand, E. W., Batchelor, J. R., Klemperer, M. R., Sanderson, A. R., Berkel, A. I. and Rosen, F. S. (1971). *Lancet*, **ii**, 571
107. Kadowaki, J., Thompson, R. I., Zuelzer, W. W., Wooley, P. V., Brough, A. J. and Gruber, D. (1965). *Lancet*, **ii**, 1152
108. Dupont, B., Andersen, V., Ernst, P., Faber, V., Good, R. A., Hansen, G. S., Henriksen, K., Jensen, K., Juhl, F., Killmann, S. Aa., Koch, C., Muller-Berat, N., Park, B. H., Svejgaard, A., Thomsen, M. and Wiik, A. (1973). *Transpl. Proc.*, **V**, 905
109. Hathaway, W. E., Githens, J. H., Blackburn, W. R., Fulginiti, V. and Kempe, C. H. (1965). *New Engl. J. Med.*, **273**, 953
110. Miller, M. E. (1967). *J. Pediat.*, **70**, 730
111. Kretschmer, R., Jeannet, M., Mereu, T. R., Kretschmer, K., Winn, H. and Rosen, F. S. (1969). *Pediat. Res.*, **3**, 34
112. Gitlin, D. and Craig, J. M. (1963). *Pediatrics*, **32**, 517
113. Hoyer, J. R., Cooper, M. D., Gabrielsen, A. E. and Good, R. A. (1968). *Medicine*, **47**, 201
114. Giblett, E., Anderson, J., Cohen, F., Pollara, B. and Meuwissen, H. J. (1972). *Lancet*, **ii**, 1067
115. Knudsen, B. B. and Dissing, J. (1973). *Clin. Genet.*, **4**, 344
116. Ochs, H. D., Yount, J. E., Giblett, E. R., Chen, S. H., Scott, C. R. and Wedgwood, R. J. (1973). *Lancet*, **i**, 1393
117. Scott, C. D., Chen, S. H. and Giblett, E. R. (1974). *J. Clin. Invest.*, **53**, 1194
118. Parkman, R., Gelfand, E. W., Rosen, F. S., Sanderson, A. R. and Hirschhorn, R. (1975). *New Engl. J. Med.*, **292**, 714
119. Spencer, N., Hopkinson, D. and Harris, H. (1968). *Ann. Hum. Genet.*, **32**, 9
120. Hirschhorn, R. (1975). *J. Clin. Invest.*, **55**, 661
121. Hopkinson, D. A., Cook, P. J. L. and Harris, H. (1969). *Ann. Hum. Genet.*, **32**, 361
122. Hirschhorn, R., Levytska, V. and Parkman, R. (1974). *J. Clin. Invest.*, **53**, 33a
123. Hirschhorn, R., Beratis, N., Rosen, F. S., Parkman, R., Stern, R. and Polmar, S. (1975). *Lancet*, **i**, 73
124. Jenkins, T. (1973). *Lancet*, **i**, 736
125. Jenkins, T. (1974). Personal communication
126. Tishfield, J. A., Creagan, R. P., Nichols, E. A. and Ruddle, F. H. (1974). *Hum. Hered.*, **24**, 1
127. Agarwahl, K. and Parks, R. E. (1975). Personal communication
128. Green, H. and Chan, T.-S. (1973). *Science*, **182**, 836
129. Gitlin, D., Vawter, G. and Craig, J. M. (1964). *Pediatrics*, **33**, 184
130. Lux, S. E., Johnston, R. B., Jr., August, C. S., Say, B., Penchaszadeh, V. B., Rosen, F. S. and McKusick, V. A. (1970). *New Engl. J. Med.*, **282**, 231
131. Gatti, R. A., Platt, N., Pomerance, H. H. and Good, R. A. (1969). *J. Pediat.*, **75**, 675

132. McGuire, T. C. and Pappie, M. J. (1973). *Infection Immunity,* **8,** 272

133. DiGeorge, A. M. (1968). *Immunologic Diseases in Man. Birth Defects: Original Article Series,* **4,** 116

134. Freedom, R. M., Rosen, F. S. and Nadas, A. S. (1972). *Circulation,* **16,** 165

135. Kretschmer, R., Say, B., Brown, D. and Rosen, F. S. (1968). *New Engl. J. Med.,* **279,** 1275

136. August, C. S., Rosen, F. S., Filler, R. M., Janeway, C. A., Markowski, B. and Kay, H. E. M. (1968). *Lancet,* **ii,** 1210

137. Cleveland, W. W., Fogel, B. J., Brown, W. T. and Kay, H. E. M. (1968). *Lancet,* **ii,** 1211

138. Steele, R. W., Limas, C., Thurman, G. B., Schuelein, M., Bauer, H. and Bellanti, J. A. (1974). *New Engl. J. Med.,* **287,** 787

139. Boder, E. and Sedgwick, R. P. (1958). *Pediatrics,* **21,** 526

140. Peterson, R. D. A., Cooper, M. D. and Good, R. A. (1966). *Amer. J. Med.,* **41,** 342

141. Fireman, P., Baesman, M. and Gitlin, D. (1964). *Lancet,* **i,** 1193

142. Hecht, F., McCaw, B. K. and Koler, R. O. (1973). *New Engl. J. Med.,* **289,** 286

143. Waldmann, T. A. and McIntire, K. R. (1972). *Lancet,* **ii,** 1112

144. Cooper, M. D., Chase, H. P., Lawman, J. T., Krivit, W. and Good, R. A. (1968). *Amer. J. Med.,* **44,** 499

145. Spitler, L. E., Levin, A. S., Stites, D. P., Fudenberg, H. H., Pirofsky, B., August, C. S., Stiehm, E. R., Hitzig, W. H. and Gatti, R. A. (1972). *J. Clin. Invest.,* **51,** 3216

146. Griscelli, C., Revillard, J. P., Betuel, H., Herzog, C. and Touraine, J. L. (1973). *Biomedicine,* **18,** 220

147. Pantelouris, E. M. (1968). *Nature (London),* **217,** 370

148. Pantelouris, E. M. (1971). *Immunology,* **20,** 247

149. Wortis, H. H., Nehlsen, I. and Owen, J. J. (1971). *J. Exp. Med.,* **134,** 681

150. Manning, D. D., Reed, N. D. and Shaffer, C. F. (1973). *J. Exp. Med.,* **138,** 488

151. Kindred, B. and Loor, F. (1974). *J. Exp. Med.,* **139,** 1215

152. Melief, C. J. M. and Schwartz, R. S. (1975). *Cancer* (in press)

153. Duquesnoy, R. J. (1972). *J. Immunol.,* **108,** 1578

154. Baroni, C., Fabris, N. and Bertoli, G. (1967). *Experientia,* **23,** 1059

155. Pierpaoli, W., Baroni, C., Fabris, N. and Sorkin, E. (1968). *Immunology,* **16,** 217

156. Duquesnoy, R. J. and Good, R. A. (1970). *J. Immunol.,* **104,** 1553

Index